A Complete Textbook of Regenerative Medicine

Pradeep Albert, M.D.
Devi Nampiaparampil, M.D., M.S.

Copyright© Pradeep Albert and Devi Nampiaparampil
All rights reserved
April 10, 2023
Cytokine Press, LLC

Thank you to all the chapter authors & illustrators who contributed their time, knowledge & efforts to this endeavor. We are indebted to our illustrators for their beautiful, informative & irreverent illustrations. They provide the clarity that our words alone cannot provide.

This book is dedicated to all those who teach and who heal.

Pradeep:
To my loving and supportive wife Esther
My children Naveen, Vikram, Sanjay, and Sandeep
My encouraging and inspirational parents
And my mentors Michael Sadler and Marc Brenner

Devi:
To my daughters Akira and Rania,
Whatever happens, my love for you will live forever.
If regenerative medicine advances quickly enough, maybe you can, too.
To my husband Hormis,
You are more traditional by nature but you lived on "the frontier" for me.
And to my parents Joseph and Mary,
You taught me I could do anything-
Whether or not it was true.

About the Editors

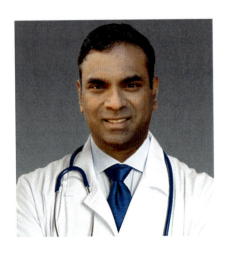

DR. PRADEEP ALBERT, M.D.

Dr. Pradeep Albert, MD, DABR, is a skilled Musculoskeletal Radiologist who founded Stem Cell University, an on-line resource for physicians and healthcare providers to access the most up-to-date information on regenerative medicine. With over 25 years of experience in Musculoskeletal Imaging/Ultrasound, he has performed over 25,000 interventional procedures and has interpreted over 350,000 imaging studies. He earned his Bachelor of Science degree with honors (Magna Cum Laude) from the State University of New York at Albany and his medical degree from Syracuse Health Science Center. He then completed his internship in Internal Medicine at Baylor College of Medicine, residency in Diagnostic Radiology at New York Medical College/ St Vincent's, and fellowship in Musculoskeletal Radiology at the University of California San Diego.

Dr. Albert is widely regarded as an expert in his field and has been instrumental in teaching students, residents, and colleagues. He is a distinguished national and international lecturer, as well as a sought-after consultant to leading institutions in the areas of Musculoskeletal Radiology, Musculoskeletal Ultrasound, Medical Informatics, and regenerative medicine. He is also the primary editor and co-author of a textbook of Regenerative Medicine (2023), and holds membership in the American College of Radiology, The American Medical Association, and The American Academy of Stem Cell Medicine. His portfolio of authored and edited publications is extensive, with over 100 lectures to his credit.

Dr. Albert has also provided imaging/ ultrasound interpretation services to prominent players in the NFL, MLB, and the NBA. He is the owner of Pure Mammography and the founder of Radsherpa, an innovative artificial intelligence company. Dr. Albert is a professor of Radiology at the New York College of Podiatric Medicine and a Clinical Professor at NYIT-College of Osteopathic Medicine. His expertise in regenerative medicine has extended to his work on stem cell legislation for the Eastern Caribbean nations.

Dr. Albert is held in high esteem in the business world and has been a featured speaker for the Radiology Business Management Association, Regenerative Medical seminars, and various technology forums on Medical Informatics and regenerative medicine. He serves on the Board of Directors for IPANS, the Independent Physicians Association of New York, and is a former board member of the Orthopaedic Foundation. Throughout his career, he has received numerous awards and honors, further testament to his exceptional contributions to his field.

DR. DEVI NAMPIAPARAMPIL, M.D., M.S.

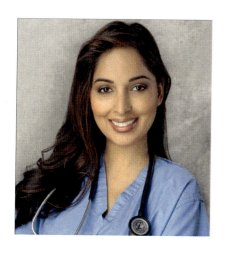

Dr. Devi Nampiaparampil has performed thousands of soft tissue and joint injections, nerve and plexus blocks, interventional spine procedures, spinal cord stimulator trials and implants, and epidural port and intrathecal pump implants in her career. She is board-certified in Pain Medicine, Physical Medicine & Rehabilitation, Sports Medicine and Hospice & Palliative Medicine. She has a private practice, Metropolis Pain Medicine, in downtown Manhattan and is a Clinical Associate Professor at NYU Grossman School of Medicine. Dr. Nampiaparampil is an elected Board member of the American Society of Interventional Pain Physicians. Every year since 2015, she has also been voted by other doctors to the Castle Connolly list of Top Doctors in the country.

Dr. Nampiaparampil graduated with honors from the seven-year combined B.A./M.D. program at Northwestern University. She double-majored in Biology and Economics and performed basic science research in Neurobiology. She completed her medical training through Harvard Medical School where she did her Medicine internship at Beth Israel Deaconess Medical Center, her Physical Medicine & Rehabilitation residency at Massachusetts General Hospital/ Spaulding Rehabilitation Hospital, and her Pain Medicine fellowship at Brigham and Women's Hospital. Afterwards, she served as the Chief of the Pain Management at the VA New York Harbor Healthcare System and established the Manhattan Veterans Affairs Hospital as a referral center for interventional pain for the Tristate region.

Dr. Nampiaparampil has over 60 publications in peer-reviewed journals including over 20 in the Journal of the American Medical Association (JAMA). Her 2008 first-author meta-analysis in JAMA highlighted the link between traumatic brain injury and chronic pain and changed how veterans returning from Iraq and Afghanistan are triaged.

Dr. Nampiaparampil served as Fox 5 NY's on-air medical contributor and has appeared in over 500 national and international news segments for Fox News Channel, Fox Business Network, CNN, MSNBC, CNBC, The TODAY Show, The Dr. Oz Show, Good Morning Britain and others.

At age 16, Devi had an infection that caused her heart, lungs, and bone marrow to fail. When she became pregnant for the first time, she worried about whether her child, Akira, would have problems with her bone marrow. That is what prompted her to start researching and writing this text. Dr. Nampiaparampil's second child, Rania, was born in 2020, early in the pandemic. The baby was born while Dr. Nampiaparampil was infected with COVID. Although Dr. Nampiaparampil had multiple risk factors for deadly complications, she came through the infection relatively unscathed. The same strain seriously harmed her other family members who had fewer risk factors. Dr. Nampiaparampil believed the baby's mesenchymal stem cells protected her. The use of stem cells to fight COVID became an area of global research at the time—before the development and distribution of vaccines or monoclonal antibodies. That experience made Dr. Nampiaparampil realize she had to complete the text regardless of pandemic-related obstacles.

Chapter Contributors (In alphabetical order)

PRADEEP ALBERT

SAIRAM ATLURI

MARC BRENNER

RICHARD CHANG

CRAIG CHAPPELL

JEREEN CHOWDHURY

PATRICK CLEARY

STRUAN COLEMAN

LISA CORRENTE

ALAN KATZ

ARLENE LAZARO

LAXMAIAH MANCHIKANTI

ANOKHI MEHTA

WILLIAM MERRITT

MILA MOGILEVSKY

DEVI NAMPIAPARAMPIL

ANNU NAVANI

SOHAN NAGRANI

BHAVI PATEL

BRIAN PEKKERMAN

ROCK POSITANO

ROCK POSITANO JR.

EMILIYA RAKHAMIMOVA

PUNEET RALHAN

COLIN RIGNEY

NORR SANTZ

BRENDAN TARZIA

VIJAY VAD

Illustrators (In alphabetical order)

NAVEEN ALBERT
Illustrator

SANDEEP ALBERT
Illustrator

SANJAY ALBERT
Illustrator

VIKRAM ALBERT
Illustrator

SADIA BHUIYAN
Illustrator

EVAN EDDLEMAN
Graphic Design & Layout

MICHAEL HARDING
Graphic Design & Layout

RYAN MARTIN
Director of Photography

TABLE OF CONTENTS

CHAPTER 1 - EVERYTHING YOU WANTED TO KNOW WITHOUT READING THE ENTIRE TEXTBOOK — 9
Pradeep Albert & Devi Nampiaparampil

CHAPTER 2 - A CLINICIAN'S UNDERSTANDING OF CURRENT REGULATIONS IN THE U.S. — 35
William Merritt, Lisa Corrente, Pradeep Albert & Marc Brenner

CHAPTER 3 - HEMOSTASIS — 38
Emiliya Rakhamimova, Jereen Chowdhury & Annu Navani

CHAPTER 4 - INFLAMMATORY PHASE — 44
Norr Santz & Devi Nampiaparampil

CHAPTER 5 - PROLIFERATIVE PHASE — 51
Anokhi Mehta & Devi Nampiaparampil

CHAPTER 6 - MATURATION PHASE — 56
Arlene Lazaro

CHAPTER 7 - PLATELET RICH PLASMA — 65
Puneet Ralhan, Mila Mogilevsky, Devi Nampiaparampil, Pradeep Albert & Alan Katz

CHAPTER 8 - EXOSOMES — 81
Pradeep Albert, William Merritt & Vijay Vad

CHAPTER 9 - MESENCHYMAL STEM CELLS: AN INTRODUCTION — 86
Devi Nampiaparampil, Pradeep Albert & Laxmaiah Manchikanti

CHAPTER 10 - BONE MARROW ASPIRATE CONCENTRATE (BMAC) — 94
Craig Chappell, Pradeep Albert, Alan Katz, Patrick Cleary & Richard Chang

CHAPTER 11 - ADIPOSE DERIVED STEM CELLS — 104
Norr Santz

CHAPTER 12 - FETAL STEM CELLS — 108
Bhavi Patel & Devi Nampiaparampil

CHAPTER 13 - STEM CELLS IN THE AMNIOTIC FLUID, PLACENTA AND WHARTON'S JELLY — 114
Brian Pekkerman & Devi Nampiaparampil

CHAPTER 14 - STEM CELLS: HISTORY & FOUNDATION — 119
Patrick Cleary & Richard Chang

CHAPTER 15 - STEM CELLS AND CANCER — 124
Sohan Nagrani

CHAPTER 16 - HYPERBARIC OXYGEN — 128
Alan Katz & Devi Nampiaparampil

CHAPTER 17 - BASICS OF NEEDLE TECHNIQUE — 137
Devi Nampiaparampil, Pradeep Albert & Sairam Atluri

CHAPTER 18 - THE SHOULDER — 140
Colin Rigney, Pradeep Albert & Devi Nampiaparampil

CHAPTER 19 - THE ELBOW — 170
Colin Rigney & Pradeep Albert

CHAPTER 20 - THE HAND AND WRIST — 201
Colin Rigney, Pradeep Albert & Devi Nampiaparampil

CHAPTER 21 - THE HIP — 234
Colin Rigney, Pradeep Albert, Devi Nampiaparampil & Struan Coleman

CHAPTER 22 - THE KNEE — 267
Colin Rigney, Pradeep Albert & Brendan Tarzia

CHAPTER 23 - THE FOOT AND ANKLE — 297
Colin Rigney, Pradeep Albert, Rock Positano & Rock Positano Jr.

APPENDIX - KINESIOLOGIC PLANES OF MOTION — 326
Pradeep Albert

CHAPTER 1
Everything You Wanted to Know Without Reading the Entire Textbook

Pradeep Albert & Devi Nampiaparampil

> **CHAPTER PREVIEW**
>
> This is the lightning round rapid fire Q&A section of the textbook. It contains the questions you are most likely to be asked by patients, students, doctors, and other members of your team. If you are pressed for time, this is the highest yield section of the book.

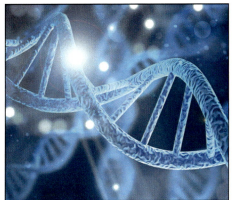

What is regenerative medicine?

A relatively new and exciting field of medicine that emphasizes using cellular therapies to regenerate and heal your body without surgical or pharmacological intervention.

This book is a practical guide to regenerative medicine. After reading this book, you will have learned about regenerative medical procedures' risks, benefits,and alternatives. We have provided: consent forms, information on how to set up your procedure suite, and tips on how to perform these procedures efficiently.

We have also included a section on injection techniques along with figures and sample images to guide those who are just starting. We also have step-by-step procedure templates that can be incorporated into your electronic medical record to speed up your charting. There are sections on how you can adapt your practice to add regenerative medicine.

There is a section on basic science. It is relevant for physicians around the world. However, it is geared towards physicians practicing in the United States, where there is significant FDA regulation of products such as platelet-rich plasma and stem cells. We will tackle other biologic products, such as exosomes, amniotic products, and other cellular therapies. We also cover the economics, regulatory framework, and malpractice issues in regenerative medicine. After reading this book, you can feel comfortable adding or expanding regenerative medicine in your practice.

Why the sudden interest in regenerative medicine?

Patients want to get better faster. Many musculoskeletal injuries are initially treated by corticosteroid therapy and then end with surgery. In the post-COVID era, patients are better informed about emerging technologies in healthcare and are beginning to learn about stem cell therapies and regenerative medicine.

Generally speaking, patients are not happy with corticosteroid injections and joint replacements alone. Viscosupplementation and other pharmacological interventions do not "fix" the underlying pathology.

The aim of regenerative medicine is to repair tissues **without surgical intervention**. Most physicians practicing in this area inject, as opposed to operate-- although regenerative injections can be performed in conjunction with surgery.

In this textbook, we will explore how these procedures work, how to perform these procedures, and whether or not (depending on your skill set) you should incorporate these procedures into your practice. We will have a discernible review of the science and a balanced look at these new technologies and procedures.

Masuko K, Murata M, Yudoh K. Anti-inflammatory effects of hyaluronan in arthritis therapy: Not just for viscosity. Int J Gen Med 2009; 2:77-81

What is PRP and how would I use it?

PRP stands for platelet-rich plasma. In a nutshell, you draw blood from a patient, spin it down in a centrifuge to separate out the various cells, extract the platelets and the growth factors attached to them, and then inject that straw-colored liquid "liquid gold" back into the patient at a site of injury. There is no standard classification for PRP, which is one of the problems. The straw colored fluid is considered Platelet Rich Plasma (PRP) if it has a higher concentration of platelets than whole blood. (Dhurat et al., 2014).

Dhurat R. and Sukesh MS. Principles and methods of preparation of platelet-rich plasma: A review and author's perspective. J Cutan Aesthet Surg. 2014; 7(4): 189-97

There are multiple kits available commercially for all platelets.

The amount of blood needed will vary based on the kit you choose to use. Generally, a commercially available kit will require 10-60cc whole blood.

There are kits that yield leukocyte-rich vs. leukocyte-poor PRP. Leukocyte-rich PRP contains white blood cells that may produce a greater inflammatory response. Leukocyte-poor formulations tend to have less of an inflammatory response (Ehrenfest et al., 2009).

Ehrenfest DMD, Rasmussen L, Albrektsson T. Classification of platelet concentrates: from pure platelet-rich plasma (P-PRP) to leukocyte- and platelet-rich fibrin (L-PRF). Trends in Biotechnology 2009; 27(3):158-67

In some kits, the platelets remain intact within the test tube and the syringe into which you draw the PRP. The platelets only become activated and initiate the clotting cascade when they hit human tissue (collagen). Other kits activate the platelets within the tube itself (with a chemical agent). We discuss platelet activation and the clotting cascade in greater detail in our Wound Healing chapters.

In High School biology class we were taught platelets were important because they stopped bleeding. Now we understand that there's more to platelets than just stopping bleeding. Whether you have a break in the skin or a fracture in the bone, the body releases substances that attract platelets to the area. Platelets initiate the biological cascade of repair by depositing a matrix for healing. When a patient has an acute painful injury, our standard treatment currently is to start anti-inflammatory a.k.a. antiplatelet agents. But maybe we shouldn't be doing that. That's an area of debate.

PRP emerged in the 1970s when veterinarians tried to heal injured racehorses with PRP which proved successful (Fortier et al., 2007). Then through the 1990s and the early 2000s, it became more popular among injured athletes who were improving without surgery. This spurred more research in the field of regenerative medicine.

Fortier LA and Smith RKW. Regenerative medicine for tendinous and ligamentous injuries of sport horses. Veterinary Clinics of North America: Equine Practice 2008; 24(1): 191-201

Beck H. (2011, December 29) Bryant's Advice for Alex Rodriguez. New York Times. Retrieved from http://www.nytimes.com

If you have a chronic injury-- implying that your platelets and your growth factors are not sufficiently effective at healing-- why would that change because you are injecting the same platelets and growth factors into the area?

PRP contains a higher concentrated number of platelets and growth factors than whole blood. Your platelets may be able to function more effectively at higher concentrations. It's hard to know. Perhaps you are a diabetic or a smoker, and your wound healing abilities have been affected. They may be lessened, but that doesn't mean they don't exist. Similarly, if you are on medications that affect platelet function, such as aspirin, over-the-counter or prescription-strength non-steroidal anti-inflammatory drugs, or blood thinners, then your ability to heal wounds effectively might be decreased (Anderson et al., 2012). A medication that can save your life-- like aspirin-- could be detrimental to your musculoskeletal system.

Anderson K and Hamm RL. Factors that impair wound healing. J Am Coll Clin Wound Spec 2012; 4(4): 84-91

How do NSAIDs affect wound healing?

Traditionally, when patients present initially with musculoskeletal injuries, we treat those with non-steroidal anti-inflammatory drugs and steroids. These drugs decrease inflammation. However, they can also negatively impact or slow down factors involved in wound healing (Anderson et al., 2012).

Anderson K, Hamm RL. J Am Coll Clin Wound Spec 2012; 4(4): 84-91

How does PRP compare to corticosteroid injections?

Cortisone injections are the bread-and-butter of musculoskeletal medicine. We have a large body of research and experience on steroid injections. They tend to help patients in the short term. Many patients just need something to help them over the hump so they can do physical therapy. Others need something that works like prescription-strength ibuprofen without all the systemic side effects.

At this juncture, cortisone will be the right choice for most patients with acute or acute-on-chronic musculoskeletal pain.

However, consider the long-term. With repeated injections, cortisone can weaken the bone locally (Hess et al., 2018). The lidocaine and bupivacaine we use to decrease the patients' pain also will destroy the sodium-potassium ATP pump (Butterworth, 1996). It has been shown to be chondrotoxic (Kreuz et al., 2018). Cortisone injections have been our best option so far in the short term. That doesn't mean they always will be. PRP has shown increased cartilage growth and decreasing synovitis in as little as 8 months after intra-articular injection in the knee suggesting it may eventually become a viable alternative (Raeissadat et al., 2020).

Hess SR, O'Connell RS, Bednarz CP et al., Association of rapidly destructive osteoarthritis of the hip with intra-articular steroid injections. Arthroplasty Today 2018; 4(2): 205-9

Butterworth J. Mechanisms of Local Anesthetic Action. Anesthesia & Analgesia 1996; 82(3):673

Kreuz PC, Steinwachs M, Angele P. Single-dose local anesthetics exhibit a type-, dose-, and time-dependent chondrotoxic effect on chondrocytes and cartilage: a systematic review of the current literature. Knee Surg Sports Traumatol Arthrosc 2018; 26(3): 819-30

Raeissadat SA, Ghorbani E, Taheri MS, et al., MRI Changes After Platelet Rich Plasma Injection In Knee Osteoarthritis (Randomized Clinical Trial). Journal of Pain Research 2020; 13: 65-73

Why aren't there stronger studies supporting PRP?

We believe that standardization is key priority to effectively studying PRP.

There are several studies that support the use of platelet-rich plasma in tendinopathy, ligament disorders, and bone and muscle dysfunction. There are two main obstacles to conducting large-scale robust studies evaluating PRP. First, there is a lack of consensus about what PRP is-- and not all studies define what type of PRP they are using. There may also be a lack of funding from pharmaceutical and device companies because PRP cannot be patented at this time.

There are several factors that vary between PRP studies. These include the platelet concentration for a given volume of PRP, the platelets' activation status (whether the platelets are starting to clot or not), and leukocyte status (whether there is an increased concentration of white blood cells in the PRP sample), and the volume of the injectate.

There are four types of PRP, two that are liquid and two that are viscous. The two liquid types can be further divided into leukocyte-rich or leukocyte-poor depending on whether white blood cells (leukocytes) are present.

If the plasma has a clotting factor that activates it outside the patient in the test tube/kit then the platelet concentrate becomes more viscous-like semi-solid consistency. These types of PRP are referred to as platelet-rich fibrin matrix (PRFM) as they are made up of fibrin. Fibrinogen turns into Fibrin when activated. These semisolid types of PRP are again classified into leukocyte-rich or leukocyte-poor depending on whether white blood cells (leukocytes) are present.

Practically speaking, the liquid types are commonly used in musculoskeletal medicine, and the semi-solid ones are commonly used in aesthetics, hair restoration, and wound healing applications. Although many studies have been done supporting the use of different types of PRP for different applications we must remember that there is no universal classification system.

These four types of PRP are listed here below.
1. Leukocyte-rich PRP: has high levels of white blood cells and is in liquid form (anticoagulated)
2. Leukocyte-poor PRP: has low levels of white blood cells and is in liquid form (anticoagulated)
3. Platelet-Rich Fibrin (PRF) or Platelet-Rich Fibrin Matrix (PRFM): has a low number of white blood cells
4. Platelet-Rich Fibrin (PRF) or Platelet-Rich Fibrin Matrix (PRFM): has a high number of white blood cells.

In vivo and in vitro are two terms you will find when reading about scientific studies. **In vivo** means with or within a living organism. **In vitro** (in glass in Latin) describes work performed outside of a living organism.

When the Platelet is activated and becomes more solid, it can be "activated" by the following mechanisms
1. With calcium inside a test tube (in vitro)
2. With thrombin inside a test tube (in vitro)
3. Inside the patient by collagen (in vivo); this is the most common method in muscoskeletal medicine.
4. PRP can also be activated mechanically by heating the sample or by mechanically damaging the platelet wall with a filter.

Dr. Albert recommends the following PRP classification system to standardize PRP.

A PRP Kit that concentrates platelets by a concentration of 3X with an injectable product of 10 CCs. Therefore, it would be documented as an Injection of 10 CC of medium concentration PRP.

A PRP Kit that concentrates platelets by a concentration of 1.4X with an injectable product of 10 CCs, Therefore, it would be classified as an injection of 10 CC of low or standard concentration PRP.

If you want to be more precise, you can add the following criterion to document the presence or absence of RBCs and WBCs.

Low or Standard Concentration	1X - 2X Platelet concentration
Medium Concentration	2X - 5X Platelet concentration
High Concentration	>5X Platelet concentration

Erythrocyte or RBC (if it's pink, it's positive, if its straw-colored, it's negative)	+/-
Leukocytes or WBC	+/-

Below are three examples that demonstrate Dr. Pradeep Albert's PRP classification system:

A PRP Kit that concentrates platelets by a concentration of 3X with an injectable product of 10 cc that is straw-colored or (erythrocyte-poor); Leukocyte-poor would be classified as a double negative (negative for RBC and WBC). Therefore, it would be documented as an Injection of 10CC of double negative medium concentration PRP.

A PRP Kit that concentrates platelets by a concentration of 1.4X with an injectable product of 10 cc pink-colored (erythrocyte-rich) PRP that is leukocyte-RICH. Therefore, it would be classified as a leukocyte-rich PRP injection with 10CC of E+ leukocyte-rich low concentration PRP.

A PRP Kit that concentrates platelets by a concentration of 6X with a straw-colored injectable product of 10 cc that is leukocyte-poor. Therefore, it would be classified as a leukocyte-poor PRP injection with 10CC of E+ leukocyte-poor high concentration PRP.

Remember that the higher concentration of PRP doesn't make the PRP better. There may be deleterious effects of high levels of PRP. This is a simple way to standardize PRP.

PRP kits look like test tubes. Can I make PRP without a kit?

We strongly advise against making your own PRP. (This is for many reasons, including time saved, sterility, and preparation error). We strongly recommend purchasing kits from companies that have met the Food & Drug Administration's standards.

Clinicians in countries outside the U.S. have proposed the following technique:

1. Obtain whole blood by drawing blood (venipuncture) in sodium citrate blood specimen collection (light blue top tubes)
2. Keep at room temperature
3. Centrifuge 6 test tubes at 900 rpm for 5 minutes
4. Aspirate the yellow fluid, including the buffy coat leaving the red blood inside the test tube
5. Discard the test tube with blood
6. You will have the straw colored liquid in the syringe from both test tubes.
7. Use this straw colored liquid as your PRP injection.

My patients don't know what stem cells are, so they ask me. I don't know what they are either. What do I tell them?

When patients ask about stem cells, they really want to know if it will help them. Here is some basic information you can share with your patients.

Stem cells are your body's raw materials. These amazing cells can make more of themselves or make more differentiated cells like those that make up your skin, blood, heart, and other organs. Stem cells help you to recover from all types of injuries and insults. Stem cells replenish dead and damaged cells by sending signals or by making more cells. You are constantly regenerating your whole body. Unfortunately, these cells diminish in number as you get older. (National Institutes of Health, 2019).

National Institutes of Health Stem Cell Information Home Page. In Stem Cell Information. Bethesda, MD: National Institutes of Health, U.S. Department of Health and Human Services, 2016 [cited March 16, 2019] Available at <//stemcells.nih.gov/info/basics/1.htm>

Think about a snake that molts and gets rid of its skin. We can see its skin regenerating at a particular point in time. In humans, this process occurs continuously in the skin, hair, blood, bone, and other cells.

CHAPTER 1 - EVERYTHING YOU WANTED TO KNOW WITHOUT READING THE ENTIRE TEXTBOOK

When do you use leukocyte-rich PRP vs. leukocyte-poor PRP?

There is no definitive answer. This table is derived from Dr. Pradeep Albert's clinical experience and can serve as a guide.

SHOULDER		
Rotator Cuff Tear	LR	5-7cc
Labral Tear	LR	5-7cc
Shoulder Arthritis	LR	5-7cc

LR = Leukocyte-Rich

LP = Leukocyte-Poor

HIP		
Hip Bursitis	LR	5-7cc
Hip Osteoarthritis	LP	5-7cc
Iliopsoas	LP	5-7cc
SI Joint	LP	5-7cc
Hamstring/Gluteus Tendon Tear	LP	5-7cc

ELBOW		
Lateral Epicondylitis	LP	5-7cc
Medial Epicondylitis	LP	5-7cc
Biceps Tendon Tear	LP	5-7cc

KNEE		
Knee Osteoarthritis	LR	5-7cc
ACL	LP	5-7cc
PCL	LP	5-7cc
MCL	LP	5-7cc
LCL	LP	5-7cc
Patella	LP	5-7cc
Meniscal Injuries	LP	2-3cc

WRIST / HAND		
De Quervain Tenosynovitis	LP	5-7cc
Stenosing Tenosynovitis "Trigger Finger"	LP	5-7cc
Triangular Fibrocartilage Complex Tear	LP	5-7cc

ANKLE		
Achilles Tendinopathy	LP	≤2cc
Plantar Fasciitis	LP	5cc
Plantar Plate Tear	LP	≤2cc
Posterior Tibial Tendon Tear	LP	≤2cc
Peroneal Tendon Tear	LP	≤2cc

SPINE		
Facet Arthritis	LR	≤2cc
Disc Disease	LP	1-2cc

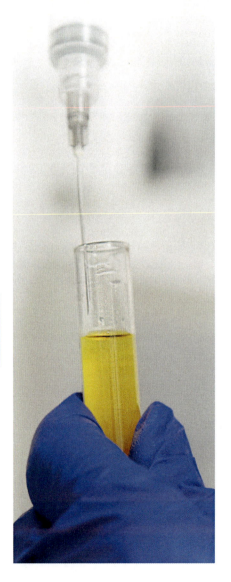

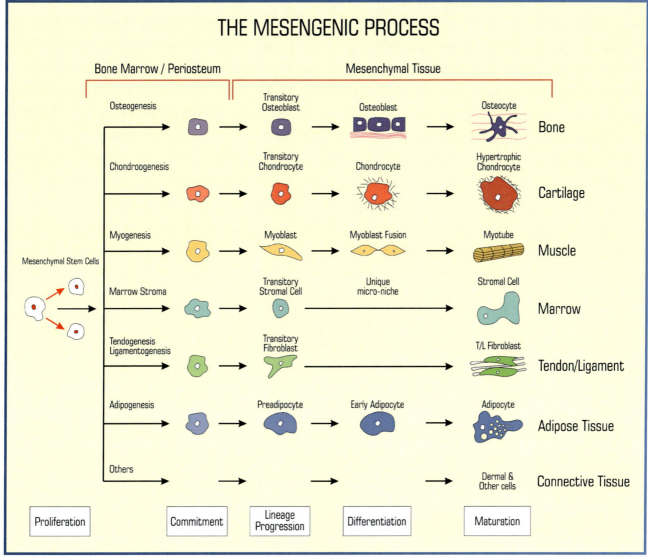

Figure 1: The Mesengenic Process

If you obtain mesenchymal stem cells (which can be obtained from adipose tissue, bone marrow, and umbilical cord) and then inject them directly into an area of injury, these cells will proliferate and improve the overall healing of damaged tissue. Do they regenerate tissue? That is controversial. Do they have a role in recovery? The answer is yes (Pittenger et al., 1999).

Pittenger MF, Mackay AM, Beck SC. Multilineage potential of adult human mesenchymal stem cells. Science 1999; 284:143-7

Stem cells travel around in our blood, but they are found in relatively low concentrations. Practically speaking, you have several options to harvest stem cells. You can get them from your own body where stem cells are abundant in specific organs and tissues. These are **autologous stem cells**. Or you can get stem cells from outside your body from other donors, including placental tissue. These are **allogeneic stem cells**.

If you are getting stem cells from your own body, you can harvest them from your bone marrow, which has a higher concentration than in blood. Bone marrow has hematopoietic stem cells, which are the precursors for blood cells. And mesenchymal stem cells, which are of interest in musculoskeletal medicine. To perform a bone marrow aspiration, your options are the anterior or posterior iliac crest, the tibia, or the calcaneus (Hyer et al., 2013). Most people will obtain these cells from the iliac crest by aspirating bone marrow. The technique is similar to a bone marrow biopsy.

Hyer CF, Berlet GC, Bussewitz BW, et al., Quantitative assessment of the yield of osteoblastic connective tissue progenitors in bone marrow aspirate from the iliac crest, tibia, and calcaneus. J Bone Joint Surg Am 2013; 95(14): 1312-6

If you are a podiatrist, your best bet is the tibia or the calcaneus. Extraction from the calcaneus is suboptimal as this can be very painful (Kuyucu et al., 2017; Hyer et al., 2013). As long as you can get bone marrow, you can obtain stem cells.

Kuyucu E, Erdil M, Kara A, et al., Difference between biomarkers of tibial bone marrow and adipose tissue. SICOT J 2017; 3-46

You can also derive stem cells from fat, where they are abundant. These are called "adipose-derived stem cells" or "adipose-derived stromal cells." In this scenario, you are doing something similar to liposuction. It is better to clarify to patients that there is no cosmetic benefit to your procedure. You are not removing enough fat to make a significant difference in the patient's stature, nor contouring the patient's body shape or tightening the skin around the harvest site (Jurgens et al., 2008). There is some controversy surrounding this. The FDA does not allow you to manipulate tissues to obtain stem cells. Therefore, if you added lipase (an enzyme that digests fat) to break down the fat and receive the "stromal vascular fraction," a liquid more likely to contain adipose-derived stem cells, you would be going against the 2019 FDA regulations. However, the FDA allows this if you use a mechanical device to get the stromal vascular fraction without "manipulating" the stem cells.

Jurgens WJFM. Oedayrajsingh-Varma MJ, Helder MN. Effect of tissue-harvesting site on yield of stem cells derived from adipose tissue: implications for cell-based therapies. Cell and Tissue Research 2008; 332(3): 415-26

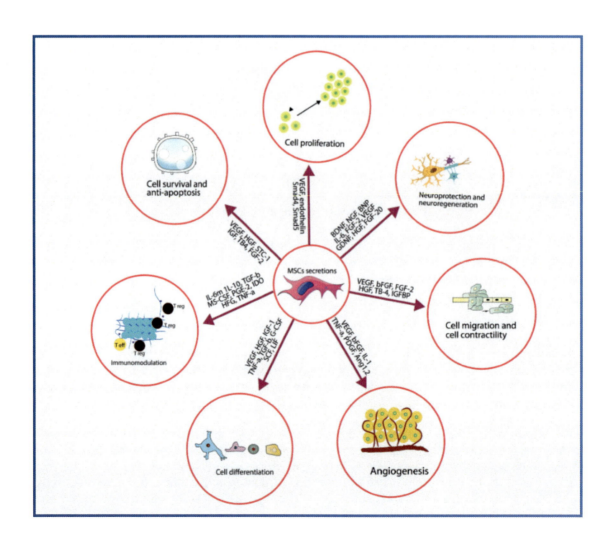

Why are Mesenchymal Stem cells now being called medicinal signaling cells?

Medicinal signaling cells (MSC), formerly referred to as mesenchymal stem cells are immunomodulatory and have the potential to migrate to injured tissue. The term "Mesenchymal Stem Cell" began in 1991 based on a belief that what happened in vitro would also occur in vivo. This turned out not to be the case (Caplan et al., 1991). Newer information lets us know that MSC's are secretory and produce a large array of cytokines and growth factors which prompted the new name, "Medicinal Signaling Cell". MSC's act as a sort of drug store at sites of injury (Al Caplan. What's in a name, Tiss Eng, A, 16:2415-2417). MSC's also participate in the recruitment of other cells needed in tissue repair. They promote the survival of existing cell repair, secrete growth factors, modulate the local environment, and decrease inflammation. They can be obtained from bone marrow referred to as bone marrow aspirate concentrate (BMAC).

The following question is for those practicing medicine outside the United States.

A salesperson from a large biologic company keeps telling me that I should use amniotic stem cells. I am confused about what the amniotic tissue is from... is it from an abortion? What is this all about? Is this even legal?

There is a difference between acellular amniotic fluid products (which do not contain stem cells), the amniotic membrane (which contains stem cells), umbilical cord and placental stem cells (which could come either from the mother or the fetus), and fetal stem cells (coming from a growing fetus).

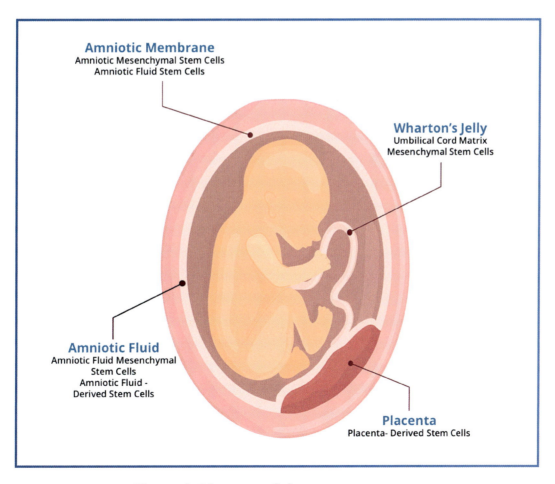

Figure 2: Diagram of the pregnant uterus

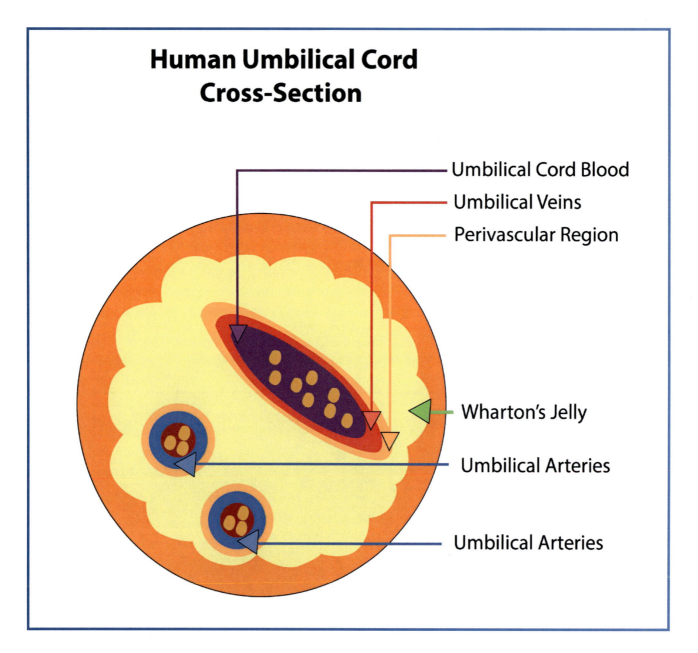

Figure 3: Cross section from the umbilical cord where stem cells can be obtained

Amniotic fluid products are **not obtained from abortions**. Amniotic fluid products are obtained postpartum (after delivery). Both the mother and the baby will have significant testing performed to ensure that their tissue products are safe.

The FDA currently has not approved any amniotic fluid or amniotic fluid-derived products for use. This does not mean they don't work. It just means they cannot be used in the United States. For those outside the U.S., this does not apply.

As of November 2017, these products were re-designated as biologic drugs, and a 36-month discretionary enforcement period was enacted. As of November 2020, these products will need an IND (Investigational New Drug) to be administered to patients (likely in a clinical trial setting). The FDA currently regulates acellular products that are now used as an injectate. They come in two forms, frozen vs. dehydrated or desiccated tissue.

So what's in the amniotic fluid products that are good for healing/repair?

There is no significant concentration of mesenchymal stem cells in amniotic fluid. However, proteins and other growth factors (sometimes called trophic factors, secretomes, cytokines, and sometimes morselized ACELLULAR membranes) are found in great abundance.

In the United States, under current guidelines, the acellular product, one that has been irradiated to remove any cells, is currently being used in wound healing and surgery (skin grafts, dural repair bone graft), etc. However, the FDA does not allow injecting these morselized amniotic products into areas of injury.

What is the difference between frozen vs. desiccated amniotic fluid?

Frozen amniotic products likely contain intact proteins called secretomes, extracellular proteins which cause cell signaling to grow, and exosomes (extracellular vesicles that contain protein which can be incorporated into cells and cause genetic changes to a cell to attract stem cells) as well as other growth factors. The idea is to freeze the amniotic fluid and the trophic factor associated with healing and growth intact without denaturing them. In the frozen form, the amniotic fluid and the morselized tissue are set and subsequently reconstituted so that the cells will not undergo apoptosis, a form of cellular death. This is different from desiccation.

Tjalsma H, Antelmann H, Jongbloed J et al., Proteomics of Protein Secretion by Bacillus subtilis: Separating the "Secrets" of the Secretome". Microbiology and Molecular Biology Reviews 2004; 68 (2): 207–233

Many cellular labs harvest stem cells from the blood in the umbilical cord vein and the Wharton's jelly of the umbilical cord.

What's the difference between a powder acellular amniotic product versus a frozen amniotic product?

<u>Currently both forms are **NOT** allowed for regenerative medicine in the United States. Outside the United States, the following sections regarding amniotic fluid products are relevant.</u>

In the powder form, mesenchymal cells and subjacent growth factors derived from the amniotic fluid are dehydrated before transport. Desiccated amniotic fluid products often come in powder form. There are no living cells in the powder form. The powder form contains only denatured proteins. Desiccated or lyophilized products may also have cryoprotectants and/or lyoprotectants to help keep proteins from denaturing during the lyophilization process. Lyophilization is a type of freeze-drying. The powder can be reconstituted when adding saline or another liquid. Desiccated products may also contain cryoprotectants and/or lyoprotectants to help keep proteins from denaturing during the lyophilization process. These powder products are often applied topically over non-healing ulcers. Some practitioners outside the US add these powders to PRP to enhance efficacy.

Both products are gamma radiated to ensure there are no longer living cells, including bacteria. The fluid is acellular, but it still has growth factors in it. Outside the US, these growth factors are applied topically or injected into areas of injury along with PRP. Amniotic products are managed almost like organ transplants in the United States. They are regulated like a tissue bank (U.S. Department of Health and Human Services, Food and Drug Administration, Center for Biologics Evaluation and Research, et al.,2017).

U.S. Department of Health and Human Services, Food and Drug Administration, Center for Biologics Evaluation and Research, et al., Regulatory considerations for human cells, tissues, and cellular and tissue-based products: minimal manipulation and homologous use: Guidance for industry and Food and Drug Administration staff, 2017 [cited March 16, 2019] Available at https://www.fda.gov/downloads/biologicsbloodvaccines/guidancecomplianceregulatoryinformation/guidances/cellularandgenetherapy/ucm585403.pdf

CHAPTER 1 - EVERYTHING YOU WANTED TO KNOW WITHOUT READING THE ENTIRE TEXTBOOK

Why do some people believe in using amniotic/placental derived mesenchymal stem cells versus using your own cells?

<u>The following section may be more relevant outside the United States, where mesenchymal stem cells are allowed.</u>

There are pros and cons to using placental tissues and amniotic fluid/placental products vs. your stem cells. Some argue that older people's stem cells are not as good or plentiful as younger stem cells. Therefore, allogeneic mesenchymal stem cells may have more extraordinary healing properties and may be helpful in older patients.

Multiple studies suggest adult stem cells (from the mother) found in amniotic fluid products are excellent for treating inflammatory disease processes such as arthritis.

Others take these adult amniotic and placental mesenchymal stem cells, expand or multiply them in a laboratory, and then inject them into areas of injury.

Some infuse them intravenously. This is not currently allowed in the United States. In the post coronavirus or COVID-19 world, many researchers inject intravenous mesenchymal stem cells to heal lung parenchyma (Liu et al., 2020).

Liu, S., Peng, D., Qiu, H. et al., Mesenchymal stem cells as a potential therapy for COVID-19. Stem Cell Res Ther 2020; 11, 169

As of 2021, researchers and physicians in other countries are performing stem cell infusions to treat post-COVID lung disease, emphysema, cardiomyopathy, help with muscle growth, and Type II diabetes. Although many of these indications are not well-researched, intravenous injections of stem cells may play a significant role in regenerative medicine.

What about applying some products topically?

In terms of placental products, the placental membrane, including the villae, can be physically applied on top of a wound (Hong et al., 2010; Choi et al., 2013). These are acellular products that are gamma radiated to ensure no bacteria on them. They are typically applied to a wound during surgery.

Hong JW, Lee WJ, Hahn SB. The effect of human placenta extract in a wound healing model. Ann Plast Surg 2010; 65(1): 96-100

Choi JS, Kim JD, Yoon HS, et al., Full-thickness skin wound healing using human placenta-derived extracellular matrix containing bioactive molecules. Tissue Eng Part A 2013; 19(3-4): 329-39

How do you multiply stem cells in the laboratory?

You can take a stem cell, put it in a Petri dish with a growth factor and growth agents, and it will multiply. The newly formed stem cells will grow and multiply in a similar fashion. There is evidence that after you multiply stem cells repeatedly, they could lose some function. This is similar to when you copy a copy of a copy on a xerox machine. The final copy may not be as good as the original.

Stem cells can also continue to multiply after you grow them in cell culture. This can be a problem if you don't want them to grow once you inject them into the body.

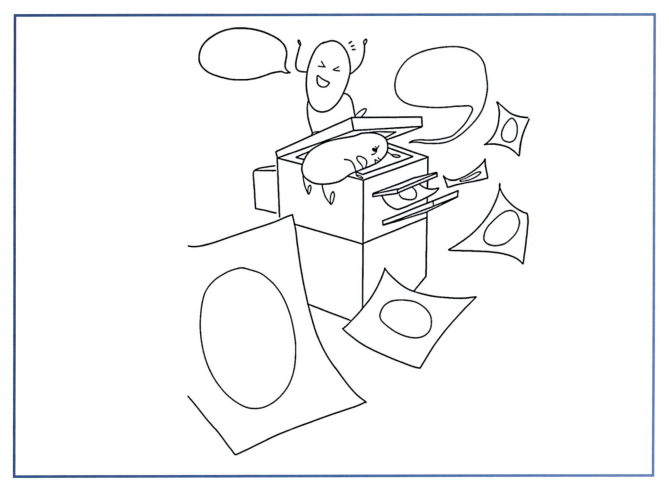

Figure 4: Multiplying expanded stem cells

Why do some people prefer fetal and amniotic stem cell products?

There are several benefits to fetal and amniotic stem cells over other types of stem cells. Both fetal stem cells and amniotic fluid stem cells are immunologically naive, which means that they are unlikely to attack their new host, the recipient (Helmy et al., 2010). In addition, both fetal stem cells and amniotic fluid stem cells can be cultured relatively rapidly and inexpensively in vitro.

At this time, there is no standard method for the isolation, culture or preservation of amniotic fluid mesenchymal stem cells. It is unclear whether stem cells should be administered into the blood or directly into the organs. The optimal timing of stem cell administration is unknown. Scientists and clinicians debate about whether stem cells should be combined with other treatment options. We still need to identify and characterize the long-term side effects of stem cell administration. In spite of these unknowns, amniotic fluid stem cells and fetal stem cells hold tremendous promise in the field of regenerative medicine.

Helmy KY, Patel SA, Silverio K, et al., Stem cells and regenerative medicine: accomplishments to date and future promise. Ther Deliv 2010; 1(5): 693-705

How do you know that you have a stem cell in whatever you collect? How can you identify it?

The best way to identify and categorize stem cells is to use an instrument called a flow cytometer. Researchers may be able to use fluorescent antibodies to attach to biomarkers that are often present on pluripotent stem cells. Most practicing physicians do not have access to flow cytometers. Unless you are doing cell counts and cultures on the specimen, you can't be 100% sure you have stem cells when you aspirate from bone marrow or from fat. When you are drilling into the iliac crest and aspirating bone marrow, If you have a large amount of aspirate there should be plenty of stem cells that are present. Just as when you extract fat. You have to be sure to aspirate the actual bone marrow (Trejo-Ayala et al., 2015).

Trejo-Ayala RA, Luna-Perez M, Gutierrez-Romero M. Bone marrow aspiration and biopsy. Technique and considerations. Revista Medica Del Hospital General De Mexico 2015; 78(4): 196-201

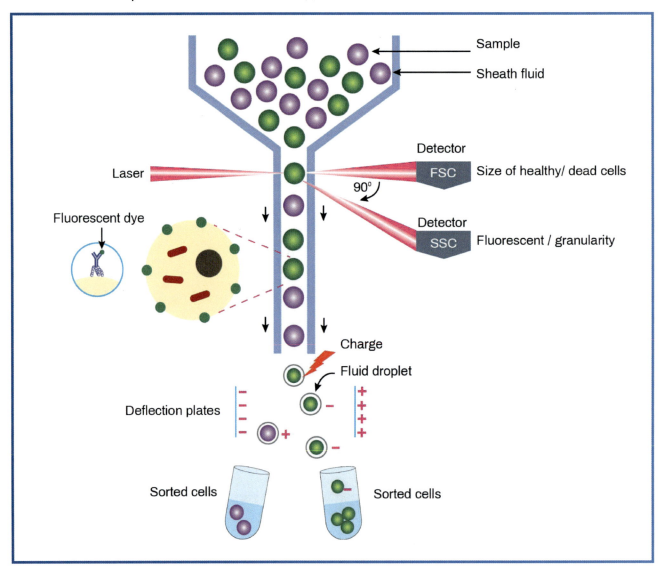

How do you convince patients coming in for something as common as shoulder pain that they should consider a procedure as invasive as bone marrow aspiration or fat harvesting for treatment?

Is this the first intervention that patients should undergo? No. There are exceptions, but our general algorithm is oral anti-inflammatories for immediate relief, corticosteroid injections and physical therapy for short-term relief, and lifestyle modification for long-term relief. If that doesn't work, consider regenerative therapies and/ or surgery. We usually recommend platelet-rich plasma over stem cells as a first step, but there are others who would disagree.

PRP and stem cells are not contraindications to future surgeries. PRP is often used as an adjunct to facilitate wound healing after surgery. Unlike cortisone injections, which may impact the timing of surgery, PRP and stem cells should not cause any delays (Mazda et al., 2018).

Mazda F, Burgstaller JM, Held U, et al., Do preoperative corticosteroid injections increase the risk for infections or wound healing problems after spine surgery? A Swiss prospective multicenter cohort study. Spine 2018; 43(15): 1089-94

Do stem cells make more sense in someone hesitant about surgery or in someone who had a failed surgery?

It can be considered in both populations. You should explain the procedure's risks, benefits, and alternatives, as with all procedures.

How does stem cell therapy affect cartilage?

In a rat model, mesenchymal stem cells injected directly into the synovium of knees that had undergone meniscectomies adhered to the lesions and regenerated the meniscus. In other animal studies, intra-articular injections of stem cells helped to heal chondral defects. Subcutaneous injections did not. It is possible that the stem cells required additional modifications to travel to the injury site (Korpershoek JV et al., 2017).

Korpershoek JV, de Windt TS, Hagmeijer MH et al., Cell-based meniscus repair and regeneration: At the brink of clinical translation? A systematic review of preclinical studies. Orthop J Sports Med 2017; 5(2): 232596711690131

How does stem cell therapy affect muscle strength?

When mice with the equivalent of muscular dystrophy received intravenous injections of stem cells, they showed increased muscle strength (Leukogeorgakis, et al., 2016). Injured muscles often heal with fibrosis and scarring, impairing contractility and function. In a rat model, mesenchymal stem cell therapy decreased fibrosis and improved muscle contractility compared to a control (Klimczak at al., 2018).

Loukogeorgakis S, Coppi P. Stem cells from amniotic fluid—potential for regenerative medicine. Best Practice & Research Clinical Obstetrics and Gynaecology 2016; 31: 45-57

Klimczak A, Kozlowska U, Krpisz M. Muscle stem/ progenitor cells and mesenchymal stem cells of bone marrow origin for skeletal muscle regeneration in muscular dystrophies. Arch Immunol Ther Exp (Warsz) 2018; 66(5): 341-54

Do you always do PRP before stem cells?

Usually, because it's lower cost, less invasive, and has more science to support it at this junction.

If the patient is coming to you specifically for stem cell injections, you should be fine as long as you go through the risks, benefits, and alternatives.

Do you plant the seeds for regenerative treatment options early on?

If patients have acute pain and fairly straightforward injuries, it may be better to stick to the tried and true standard treatment options.

If patients have acute on chronic conditions, you may briefly want to mention regenerative options as you are outlining the algorithm of treatment options.

If patients are not responding to the standard therapies and are progressing towards more invasive treatment strategies, then it is reasonable to mention PRP or stem cell injections.

If a patient seems skeptical, you don't have to sell them on it. This is true for any treatment intervention. We have patients whose histories, physical exam findings, and imaging studies suggest isolated inflammation areas that would respond well to steroids. But if the patients are biased against cortisone injections, it's improbable that steroid injections will yield a positive outcome (Manchikanti et al., 2017). The same is valid here. In our experience, the patients' "pre-test" expectations are highly predictive of the patients' "post-test" satisfaction rates.

Manchikanti L, Boswell MV, Kaye AD. Therapeutic role of placebo: evolution of a new paradigm in understanding research and clinical practice. Pain Physician 2017; 20: 364-86

Do you steer certain patients towards stem cells vs. PRP?

Based on our experience, older patients, smokers, and diabetics have less success with PRP. These patients are excellent candidates for stem cell procedures which may not produce the desired result.

Philosophically, one might argue that PRP allows existing cells to repair an injured area because it consists of growth factors. Stem cells arguably bring new cells into an injured area for soft tissue regeneration. Are you providing a withering plant with sunlight and water? Or are you planting a new seed in the soil? For many reasons, these studies have been hard to conduct. But that is the theoretical difference.

Is the goal with these procedures to achieve healing-- as evidenced advanced imaging-- or is the goal pain relief?

If you perform advanced imaging on a patient after she reaches a certain age, you will see osteoarthritic and other wear-and-tear changes throughout her body. That does not mean the patient has pain everywhere. In many patients, the pain does not necessarily correlate to imaging findings. Therefore, it is essential to manage the patient's expectations.

In Dr. Albert's experience as a musculoskeletal radiologist, doctors and patients are always looking for improvement in imaging (usually MRI). On an early MRI, a patient with an acute injury might have bone marrow edema. In the hip, the amount of bone marrow edema, as measured by MRI, correlates with the severity of pain, radiographic findings, and several microfractures (Taljanovic et al., 2008). The edema serves as both doctors' and patients' MRI markers for the injury. Some people will assume the injury has resolved if the bone marrow edema resolves. However, the thing to keep in mind is that, even if you do nothing, time itself can make the edema pattern resolve. It's not necessarily something you have done (Roemer et al., 2009).

Taljanovic MS, Graham AR, Benjamin JB, et al., Bone marrow edema pattern in advanced hip osteoarthritis: quantitative assessment with magnetic resonance imaging and correlation with clinical examination, radiographic findings, and histopathology. Skeletal Radiology 2008; 37(5): 423-31

Roemer FW, Guermazi A, Javaid MK, et al., Change in MRI-detected subchondral bone marrow lesions is associated with cartilage loss: the MOST study. A longitudinal multicentre study of knee osteoarthritis. Annals of the Rheumatic Diseases 2009; 68: 1461-5

With many acute-on-chronic musculoskeletal injuries, it is rare that the imaging findings directly correlate with the patient's pain and function (Jensen et al., 1994). Therefore, when it comes to regenerative therapies, you don't want to set the expectation that before-and-after MRIs are the gold standard for healing. If patients pay out of pocket for these therapies and still have pain afterward, they will probably not be happy if you point at the MRI and say the problem has been resolved.

Jensen MC, Brant-Zawadzki MN, Obuchowski N, et al., Magnetic resonance imaging of the lumbar spine in people without back pain. New England Journal of Medicine 1994; 331: 69-73

Similarly, histologic analysis is impractical. A biopsy can tell you how many chondrocytes are in a high-power field. It can also tell you about the water content in the cartilage (Lin et al., 2016).

Lin Y, Hall AC, Smith IDM, et al., Mapping chondrocyte viability, matrix glycosaminoglycan, and water content on the surface of a bovine metatarsophalangeal joint. Cartilage 2016; 7(2): 193-203

In Dr. Nampiaparampil's experience as a pain management specialist, there are also challenges in tying improvement to pain. First, pain is a challenging thing to measure. One patient can rate his discogenic low back pain as a 10/10, and another patient to rate their acute postoperative pain as 4/10. The patient's assessment and expectations of how severe the pain is will play a significant role here. Second, there is a recall bias. A patient's pain may improve, but it's hard to gauge the improvement if they don't remember exactly how bad it felt earlier. Third, other factors, besides the severity of the injury, affect patients' perception of pain. These include relatively common psychological comorbidities such as depression and anxiety, insomnia, coping skills, community and societal support systems, and financial stressors (Andersson et al., 1999).

Andersson HI, Ejlertsson G, Leden I, et al., Impact of chronic pain on health care seeking, self-care, and medication. Results from a population-based Swedish study. J Epidemiol Community Health 1999; 53: 503-9

A decade ago, if a patient in any setting said his pain score was above a 3/10, based correctly or incorrectly on the standards set by the Joint Commission on Accreditation of Healthcare Organizations (JCAHO), many doctors would have felt pressured to intervene, and to escalate the potency and dosage of medications. These measurement difficulties may have contributed to the opioid crisis we are dealing with today (Skeptical Scalpel, 2016).

Skeptical Scalpel. The Joint Commission deserves some blame for the opioid crisis. Missouri Medicine 2016; 113(6):449

Therefore, we recommend assessing patients' function pre-procedure, helping them to identify the concrete goals that they are aiming for, discussing the likelihood of achieving those outcomes, and then reassessing their function about six to twelve weeks after the procedure.

If a patient with ankle pain couldn't run more than a mile before, and now he can, that is a concrete outcome that you can point to. If a patient couldn't carry his bag to work before the procedure, and now he can, that is a clear outcome. We have patients whose primary goal is to play golf. We have others who want the procedure because their jobs depend on it. Either way, in our experience, helping patients to focus on specific goals usually leads to better outcomes and better patient satisfaction. Sometimes it helps to ask a loved one if they have noticed any improvements or less complaints. You'll be surprised how often people watching the patient notice improvement when the patient does not.

Why would transplanting stem cells from one body area to an injury make a difference? If you already have stem cells in your body, why aren't they already repairing the injured area? Doesn't that imply there may be something wrong with their function?

When we are young, we sustain a variety of injuries. All types of things happen, but somehow, we regenerate and grow. As we get older, we see more signs of wear and tear both clinically, histologically, and on imaging. Is it because our stem cells are declining in number or function? It's unclear (Ahmed et al., 2017).

Ahmed ASI, Sheng MHC, Wasnik S. Effect of aging on stem cells. World J Exp Med 2017; 7(1): 1-10

At present, we measure aging in units of time. But some scientists argue that we should use the telomere length instead. Telomeres are brackets on the ends of chromosomes. Every time your stem cells replicate, the telomeres get shorter and shorter (Levy et al., 1992).

Levy MZ, Allsopp RC, Futcher AB, et al., Telomere end-replication problem and cell aging. Journal of Molecular Biology 1992; 225(4): 951-60

If you recall the Dolly the sheep cloning experiment, Dolly died just six years after birth. That's because, rather than replicating the telomeres of a new baby, they replicated the telomeres of an advanced age sheep (Xu et al., 2003).

Xu J and Yang X. Will cloned animals suffer premature aging- the story at the end of clones' chromosomes. Reprod Biol Endocrinol 2003; 1:105

I'm not injured right now. I think my stem cells and growth factors are working well. Can I harvest my stem cells now, hold on to them, and inject them back if I get injured?

That's called tissue banking. Theoretically, it might make the most sense. But right now, it would go against the "minimal manipulation" laws in the U.S. For this to work, you would have to culture the cells, grow the cell lineage, and then inject the cells back into the area of injury. Under the current laws, you have to harvest the cells and inject them into the area of injury almost immediately (U.S. Department of Health and Human Services et al., 2017).

U.S. Department of Health and Human Services, Food and Drug Administration, Center for Biologics Evaluation and Research, et al., Regulatory considerations for human cells, tissues, and cellular and tissue-based products: minimal manipulation and homologous use: Guidance for industry and Food and Drug Administration staff, 2017 [cited March 16, 2019] Available at https://www.fda.gov.downloads/biologicsbloodvaccines/guidancecomplianceregulatoryinformation/guidances/cellularandgenetherapy/ucm585403.pdf

Cancer cells seem to function as stem cells in that they can replicate and regenerate. If a patient has a history of cancer, should you avoid these procedures? Isn't there a chance that you could spread cancer?

If a patient is currently being treated for cancer or is undergoing active surveillance, you should talk to the patient's oncologist. To discuss the risks and benefits of the procedure, you need to address any hematologic abnormalities, infectious risks, medication effects, and life expectancy.

If the patient has a remote history of cancer or a very localized cancer-like skin cancer that is being addressed, can you spread it by doing a PRP injection or stem cell procedure?

PRP has not been associated with malignancy. Screening for malignancy in patients with prior malignancies may be helpful before Stem Cell therapies.

Can autoimmune disorders, such as lupus or diabetes affect the success rates of regenerative procedures?

It is possible that these patients may have altered wound healing, to begin with. In our experience, patients with diabetes have slightly poorer outcomes from PRP than those without it.

On the other hand, early research suggests PRP may be beneficial in certain autoimmune conditions such as rheumatoid arthritis (Tong et al., 2017).

Tong S, Zhang C, Liu J. Platelet-rich plasma exhibits beneficial effects for rheumatoid arthritis mice by suppressing inflammatory factors. Mol Med Rep 2017; 16(4): 4082-8

Consider the patients' medication regimen with lupus, rheumatoid arthritis, and other autoimmune disorders. The patients' medications may alter platelet function and decrease the success rate of a PRP procedure.

Why is the U.S. so hesitant to study regenerative therapies?

There are unethical, fraudulent, and dangerous players in the world of regenerative medicine. In this time of information overload, it's difficult for patients, health care providers, and regulators to decipher it all. As a result, the U.S. government is behaving cautiously. Looking at its history, the FDA appears to prioritize safety.

Some people also believe that the FDA may be siding with the pharmaceutical industry to classify stem cells as a drug rather than a patient's property. This is not an easy differentiation. Pharmaceutical companies would argue that any cellular product is a drug. Others would disagree.

Pharmaceutical companies may financially benefit if stem cells are considered a drug. This is both a good thing and a bad thing. If regenerative medicine products are classified as drugs, there are more stringent requirements that could improve the safety of these treatments. However, they can more easily be blocked by legislation. This leaves us with a more considerable debate about intellectual property and ownership of your cells.

Why do you have to inject PRP and stem cells into the area of injury? Why not create a minor injury adjacent to the original one-- and draw growth factors and stem cells to the site?

Some people do this. They dry needle the area (Furlan et al., 2005). Others inject saline or other substances. This is called prolotherapy. Prolotherapy advocates argue that the act of needling itself is what facilitates healing. (Dagenais et al., 2007).

Fulan A, van Tulder M, Cherkin D. et al., Acupuncture and dry-needling for low back pain: an updated systematic review within the framework of the Cochrane collaboration. Spine 2005; 30(8): 944-963

Dagenais S, Yeland MJ, Del Mar C, and Schoene ML. Prolotherapy injections for chronic low back pain. Cochrane Database Syst Rev 2007; 18(2): CD004059

There are pros and cons to dry needling and prolotherapy, which are outside of the scope of this text. Compared to platelet-rich plasma and stem cells, keep in mind that if you're dry needling a tendon-- as opposed to injecting growth factors directly into the tendon-- you do have a risk of injuring the tendon or causing a tendon rupture (Pedowitz et al., 2013).

Pedowitz D and Kirwan G. Achilles tendon ruptures. Curr Rev Musculoskeletal Med 2013; 6(4): 285-93

In the United States, in musculoskeletal medicine, you are allowed to use "minimally manipulated" stem cells for injections. What does that mean?

Whether you are using bone marrow or fat to obtain stem cells, you have to separate the stem cells from all of the other substances you aspirated. Most people use some type of centrifuge system. Because you are not altering the cells or growing new ones- you are just isolating them and then injecting them- that is allowed (U.S. Department of Health and Human Services et al., 2017, Golish et al., 2018).

However, if you tried to grow and multiply cell strains in cell culture media, and then inject them, that would not be allowed. Outside of the United States, one can culture and grow stem cells for injection.

U.S. Department of Health and Human Services, Food and Drug Administration, Center for Biologics Evaluation and Research, et al., Regulatory considerations for human cells, tissues, and cellular and tissue-based products: minimal manipulation and homologous use: Guidance for industry and Food and Drug Administration staff, 2017 [cited March 16, 2019] Available at https://www.fda.gov.downloads/biologicsbloodvaccines/guidancecomplianceregulatoryinformation/guidances/cellularandgenetherapy/ucm585403.pdf

Golish SR, Watson T, and Mihalko WM. New FDA guidances tighten regulation of stem cells.

Can you inject someone else's stem cells into someone who is younger and healthier at an area of injury?

Yes, that is considered an allogeneic stem cell injection. This is not FDA approved. You can perform this procedure outside the United States, and these procedures are very promising. The actual amount of stem cells you can inject is much higher than you can get from bone marrow or fat. You can inject hundreds of millions of cells into areas of injury instead of several thousands.

The downside of this is that, in theory, based on the bone marrow transplant literature, if you inject someone else's stem cells into a patient, you could potentially see either a rejection of the new stem cells by the recipient's cells or graft-vs-host disease, where the stem cells attack the recipient's cells. This is because stem cells and the immune system are closely linked (Nauta et al., 2006).

Nauta A, Westerhuis G, Kruisselbrink AB, et al., Donor-derived mesenchymal stem cells are immunogenic in an allogeneic host and stimulate donor graft rejection in a nonmyeloablative setting. Blood 2006; 108: 2114-20

Many physicians worldwide are successfully trying mesenchymal stem cells from the umbilical cord. These cells are not immunogenic and can be incorporated into the body without graft vs. host disease. Some promising studies demonstrate that embryonic stem cells may have a healing effect. However, this is currently banned in the United States.

FDA. Statement from FDA Commissioner Scott Gottlieb, M.D., and Director of FDA's Center for Biologics Evaluation and Research Peter Marks, M.D., Ph.D., cautioning consumers against receiving young donor plasma infusions that are promoted as an unproven treatment for varying conditions. FDA Newsroom February 19, 2019 [cited March 23, 2019] Available at: https://www.fda.gov/NewsEvents/Newsroom/PressAnnouncements/ucm631568.htm

Can you apply PRP or stem cells to a surgical wound site?

During surgery, it is a prevalent practice to harvest bone marrow from the iliac crest and apply it to the fusion site. This is an FDA-approved use of bone marrow (Hustedt et al., 2014; Mroz et al., 2010).

Hustedt JW and Blizzard DJ. The controversy surrounding bone morphogenetic proteins in the spine: A review of the current research. Yale J Biol Med 2014; 87(4): 549-61

Mroz TE, Wang JC, Hashimoto R, et al., Complications related to osteobiologics use in spine surgery: A systematic review. Spine 2010; 35(9): S86-104

In the same way, PRP can be applied to a surgical site. In terms of FDA regulations, the FDA "clears" devices for use if they are substantially similar to devices that have already been approved. PRP is regulated by the device used to create it. The centrifuges used to separate and concentrate PRP are similar to a centrifuge previously approved by the FDA (https://www.accessdata.fda.gov/cdrh_docs/pdf/K994148.pdf). PRP gel is considered substantially similar to a previously cleared cleared moisturizing gels that can be applied to wounds (https://www.accessdata.fda.gov/cdrh_docs/pdf8/K082333.pdf).

Jones IA, Togashi RC, and Vangsness CT. The economics and regulation of PRP in the evolving field of orthopedic biologics. Curr Rev Musculoskeletal Med 2018; 11(4): 558-65

What about cord blood banking? Why is that allowed and not stem cell banking?

The blood in the umbilical cord is a baby's blood, 50% genetically the biological mother's blood and 50% genetically the biological father's blood. The cord blood is being stored for future use to treat certain blood cancers and some inherited metabolic and immune disorders. This is an FDA-approved use. (https://www.fda.gov/biologicsbloodvaccines/resourcesforyou/consumers/ucm236044.htm).

If babies' had their blood stored 25 years ago, and they are now at an age where they are developing chronic injuries, they could potentially try using the stored cord blood for healing. But it is an area that is still being studied.

U.S. Food and Drug Administration. Cord blood banking: Information for consumers March 27, 2018 [cited March 23, 2019] Access at: https://www.fda.gov/biologicsbloodvaccines/resourcesforyou/consumers/ucm236044.htm

What are exosomes?

Cells are constantly talking to each other in their local environment and between different body parts. There are many different communication methods that cells use; ions, lipids, steroids, peptides, proteins, vesicles, and exosomes are all part of the language of cells communicating. Exosomes are complex messages between cells that may contain a host of different components.

Exosomes are tiny membrane-bound particles that can contain surface receptors, proteins, mRNA, and other bioactive molecules. These little "sacs" of molecules are extruded from the cell's membrane in a conserved generation process. The messages within the sacs are selected by the cell for export.

Exosomes carry the messages of what a particular cell is doing or needing. Exosomes can also carry messages to tell a cell or a tissue what to do, such as "grow faster," "bring more blood," or "grow bone."

Different cell types communicate different messages through exosomes. Exosomes from bone tissue can help with the mineralization of bone, while exosomes from stem cells or amniotic fluid can help with inflammation and regrowth. Most medically used exosomes are from amniotic fluid or lab expanded mesenchymal stem cells.

Amniotic fluid contains exosomes and can be collected simultaneously as birth tissues, during or before a cesarean section delivery. When stem cells are grown out in large numbers, they continually produce exosomes. These exosomes can be collected from the growth media that the stem cells are grown in. Exosome therapy is not FDA-approved in the United States.

Edgar JR. Q+A. What Are Exosomes, Exactly? BMC Biology 2016; 14: 46

When do you recommend PRP vs. stem cells vs. amniotic and placental products?

PRP has the most evidence behind it and is usually the first regenerative therapy we will consider. Stem cells are the next choice. You can obtain stem cells from fat, bone or get them from amniotic tissue.

Outside the United States, allogenic mesenchymal stem cells, exosomes, and trophic factors are treatments of choice. A viable option is to use amniotic products or growth factors. These can be used in older patients or patients who can not undergo a rigorous harvesting process. Patients that are frail and osteopenic may benefit from this therapy.

Should I practice regenerative medicine?

Regenerative medicine is not really its own specialty. Multiple disciplines are involved in pain management, physiatry, sports medicine, family medicine, orthopedic surgery, rheumatology, podiatry, and interventional radiology. If you see patients who are in chronic pain, or if you treat a musculoskeletal disease of any type, you can practice regenerative medicine. Your specialty should not limit you from practicing regenerative medicine. There are currently no board certifications required to practice regenerative medicine.

If I am doing well in my practice, why would I want to start doing something new, especially when there is more potential for problems?

The short answer is that many patients are looking for regenerative medicine therapies. Your patients are looking on the Internet to research what platelet-rich plasma is and what stem cell procedures are. Suppose you are an orthopedic surgeon and you only perform shoulder surgeries. In that case, there are specific subsets of patients, with partial rotator cuff tears, for example, that you may treat non-operatively. You may send them to physical therapy, thinking that is their only option. These patients may also have regenerative medicine treatment options as well. You may eventually lose those patients because you are not offering that procedure, but perhaps another orthopedic surgeon can provide the surgical options you offer AND can offer guidance on regenerative treatment options.

What about my referring physicians? If they do not believe in this, I can lose my referring providers by suddenly offering treatments that are not part of the established medical guidelines.

When Dr. Albert gives his lectures, one of the common questions he gets asked is, "What are the contraindications to these procedures?" And people have joked, "A patient without a credit card."

Ethically, you have to tell your patients as well as the physicians who are referring them to you what the indications and contraindications are, how these procedures work, and who they work for and do not work for. This is important. The reality is that a physician who is not well-informed about regenerative procedures can be dangerous. These are medical procedures that have indications and contraindications. If you understand the basic science behind them, you will understand who to do these procedures on and who not to do them on.

Referring physicians, like patients, need to be educated about what regenerative medicine is. Platelet-rich plasma and stem cell injections are not done in the backroom dark web of medical practices. There are multiple peer-reviewed articles that detail the science behind these procedures for musculoskeletal injuries.

How do I present this to patients? Normally, I offer anti-inflammatory options as a first resort. PRP is philosophically very different. How do I present all the options to my patients?

The idea is to get the patient feeling better. If you have osteoarthritis of the knee, you start with lifestyle modification exercise, lose weight and strengthen your core. You may add an oral anti-inflammatory initially or send them to physical therapy. Eventually, you may progress to corticosteroid injections or surgery. This is just an adjunct. It's not going to replace any of those things. Regenerative medicine is not a miraculous remedy that will completely transform your practice overnight.

We have to talk about the risks and benefits of different options. For example, with knee osteoarthritis, we will discuss two types of platelet-rich plasma, leukocyte-rich and leukocyte-poor, and which one is better. If a patient has poorly controlled Type II diabetes, and you are constantly injecting them with steroids, they may be on their way to avascular necrosis and a knee replacement. Maybe platelet-rich plasma can reduce knee pain (Dai et al., 2017) without affecting blood glucose levels like cortisone. This book is not there to replace standard interventions but rather, to complement what you are already doing. The purpose is to improve patient outcomes.

Dai WL, Zhou AG, Zhang H, et al., Efficacy of platelet-rich plasma in the treatment of knee osteoarthritis: A meta-analysis of randomized controlled trials. Arthroscopy: The Journal of Arthroscopic & Related Surgery 2017; 659-70.e1

Is this something to suggest to new patients rather than follow-ups, or vice versa? It's awkward to bring up something that is not covered by insurance.

When a patient presents with musculoskeletal symptoms, we give them options and weigh those options. If someone with several comorbidities comes in for chronic knee osteoarthritis and is on his way to getting a knee replacement, maybe platelet-rich plasma is a better treatment option. You offer different options. Patients are intelligent and educated and can do a significant amount of research on their own. Just because something is not covered by insurance, please do not assume that the insurance company has the patients best interest in mind.

Do you encourage them to look up this information? How do you prepare your staff if patients ask about regenerative medicine?

We encourage patients to research anatomy, physiology, and treatment interventions as much as possible. An educated, informed patient could be your best patient because their expectations align with reality. Educate your staff as well on what you are trying to accomplish. They can execute your vision.

When it comes to written materials, remember that things change. You can always include links to the FDA website, where regulatory updates will be available. You have to keep up to date for the sake of lawsuits for malpractice and audits for fraud. This is true for anything in medicine. The standard is constantly evolving. As long as you are not making false claims, and as long as you stay connected to other physicians practicing in the same area, you can adapt. Orthopedic surgeons had to adapt when arthroscopic surgery became more common than open surgery. Sports medicine doctors had to adapt when it became more accepted to perform ultrasound-guided physical examinations with the advent of ultrasound. Things will continue to change.

It sounds like patients turn to regenerative medicine when all other treatments have failed. But sometimes, patients who fail all other treatments are more likely to fail this one as well. How do you navigate that?

We should give the patients our assessment of the risks and benefits for any procedure. This includes our estimate of the likelihood of success. That way, the patient can make an informed decision and partner with you. If you believe the risks outweigh the benefits, don't offer to perform these procedures.

When would be the ideal time to get into this? Is it when you are established and have a steady stream of patients? Or is it something you should decide as soon as you start so you can then build it up from the beginning?

This book is written for people in all phases of the physician life cycle: those in residency, those early into the attending years, and those who have been in practice for decades. Only now are physicians really hearing about platelet-rich plasma and stem cells. Professional athletes have these procedures done, so it is becoming common knowledge. If you are starting out, you can incorporate it into your standard practice. If you have been practicing for 30 years, it is also an excellent time to look into these options.

Our goal is to minimize any anxiety that you have. This book will cover all the basics so that you can get started.

If you're just starting out, what are the best places to inject?

We recommend starting with the area you are most comfortable with in terms of technique. Some sports medicine specialists may feel more comfortable with a knee joint injection than a scapholunate ligament tear. Also, consider the risks associated with the area of injury. You may want to start with an area of the body with no major nerves or blood vessels right next to the area you are injecting.

In terms of outcome, there is more research right now to support PRP injections for lateral epicondylitis, rotator cuff injuries, and knee osteoarthritis. If you're looking for the first few patients to sing your praises, you may be better off starting with those injuries.

Also, consider the patient's other options. If a runner has a partial tear in the Achilles tendon, you may get more positive feedback starting with them than with a patient who has knee osteoarthritis.

Interventional pain management specialists tend to do spine injections. There has been growing research supporting PRP in the epidural space (Bhatia et al., 2016), in the facet joints (Wu et al., 2017), or in the discs (Monfett et al., 2016). However, current research does not include high-quality studies. The same is true of trigger point injections with PRP (Bubnov et al., 2013).

Bhatia R and Chopra G. Efficacy of platelet-rich plasma via the lumbar epidural route in chronic prolapses intervertebral disc patients- a pilot study. J Clin Diagn Res 2016; 10(9): UC05-UC07

Wu J, Zhou J, Liu C, et al., A prospective study comparing platelet-rich plasma and local anesthetic (LA)/ corticosteroid in intra-articular injection for the treatment of lumbar facet joint syndrome. Pain Pract 2017; 17(7): 914-24

Monfett M, Harrison J, Boachie-Adjei K, et al., Intradiscal platelet-rich plasma (PRP) injections for discogenic low back pain: an update. International Orthopaedics 2016; 40(6): 1321-8

Bubnov R, Yevseenko V, Semeniv I. Ultrasound guided injections of platelets rich plasma for muscle injury in professional athletes: comparative study. Medical Ultrasonography 2013; 15 (2): 101-5

I believe in some aspects of regenerative medicine, but not all of it. Do I have to go all-in? How do I make this transition?

You can take what you want to take from this book. If you are skeptical about some of these things, that is fine. No one is forcing you to do these procedures. Look into the science behind it. Some of your colleagues may be more aggressive. Stay in your own lane. Do what you think works. If you do not believe that something works, don't do it. It's just like practicing conventional medicine.

If you are transitioning into doing PRP or stem cell procedures should you offer a discounted price during your training period? How do you get the practice you need without turning off patients?

You have to explain the indications and contraindications to the procedure as well as set expectations. If you are asking patients to serve as volunteers for demonstrations at courses or conferences, you can offer them a lower price or perform the procedure for free. That is because the patient is working for you to some extent.

But if the patient is having the procedure in your office, as any other patient would, it is better not to discount your work. Physicians who accept conventional insurance rates often feel apologetic about taking money from patients. But consider the context. When you perform bread-and-butter procedures, you don't reduce your fee for the insurance company because you're running late or your medical assistant called out sick. Those factors detract from the patient experience. You should be all in when you are doing something you believe in. If a regenerative procedure does not work for a particular patient, just explain that it did not work. That is it. If you start giving discounts, refunding money, and charging everyone different prices, you will run into trouble. This is not going to work for you. You have to be fair. The best way to do that is to charge a uniform fee for everyone from the start.

What if you previously told patients you didn't believe in platelet-rich plasma and stem cells? Won't you sound like a hypocrite if you suddenly present these options to patients?

Many things change in medicine. It's okay if you stated that these procedures don't work and now you want to try them. As long as you are honest and explain that you have changed your mind, patients understand. Learning something new, changing your mind, and adapting to new circumstances are not signs of weakness.

Are some of these products easier to use when you are just starting out?

In terms of ease of use, platelet-rich plasma and amniotic fluid are the easiest transitions because they are injections. If you know how to inject steroids, you should have the technical skills to inject these products.

In terms of practice logistics, platelet-rich plasma is low cost, easy to obtain, and easy to inject. Amniotic fluid is easy to obtain and comes in a kit that is easy to order. However, because the fluid is not coming directly from the patient, there is a greater risk of infection or adverse reaction.

In terms of peer pressure and acceptance from others in the medical community, platelet-rich plasma has the most scientific evidence behind it.

How do you describe the risks and benefits to PRP vs. stem cells vs. amniotic fluid injections?

With any injection, there is a risk of bleeding, infection, soreness or worsening pain, anxiety, lightheadedness, and nausea. We must go through the risks specific to the anatomic location, including nerve or blood vessel injuries. For bone marrow aspirates, for example, there are risks that come from drilling into the iliac crest (Malempati et al., 2009). Then we get into the risks that are specific to these regenerative therapies. Generally, if you use the patient's own cells and growth factors, there should not be any allergic or immune reaction risks. The patient will not have a reaction to their own blood products. However, in very rare cases, the patient may have a reaction to inactive ingredients used in preparing the PRP (Latalski et al., 2019).

Malempati S, Joshi S, Lai S, et al., Bone marrow aspiration and biopsy. N Engl J Med 2009; 361: e28
Latalski M, Walczyk A, Fatyga M, et al., Allergic reaction to platelet-rich plasma (PRP): Case report. Medicine 2019; 98(10): e14702

CHAPTER 1 - EVERYTHING YOU WANTED TO KNOW WITHOUT READING THE ENTIRE TEXTBOOK

How is this industry regulated? What can you do and what can't you do?

The Food and Drug Administration (FDA) regulates food and drugs. Platelet-rich plasma, bone marrow aspirate, and adipose-derived stem cells are neither food nor drugs. They are considered Human Cells, Tissues, and Cellular- and Tissue-Based Products (HCT/Ps). HCT/Ps can be regulated as either minimally-manipulated tissue allografts intended for homologous use (regulated solely under Section 361 of the PHS Act) or as biologics (regulated under Section 351 of the PHS Act). Many amniotic fluids and exosome products will be advertised as "361 products." However, this is misleading. As of November 2017, amniotic fluid and exosome products are considered either secreted products (and thus not an HCT/P) or overly manipulated. The FDA granted these products a 36-month discretionary enforcement period which ends in November 2020. After November 2020, amniotic fluid and exosome products are considered biologics ("351 products"). They must have an approved Investigational New Drug (IND) application to be used in clinical trials and an approved Biologics Licensing Application (BLA) to market and sell to doctors. The FDA has granted certain "351 products" the ability to be sold concurrently while being investigated in clinical trials, but this can be considered relatively rare and is heavily restricted.

https://www.fda.gov/regulatory-information/search-fda-guidance-documents/regulatory-considerations-human-cells-tissues-and-cellular-and-tissue-based-products-minimal [Cited on 7/1/20]

Sometimes, people apply the FDA's "off-label" use guidelines to biologics. For example, the anticonvulsant Neurontin (gabapentin) is FDA-approved for treating pain from postherpetic neuralgia (https://www.accessdata.fda.gov/drugsatfda_docs/label/2017/020235s062,020882s045,021129s044lbl.pdf).

Because the drug can work for one form of neuropathic pain, we often use it for other more common neuropathic pain syndromes such as diabetic neuropathy (Backonja et al., 1998), cervical and lumbar radiculopathies (Woods et al., 2015; Cohen et al., 2015), and nerve entrapment syndromes (Hahn, 2011). Many doctors use it for low back pain (Atkinson et al., 2016). Otolaryngologists use it for chronic cough (Ryan et al., 2012). The medication is used to treat a wide variety of conditions.

https://www.accessdata.fda.gov/drugsatfda_docs/label/2017/020235s062,020882s045,021129s044lbl.pdf. [Cited on 3/25/19]

Backonja M, Beydoun A, Edwards KR, et al., Gabapentin for the symptomatic treatment of painful neuropathy in patients with diabetes mellitus: A randomized controlled trial. JAMA 1998; 280 (21): 1831-6

Woods BI and Hilibrand AS. Journal of Spinal Disorders and Techniques 2015; 28(5): E251-9(9)

Cohen SP, Hanling S, Bicket MC, et al., Epidural steroid injections compared with gabapentin for lumbosacral radicular pain: A multicenter randomized double-blind comparative efficacy study. BMJ 2015; 350: h1748

Atkinson JH, Slater MA, Capparelli EV, et al., A randomized controlled trial of gabapentin for chronic low back pain with and without a radiating component. Pain 2017; 157(7): 1499-1507

Hahn. Treatment of ilioinguinal nerve entrapment- a randomized controlled trial. Acta Obstetricia et Gynecologica 2011; 955-60

Ryan NM, Birring SS, Gibson PG. Gabapentin for refractory chronic cough: A randomised, double-blind, placebo-controlled trial. The Lancet 2012; 380 (9853): 1583-9

The FDA approves the use of a medication for one purpose, but doctors can use it for whatever they want (once it is on the market). That is called off-label use. PRP injections (are) effective at healing cancellous bone (Sethi et al., 2008). PRP gel is considered similar to previously cleared moisturizing gel that can be applied to wounds (https://www.accessdata.fda.gov/cdrh_docs/pdf8/K082333.pdf). Therefore, we can use PRP for wound healing. However, this would be considered off-label use.

Sethi PM et al., Evaluation of autologous platelet concentrate for intertransverse process lumbar fusion. Am J Orthop 2008; 37:E84-90

Jones IA, Togashi RC, and Vangsness CT. The economics and regulation of PRP in the evolving field of orthopedic biologics. Curr Rev Musculoskeletal Med 2018; 11(4): 558-65

Then there's the issue of medical devices, which are devices that are used to harvest these regenerative substances from a patient's body and then transform them into a more concentrated and usable form. When the technology from an existing medical device, such as a centrifuge for separating out cells in a tube of blood, is being significantly altered, the manufacturer must submit an application to the FDA called a 510(k). If the technology is not considered significantly different, the manufacturer can obtain an exemption. That means the product can be used-- even if it's for a different purpose than originally intended. That means that a centrifuge can potentially be used to separate out platelets, for PRP injection, from other cells in a tube of blood. Centrifuges that prepare and concentrate platelets are not considered substantially different from existing medical devices (https://www.accessdata.fda.gov/cdrh_docs/pdf/K994148.pdf).

Jones IA, Togashi RC, and Vangsness CT. The economics and regulation of PRP in the evolving field of orthopedic biologics. Curr Rev Musculoskeletal Med 2018; 11(4): 558-65

A drug is made with ingredients, each in the same proportion, for use in a specific subset of people. If Dr. Nampiaparampil buys brand name Drug X from a major pharmacy in California and Dr. Albert buys brand name Drug X from a Mom-and-Pop pharmacy in New York, those two drugs should be interchangeable. The FDA holds pharmaceutical companies to this standard (FDA, 2018).

FDA. Current good manufacturing practice (CGMP) regulations. Updated November 1, 2018 [Cited March 25, 2019] Accessed at https://www.fda.gov/drugs/developmentapprovalprocess/manufacturing/ucm090016.htm

Although we are currently applying standards used for drugs and devices to these biologic products, biologics are fundamentally different. They are tailored to individual patients. Let's suppose interleukin-1 heals all things. Interleukin-1 should be the same from person to person. But let's say that, to be effective, interleukin-1 must combine with an antibody that only the patient has. That is a lot harder to produce-- and even harder to regulate. At present, the government is applying tissue banking laws to these products.

CHAPTER 2: A Clinician's Understanding of Current Regulations in the U.S.

William Merritt, Lisa Corrente, Pradeep Albert & Marc Brenner

CHAPTER PREVIEW

This chapter covers general regulatory considerations regarding the use of regenerative therapies in the United States.

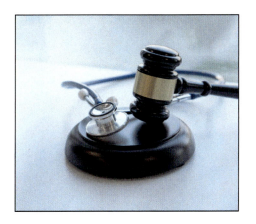

How are regenerative medicine products regulated? What can you do and what can't you do? The Food and Drug Administration (FDA) regulates foods, drugs, medical devices, and cosmetics. Bone marrow aspirate, stem cells, and platelet rich plasma don't obviously fit into those categories. Traditionally, pharmaceutical companies make medicines that are not unique to each person, however many of these biologic treatments can be unique to a donor/patient. We are entering a whole new age of biologics.

Let's say that Interleukin 1 heals all things. Interleukin 1 is the same from person to person; but Interleukin 1 combined with something else that only you make or combined with an antibody that only you have, is a lot harder to regulate and to produce.

Manufacturers use medical devices to extract cellular tissue and blood products. These devices process your own tissue. As long as it's minimally manipulated, the FDA allows you to use it clinically!

What is a HCT/P?

A HCT/P is a product that is derived from human cells or tissue. HCT/Ps can be sourced from the same patient being treated (autologous) or from a donor (allogeneic). HCT/Ps are regulated by the FDA. Autologous HCT/Ps have much more regulatory leeway as you are taking a patients own cells using them in their own body. These HCT/Ps are typically sourced and used during the same medical procedure.

Allogeneic HCT/Ps are under much closer regulatory scrutiny since they are sourced from a donor, further processed by a manufacturer, stored, and distributed before use in a patient. Allogeneic treatments include organs for transplant, bone chips, ligaments, amniotic membrane, etc.

Is a HCT/P a tissue, biologic drug, or device?

The short answer is that a HCT/P can be regulated as any one of those or a combination of them. Most often in the regenerative medicine space you will hear about "Section 361" products or "Section 351" products. These references are to sections of the Public Health and Safety (PHS) Act. A HCT/P solely regulated under Section 361 of the PHS Act is considered a tissue and does not need market approval from the FDA, but it has to meet a somewhat confusing set of criteria to be considered a tissue:

1. The HCT/P is minimally manipulated;
2. The HCT/P is intended for homologous use only; homologous means repair
3. The HCT/P is not combined with other materials (other than water, and/or preservatives as long as they don't raise safety concerns); AND

4. Either:
    a. The HCT/P does not have a systemic effect and is not dependent upon the metabolic activity of living cells to function
    b. The HCT/P has a systemic effect or is dependent on upon the metabolic activity of living cells to function and:
        v. It is for autologous use;
        vi. It is for allogeneic use in a first- or second-degree blood relative;
        vii. Or it is for reproductive use.

The last criteria describes how autologous HCT/Ps have more regulatory leeway than allogeneic HCT/Ps.

If a HCT/P does not meet the criteria to be considered a tissue, it is typically considered to be a "Section 351" HCT/P and is regulated as a biologic drug.

Less commonly, HCT/Ps can be regulated as devices. This is limited to a few products: demineralized bone in a handling agent, corneal lenticules, preserved umbilical cord vein grafts, human collagen, and femoral veins intended as A-V shunts. Combining cultured cells with human collagen would be considered a combination device and be subject to regulation and market approval for both the device and drug components of the combination device.

How does the FDA define minimal manipulation?

FDA defines "minimal manipulation" as: "1) For structural tissue, processing that does not alter the original relevant characteristics of the tissue relating to the tissue's utility for reconstruction, repair, or replacement; 2) For cells or nonstructural tissues, processing that does not alter the relevant biological characteristics of cells or tissues."

How does the FDA regard homologous use?

Homologous use reflects the repair, reconstruction, replacement, or supplementation of a recipient's cells or tissues with human cells, tissues, and cellular and tissue-based product (HCT/ P) that perform the same basic function or functions in the recipient as in the donor. This criterion reflects the Agency's conclusion that there would be increased safety and effectiveness concerns for human cells, tissues, and cellular and tissue-based product that are intended for a non-homologous use, because there is less basis on which to predict the product's behavior, whereas HCT/Ps for homologous use can reasonably be expected to function appropriately.

How is PRP regulated?

PRP is regulated as an autologous blood product, not a HCT/P. However, the devices used to spin down the blood are regulated as medical devices and are typically approved via a 510(k). The 510(k) device approval pathway requires that a device be substantially equivalent to a previously approved predicate device. In the case of PRP, the original device was intended to make PRP for use with bone graft materials. This means they have shown that PRP injection helps with cancellous bone for bone healing and calling everything else "off-label" use. Essentially, the FDA says that the device is approved for bone graft healing. You can use it for other purposes (as a medical doctor) whether you want to make someone's skin look good or for hair growth, etc. The analogy is that some anticonvulsants are approved for epilepsy, but we can also use them for mood stabilization.

How are stem cells regulated?

Stem cells are considered a HCT/P. The criteria for evaluating how they are regulated (tissue or biologic drug) is described previously in this chapter.

What cells can I inject without breaking the law?

Essentially, the vast majority of allogeneic stem cells are considered biologic drugs unless sourced from a donor that is blood related to the patient. Hematopoietic stem cells derived from cord blood are an exception with FDA approval for use in patients with hematopoietic disorders.

How is bone marrow aspirate regulated?

Bone marrow aspirate is regulated in a similar fashion to PRP. The device to process bone marrow aspirate has 510(k) approval, but the use of bone marrow aspirate is typically off-label and at the discretion of the doctor.

FDA drug approval is slow and expensive, are there any alternatives?

With the growing evidence that stem cell-based therapies can be effective for a number of indications, the pace at which the FDA approval process moves can be frustrating for doctors, patients, and biotechnology companies. There are clinics outside of the United States that are legally able to perform stem cell therapies.

The FDA and Congress have also acknowledged that the market approval process is potentially holding back valuable regenerative therapies and have begun to take action.

The U.S. Food and Drug Administration recently announced a comprehensive policy framework for the development and oversight of regenerative medicine products, including cellular therapies. "We're at the beginning of a paradigm change in medicine with the promise of being able to facilitate regeneration of parts of the human body, where cells and tissues can be engineered to grow healthy, functional organs to replace diseased ones; new genes can be introduced into the body to combat disease; and adult stem cells can generate replacements for cells that are lost to injury or disease. This is no longer the stuff of science fiction. This is the practical promise of modern applications of regenerative medicine," said former FDA Commissioner Scott Gottlieb, M.D. "But this field is dynamic and complex. As such, it has presented unique challenges to researchers, health care providers, and the FDA as we seek to provide a clear pathway for those developing new therapies in this promising field, while making sure that the FDA meets its obligation to ensure the safety and efficacy of the medical products that patients rely upon. Alongside all the promise, we've also seen products marketed that are dangerous and have harmed people."

The 21st Century Cures Act (Cures Act) created what's known as the Regenerative Medicine Advanced Therapy (RMAT) designation (previously known as the RAT designation), which can be used to speed the review of cell therapies, therapeutic tissue engineering products, human cell and tissue products or any combination product using such therapies or products. Advantages of the RMAT designation include all the benefits of the fast track and breakthrough designations, including early interactions between the agency and sponsors.

But as opposed to the breakthrough designation, the RMAT designation does not require evidence to indicate that the drug may offer a substantial improvement over available therapies.

And like breakthrough designations, RMAT designations do not mean the product will be approved and do not change the statutory standards for demonstration of safety and effectiveness needed for approval. In addition to creating the RMAT, Section 3034 of the Cures Act also mandates that FDA issue guidance clarifying how FDA will evaluate devices used in the recovery, isolation or delivery of RMATs.

CHAPTER 3 Hemostasis

Emiliya Rakhamimova, Jereen Chowdhury & Annu Navani

> **CHAPTER PREVIEW**
>
> When an injury occurs, blood vessels underneath the skin are immediately damaged and the blood inside of the vessels begins to leak out. This chapter describes the processes of vasoconstriction and vasodilation as well as how platelets form plugs and clots. The chapter also goes over the intrinsic and extrinsic clotting cascades.

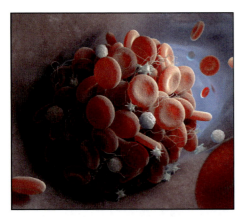

Throughout life, the human body must withstand and repair a large number and variety of injuries to the skin and its underlying tissue. This ability of the body to heal itself is vital to our survival. Human beings require a stable internal environment to stay alive regardless of the ever-changing conditions outside of our bodies. Therefore, any breach of the skin, which forms the outermost protective barrier between our internal environment and the external world, can pose a potential threat to the survival of the entire organism (Ratnoff, 1993).

The body reacts to any wound, big or small, in a highly-coordinated manner with the purpose of keeping its inner contents in and any external threats out. To do this, the body must be able to heal the wound as quickly as possible. This is to minimize the amount of blood flowing outwards as well as to minimize the harmful, infection-causing agents, known as pathogens, that may be flowing in (Thomsen et al., 2006).

In order to re-establish the separation between its internal and external environments, the body forms a clot at the site of the injury. The clot functions as a temporary mechanical plug that quickly stops the blood from flowing out of the body until the damaged cell tissue can be repaired. Simultaneously, endothelial cells, which line the inside of blood vessels, release substances, such as prostacyclin and nitric oxide, to prevent the clot from occluding the damaged vessel (Broos et al., 2011) The clot will be broken down once the damaged cells have been replenished and are capable of keeping the skin closed on their own again.

When an injury occurs, blood vessels underneath the skin are immediately damaged and the blood inside of the vessels begins to leak out. When circulating platelets get exposed to collagen underlying the inner blood vessel wall, the blood vessel narrows in a process known as vascular constriction, or vasoconstriction. This vasoconstriction process is controlled by substances known as thromboxane and serotonin. When the vessels become narrower, blood flows through them at a smaller volume, which decreases the amount of blood leaking out of the damaged vessel wall and the body. At the same time, elsewhere in the wound space, platelets and other cells release histamine. Histamine causes the blood vessels to expand, in a process called vasodilation. This enables the movement of healing factors towards the site of injury (Steed, 1997).

Vascular constriction slows the loss of blood (Broughton et al., 2006). Clots are more effective at preventing blood loss. Clot formation at the site of injury is known as hemostasis. If this mechanism were not in place, a significant amount of blood would be lost with injuries as minor as papercuts.

Hemostasis is divided into two stages known as primary and secondary hemostasis. In both stages, a series of chemical reactions take place due to the activation of the protein thrombin (a.k.a. Factor IIa; "a" for activated). There are 13 proteins involved in the clotting cascade that is part of hemostasis.

Thrombin (Factor IIa) belongs to a class of proteins known as enzymes, which become activated in order to allow specific chemical reactions to take place. In normal physiology, thrombin (Factor IIa) is only produced in the event of tissue damage, thereby safeguarding against unnecessary blood clotting in the absence of injury. Therefore, thrombin (Factor IIa) is a coagulation factor, or blood clotting agent, that should only be activated to prevent blood loss (Coughlin, 2000).

In primary hemostasis, thrombin (Factor IIa) begins to accumulate at the site of the injured blood vessel. As it accumulates, it also releases chemicals that function as messengers to recruit and activate specialized disc-like cells in the blood known as platelets. Platelet cells have no nucleus, are the smallest in size out of all the different blood cells, and are actually fragments of larger cells found in the bone marrow (Mason, 2007). Inside of a platelet there are many small intracellular compartments, termed granules for their appearance, which in turn contain various chemicals that can be released that aid communication between platelets themselves or between platelets and other types of cells.

The primary function of platelets is to come together at the site of tissue damage in order to seal small breaks in blood vessels by forming a platelet clot. Platelet cells are able to aggregate in large numbers by releasing chemical messengers from their granules, which signal even more platelets to become activated. Upon activation, platelets begin to change shape by flattening themselves out in order to cover more surface area at the damaged tissue. Their increased surface area also exposes sites on the platelet to which other platelets can adhere, thereby causing aggregation. Proteins known as selectins play a role in this process. The adhesive properties of platelets make them beneficial in wound healing and harmful in disease processes such as atherogenesis or atherosclerosis (Gawaz, 2005).

Once they are at the site of injury and adhering to each other, platelets also become immobile so that the mechanical plug that they are creating does not move from the place while the tissue is being repaired. This platelet clot may be sufficient for very minor bleeding, but more often than not, this initial aggregate of platelets provides the physical foundation for a more stable clot that will be formed during secondary hemostasis. Platelets on their own are not sufficient to seal extensive breaks in blood vessels and prevent bleeding, because the platelet clot that they create is not very stable.

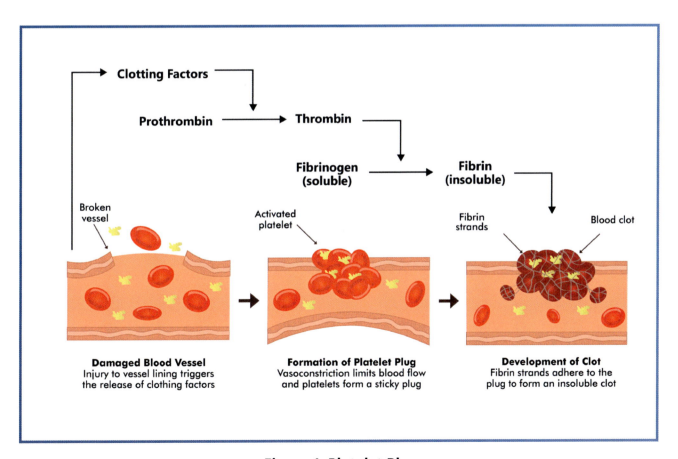

Figure 1: Platelet Plug

Secondary hemostasis serves to complete the process of blood clotting with the production of an insoluble protein known as *fibrin (a.k.a. Factor Ia; again "a" for activated)*. Fibrin (Factor Ia) and other blood clotting proteins stabilize the clot that was initiated by the platelets. The product is known as the fibrin clot. Blood clotting proteins such as fibrin (Factor Ia) stabilize the clot through their interaction with collagen (Mosesson, 2005).

Inactivated platelets circulating through the blood have a discoid appearance. Once they become activated by thrombin (Factor IIa), the platelets change shape. Activated platelets have elongated pseudopods that provide more surface area for fibrin strands to adhere to (Hantgan, 1985).

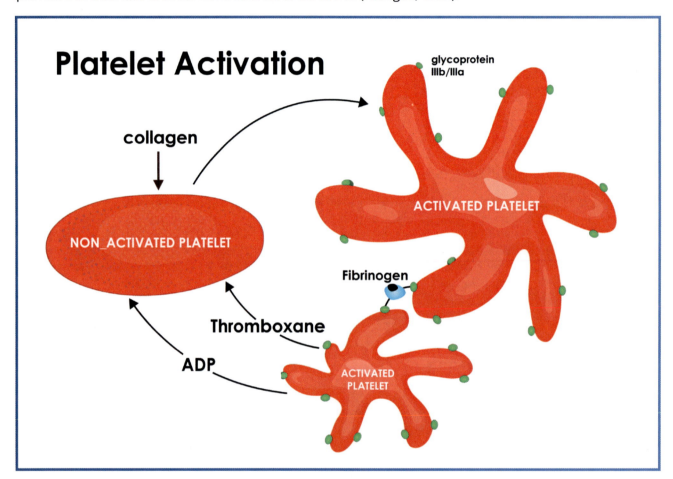

Figure 2: Platelet Activation

Thrombin (Factor IIa) is responsible for the reaction that makes fibrin (Factor Ia) out of a larger, soluble protein found in the blood known as *fibrinogen (a.k.a. Factor I; notice no "a" because this is inactivated fibrin)*. This process can take place through either the intrinsic or extrinsic pathway, which are both series of chemical reactions involving blood clotting proteins (Davie et al., 1991).

The intrinsic pathway gets its name from the fact that it does not require the participation of substances extrinsic to the blood. This pathway begins when the blood clotting proteins come in contact with the collagen of the basal lamina of the blood vessel. The basal lamina is a network of collagen and other proteins, and is attached to epithelial cells. The basal lamina supports the overlying epithelium and separates it from cells of other tissues. If trauma takes place and causes damage to endothelial cells lining the blood vessels, the underlying collagen of the basal lamina becomes exposed to the proteins circulating in the blood. The circulating blood clotting proteins then begin to activate each other in what is known as the clotting cascade (Gawaz, 2005).

The intrinsic pathway cascade begins when Factor XII comes in contact with tissue factor (a.k.a. Factor III) in the exposed surface of the basal lamina and gets activated. Factor VIIa catalyzes the conversion of Factor IX to Factor IXa (Mayer, 2008).

Together, tissue factor (Factor III), Factor VII, Factor VIII, and Factor IX convert Factor X into Factor Xa (Rosing et al., 1985). von Willebrand Factor (vWF) stabilizes Factor VIII during this process (Peyvandi, 2011).

Activated Factor X converts prothrombin (Factor II) to thrombin (Factor IIa). This pathway to thrombin is also known as the final common pathway.

Thrombin (Factor IIa) activates Factor XIII to Factor XIIIa (a.k.a. fibrin stabilizing factor), which links fibrin proteins together and renders a clot near the vicinity of the exposed basal lamina (Ariens, 2002).

Extrinsic coagulation occurs when trauma causes damage to both endothelial cells and the basal lamina. The plasma containing the coagulation factors leaves the blood vessels and comes in contact with external proteins. The peripheral cells have proteins, known as tissue factor (Factor III), embedded in their membranes. Tissue factor can activate Factor VII, which is present in plasma that has leaked out from the damaged blood vessels. Consequently, Factor VIIa activates Factor X.

From there on, the steps in the extrinsic and intrinsic pathways are similar. Activated Factor X is able to convert prothrombin into thrombin (factor II). Thrombin (factor II) converts fibrinogen to fibrin, and again brings us to the fibrin clot.

Let's do a brief synonym recap, so this makes more sense:

"~" means "equivalent to"

Factor I ~ Fibrinogen
Factor II ~ Thrombin
Factor III ~ Tissue factor
Factor IV ~ Thromboplastin ~ Thrombokinase
Factor V
Factor VI
Factor VII
Factor XIII ~ Anti-hemophilic factor
Factor IX ~ Christmas factor
Factor X
Factor XI
Factor XII ~ Hageman factor
Factor XIII ~ Fibrin stabilizing factor
"a" after any factor name ~ "activated" version of that factor

Clinically, abnormalities in the intrinsic pathway lead to abnormalities in the PTT. Abnormalities in the extrinsic pathway cause abnormalities in the PT/ INR. Absent or abnormal vWF can lead to life-threatening bleeding (Peyvandi, 2011). Absent or abnormal Factor VIII is known as hemophilia A. Absent or abnormal Factor IX is known as hemophilia B. And absent or abnormal factor XI is known as hemophilia C (White, 2001).

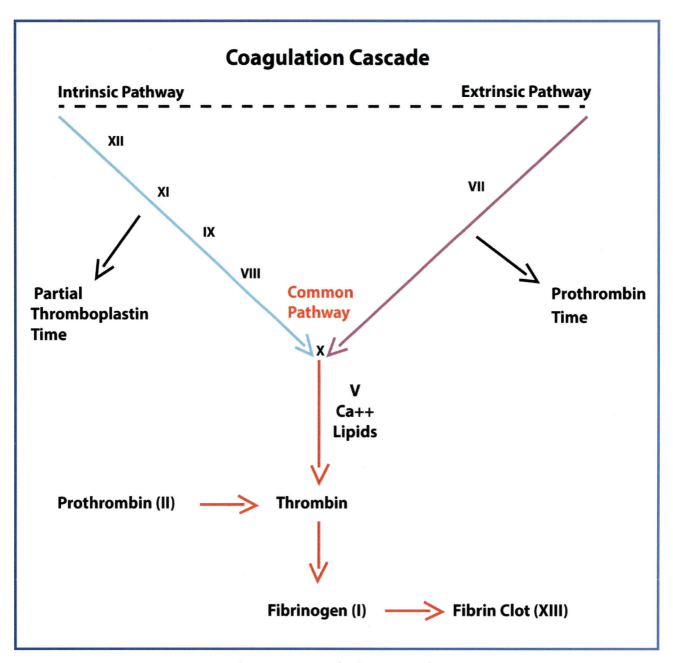

Figure 3: Coagulation Cascade

References:

Ratnoff, OD. Blood. In Physiology 3rd Edition. Ed. Berne & Levy Mosby Year Book. St. Louis, MO 1993

Thomsen, TW, Barclay DA, Setnik GS. Basic laceration repair. N Engl J Med 2006; 355: e18

Broos K, Feys HB, DeMeyer SF, et al., Platelets at work in primary hemostasis. Blood Reviews 2011; 25(4): 155-67

Steed DL. The role of growth factors in wound healing. Surgical clinics of North America 1997; 77(3): 575-86

Broughton G, Janis J, Attinger C. Wound healing: An overview. Plastic and Reconstructive Surgery 2006; 117(7S): 1e-S-32e-S

Coughlin SR. Thrombin signalling and protease-activated receptors. Nature 2000; 407: 258-64

Mason KD, Carpinelli MR, Fletcher JI, et al., Programmed anuclear cell death delimits platelet life span. Cell 2007; 128(6): 1173-86

Gawaz M, Langer H, May AE. Platelets in inflammation and atherogenesis. J Clin Invest 2005; 115(12): 3378-84

Mosesson MW. Fibrinogen and fibrin structure and functions. Journal of Thrombosis and Haemostasis 2005; 3(8)

Hantgan RR, Taylor RG, Lewis JC. Platelets interact with fibrin only after activation. Blood 1985; 65: 1299-1311

Davie EW, Fujikawa K, Kisiel W. The coagulation cascade: initiation, maintenance, and regulation. Biochemistry 1991; 30(43): 10363-70

Mayer SA, Brun NC, Begtrup K, et al., Efficacy and safety of recombinant activated Factor VII for acute intracerebral hemorrhage. N Engl J Med 2008; 358: 2127-37

Rosing J, Van Rijn JL, Bevers EM et al., The role of activated human platelets in prothrombin and factor X activation. Blood 1985; 65: 319-332

Peyvandi F, Garagiola I, Baronciani L. Role of von Willebrand factor in the haemostasis. Blood Transfusion 2011; 9 (Suppl 2): s3-s8

Ariens RAS, Lai T, Weisel J. et al., Role of factor XIII in fibrin clot formation and effects of genetic polymorphisms. Blood 2002; 100:743-54

White GC. Rosendaal F, Aledort LM, et al., Definitions in hemophilia: Recommendation of the Scientific Subcommittee on Factor VIII and Factor IX of the Scientific Standardization Committee of the International Society on Thrombosis and Haemostasis. Thromb Haemost 2001; 85: 560

CHAPTER 4 Inflammatory Phase

Norr Santz & Devi Nampiaparampil

> **CHAPTER PREVIEW**
>
> The inflammatory phase enables the body to keep bacteria, fungi, and other parasites external to the organism, to remove dead cells, and to set the stage for tissue restoration. It is characterized by vasodilation and increased vascular permeability. The inflammatory phase is intended to protect against infection and injury, but it can also be a destructive process that harms tissues.

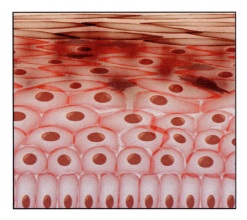

As discussed in the previous chapter, the body responds to wounds with two goals in mind: first to keep things that belong inside the body- in, and second, to keep things that belong outside the body- out. To accomplish these goals, the body must be able to heal the wound as quickly as possible. The inflammatory phase enables the body to keep bacteria, fungi, and other parasites outside of the organism (Thomsen et al., 2006), to remove dead cells, and to set the stage for tissue restoration (Koh et al., 2011).

Trauma-- or the development of a wound--can initiate acute inflammation. Foreign bodies, infection and tissue necrosis can also precipitate acute inflammation. The body attempts to eliminate the invading pathogens and to clear the necrotic debris.

The inflammatory phase is the second phase in the wound healing process. This phase overlaps with the first phase of wound healing, the hemostasis phase, which begins immediately after the injury. The hemostasis phase is dominated by vasoconstriction and platelet aggregation. The inflammatory phase is identified by vasodilation and increased vascular permeability.

Vasodilation is a process that enlarges the diameter of the blood vessel. It opens up. We need vasodilation in order to improve blood flow to the site of injury. During the inflammatory phase, platelets, basophils (a type of white blood cell), and mast cells (immune cells that live in connective tissue) all release a chemical known as histamine. Histamine triggers vasodilation (Steed, 1997).

Vascular permeability has to do with the border between the blood vessel and the cell (the intracellular space), and between the blood vessel and the extracellular space (a.k.a. the interstitial fluid, the third space). If you have a less permeable border, substances cannot pass back and forth easily. If you have a highly permeable border, you will get more movement back and forth (Park-Windhol et al., 2016). During wound healing, we want a more permeable border for two reasons, First, healing factors can exit the bloodstream and get to the wound. Second, waste products and dead cells can be carried from the wound into the bloodstream. Then they can be removed altogether (Nagy et al., 2008).

There are three distinct classes of permeability: basal vascular permeability (what we have at baseline), acute vascular permeability (what we see during an acute injury), and chronic vascular permeability (what we see in pathologic inflammation; it is the inflammation associated with chronic disease). Typically we see increased vascular permeability in acute and chronic inflammation, wound healing, and cancer (Nagy et al., 2008).

While the coagulation cascade is in motion, other reactions are occurring at the site of the wound as well. The phospholipids in cell membranes produce arachidonic acid (Moncada et al., 1979). Depending on the chemical reaction, arachidonic acid can then produce either prostaglandin E2 (PGE2), prostacyclin, thromboxane (TXA2), or leukotrienes (Ricciotti et al., 2011).

CHAPTER 4 - INFLAMMATORY PHASE

The COX-1 and COX-2 enzymes are involved in the synthesis of PGE2, prostacyclin, and thromboxane. The cyclooxygenase (COX-1 and COX-2) inhibitors, which are both non-steroidal anti-inflammatory drugs (NSAIDs) act here (Cannon et al., 2012).

Prostaglandins are vasodilators. In conjunction with histamine, they increase vascular permeability. Two other players, bradykinin and the complement system, also increase vascular permeability. Bradykinin is a byproduct of a system known as the kinin/ kallikrein pathway. It is a pathway involved in both inflammation and blood pressure regulation (Kaplan et al., 2002). Factor XII of the clotting cascade (a.k.a. the Hageman factor) plays a role here (Golias et al., 2007). The complement system "complements" the immune system and the inflammatory response.

The key proteins to know in the complement system are: C3a (which triggers mast cells to release histamine), C5a (which attracts neutrophils), and C3b (which attaches to unwanted substances and then induces neutrophils to phagocytose them). Complement is also involved in the formation of a complex: the membrane-attack complex (MAC), that sits on the surface of a pathogen and then eats a hole through the cell surface to allow for necrosis (Muller-Eberhard, 1986).

As the permeability of the blood vessel increases, fluid from the blood vessel invades the extracellular space. This causes swelling (i.e. edema). This is what we see with the naked eye. Microscopically, we will see inflammatory white blood cells known as neutrophils, monocytes, and macrophages (Landen et al., 2016). These cells help clear pathogens so healing can begin.

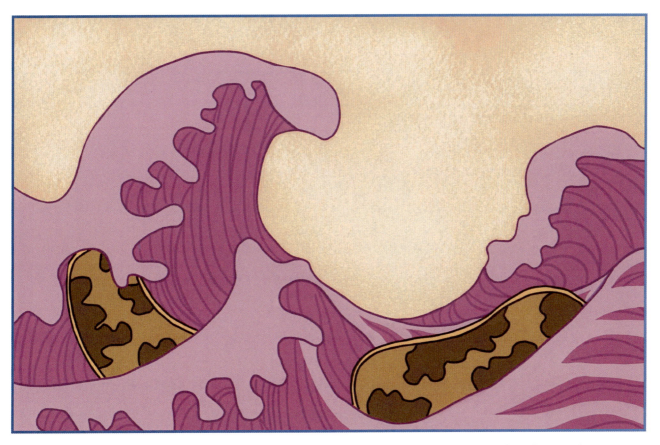

Figure 1: Macrophages, with their elongated pseudopods, engulfing bacteria

White blood cells are descended from hematopoietic stem cells in the bone marrow. There are various types of white blood cells: neutrophils (a.k.a. polymorphonuclear neutrophils or polymorphonuclear leukocytes), monocytes, mast cells, lymphocytes, basophils, and eosinophils. When monocytes leave the bloodstream to live in other tissues, they are called macrophages. Both neutrophils and monocytes (and macrophages) are phagocytes. This means they can engulf pathogens. These cells are also classified as "granulocytes" because they contain granules in their cytoplasm. In neutrophils, monocytes, and macrophages, these granules are reservoirs containing digestive and hydrolytic enzymes. These reservoirs are also known as lysosomes. They are enzymes that can destroy pathogens-- as well as tissues (Dale et al., 2008).

Neutrophils, monocytes and macrophages (altogether known as phagocytes) engulf bacteria and other pathogens into containers called phagosomes. They can also be described as "membrane-bound vesicles." Inside these phagosomes, the bacteria and debris are digested and destroyed (Koh, 2011).

Let's do a brief synonym recap, so this makes more sense:

"~" means "equivalent to"

Monocyte (in blood) ~ macrophage (in tissue)
Neutrophils, monocytes, macrophages, mast cells ~ granulocytes
Neutrophils, monocytes, macrophages, mast cells, lymphocytes, basophils, eosinophils ~ granulocytes
White blood cells
Neutrophils, monocytes, macrophages ~ phagocytes
Phagocytes are a type of granulocyte
Lysosome ~ phagosome (when found in a neutrophil, monocyte, or macrophage)

Extracellular space ~ interstitial space ~ third space

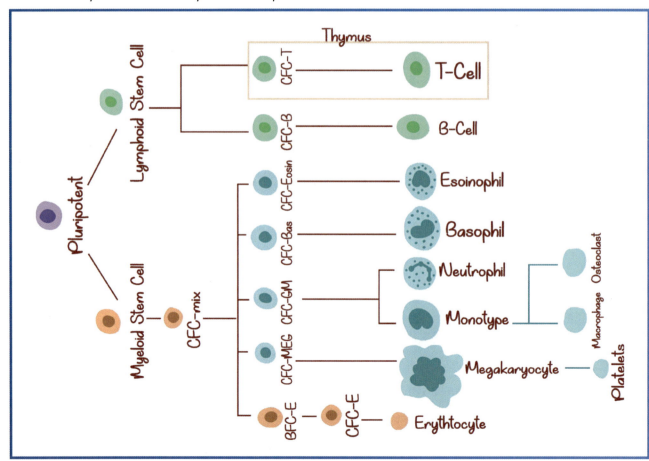

Figure 2: The family tree for blood cells

CHAPTER 4 - INFLAMMATORY PHASE

How do neutrophils, monocytes, and macrophages know what to do? Because of "danger signals." There are two classes of danger signals: damage-associated molecular patterns (DAMPs) and pathogen-associated molecular patterns (PAMPs). DAMPs are molecules found on human cells that are released when they die. PAMPs are molecules found on bacteria. They are molecules that should not be found inside the human body (Tang et al., 2012).

The danger signals are identified by agents that patrol human cells, like border control agents. These types of agents are called pattern recognition receptors. One key pattern recognition receptor is CD14. It is present on the surface of macrophages. CD14 recognizes a PAMP on the outer membrane of bacteria and then signals the macrophage to engulf, or phagocytose, the bacteria (Park et al., 2013).

The pattern recognition receptors also promote the release of substances that attract more inflammatory cells and chemicals, called cytokines and chemokines, which allow the inflammatory response to continue (Lawrence et al., 2009). Macrophages, in particular, produce tumor necrosis factor a (TNF-a) and interleukins 1b and 6 (IL-1b and IL6) that amplify inflammation (Guo et al., 2010).

Macrophages, which are monocytes in tissues, can take one form or another. These are known as the M1 form (or phenotype) or the M2 appearance (or phenotype). When wound healing begins, macrophages are primarily in an M1 phenotype. As M1s, their functions are to scavenge for cell debris, perform phagocytosis, and produce pro-inflammatory substances.

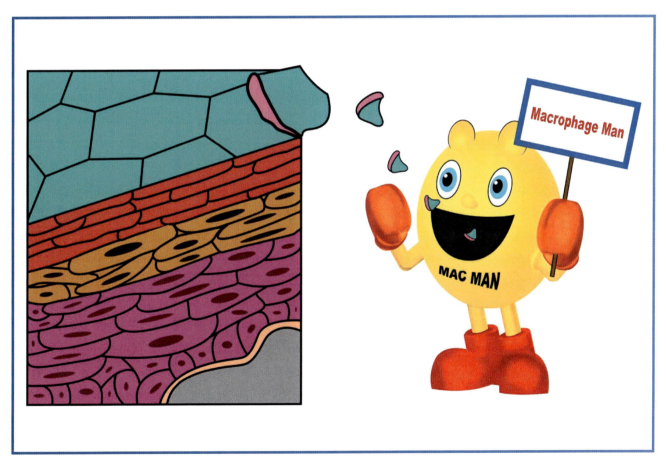

Figure 3: Macrophages are a key component of the clean up crew for wounds.

As wound healing progresses, macrophages switch to the M2 form. At this point, they produce anti-inflammatory substances and growth factors. These influence the production of cells known as fibroblasts, which usher in the next phase of wound healing (Gaffney et al., 2017).

Macrophages also help remove dead neutrophils. Neutrophils never escape back from a wound into a blood vessel. They always go where needed-- and die in the line of duty. If neutrophils stay in the interstitial space too long, they can cause tissue damage and delay healing. This is because the enzymes in neutrophils can break down proteins integral to healing such as clotting factors, complement, and cytokines. They can also produce free radicals, molecules with at least one unpaired electron. For that reason, they are quick to react with lipids, proteins, and genetic material such as DNA. This is known as "oxidative stress." After neutrophils serve their purpose fighting bacteria, macrophages influence them to commit "cellular suicide" in a process known as apoptosis. Apoptosis is a programmed cell death, a mechanism for cells to self-destruct when stimulated by the appropriate trigger (Dale et al., 2008).

Mast cells also have receptors on their cell surfaces. These receptors can attach to pattern recognition receptors. They can also attach to complement protein receptors. When they get activated, they release histamine, which again leads to vasodilation and increased vascular permeability (Krystel-Whittemore et al., 2015).

Generally, there are two kinds of immunity: innate and adaptive immunity (Medzhitov et al., 2000). Innate immunity involves the human body's nonspecific defenses. Innate starts with the physical barriers to infection, including the skin. There are also cells and chemicals circulating in the blood that protect against infections. Neutrophils, monocytes and macrophages are involved in innate immunity. Another type of white blood cell, known as a mast cell, is also involved. Mast cells also have granules inside them. Their granules contain both histamine and heparin (Galli et al., 2005). If mast cells are activated, they can release these contents selectively or suddenly. If they are released suddenly, clinically, we can see anaphylaxis (Metcalfe et al., 1997). The complement system is another major player in innate immunity. The complement system is a group of inactive proteins that are pro-inflammation. They "complement" or help with inflammation. Three pathways activate complement. These are the classical pathway, the alternative pathway, and the mannose-binding lectin pathway. Briefly, the classical pathway involves a specific complement factor known as C1. The alternative pathway is activated by the pathogen itself and the mannose-binding lectin pathway is initiated by a sugar, mannose (Zipfel et al., 2009).

Adaptive immunity produces a very specific response to a pathogen. It is also called "acquired" immunity. It is the basis for vaccines. Once the cells involved in adaptive immunity have been trained, they can decrease the likelihood that the organism is infected by a particular pathogen. For example, a person who is vaccinated against measles may develop lifelong (adaptive) immunity to measles, and thereby have some protection from the virus. That same individual would not have any protection against a different virus, such as HIV, however. The main cell lines involved in adaptive immunity are the lymphocyte-derived T- and B- cells (Medzhitov et al., 2000).

In wound healing, all of these mediators result in the four cardinal signs of inflammation: redness or erythema (rubor), warmth (calor), swelling (tumor), and pain (dolor).

Rubor:
Wounds are red because of the vasodilation that results in increased blood flow. The key mediators of vasodilation are histamine (from mast cell release), prostaglandins (from the phospholipid cell membrane), and bradykinin (from the kinin system).

Calor:
The wounds may also be warm. This is also because of vasodilation. The body may feel warm as well-- such as in a fever. In response to bacteria and other pathogens, macrophages release chemicals called cytokines into the blood. The cytokines known as interleukin-1 (IL-1) and tumor necrosis factor (TNF) travel to the hypothalamus, the part of the brain that regulates body temperature. There, they activate the cyclooxygenase pathway responsible for the production of prostaglandins. Prostaglandin E2 (PGE2) raises the body's set point for temperature.

CHAPTER 4 - INFLAMMATORY PHASE

Tumor:
The increased vascular permeability leads to fluid traveling across the border from the blood into the extracellular space.

Dolor:
Both bradykinin and prostaglandin E2 cause pain directly. The stretching of nerve endings, from swelling, can also indirectly lead to pain.

The inflammatory phase is intended to protect against infection and injury, but it can also be a destructive process that causes harm to tissues. If the body cannot stop the process once it has started, or if the body is unable to clear damaged tissue and foreign substances, there will be a problem. If there is prolonged severe and excessive inflammation, that can delay healing or cause scarring. This occurs in diabetic wounds, for example (Landen et al., 2016).

Macrophages, fibroblasts and fatty acids are involved in the transition from the inflammatory phase to the next phase: proliferation (Landen et al., 2016). There may be opportunities to accelerate wound healing and reduce scarring during this transition. We will discuss this further in later chapters of the text.

Fibroblasts regulate the wound environment. They often decrease cytokine levels. The decrease in cytokines triggers inflammatory cells to go through programmed cell death, or apoptosis. This often occurs at the peak of the inflammatory response, and then triggers decrease, and ultimately a resolution of the inflammation (Landen et al., 2016).

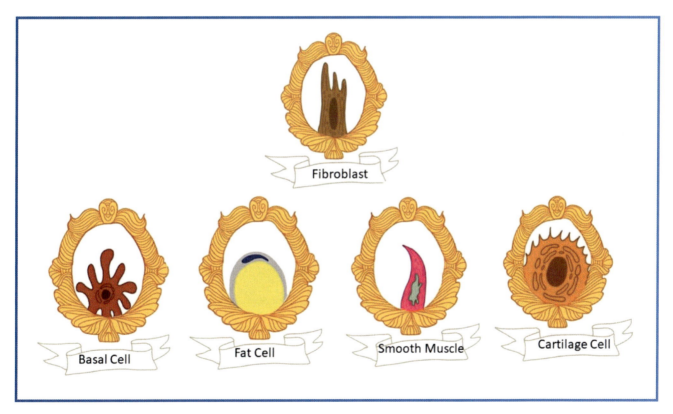

Figure 4: The fibroblast family tree

References:

Thomsen, TW, Barclay DA, Setnik GS. Basic laceration repair. N Engl J Med 2006; 355: e18

Koh TJ and DiPietro LA. Inflammation and wound healing: the role of the macrophage 2011; 13: e23

Steed DL. The role of growth factors in wound healing 1997; 77(3): 575-86

Park-Windhol C and D'Amore PA. Disorders of vascular permeability. Annual Review of Pathology: Mechanisms of Disease 2016; 11:251-81

Nagy JA. Benjamin L, Zeng Huiyan et al., Vascular permeability, vascular hyperpermeability and angiogenesis. Angiogenesis 2008; 11(2): 109-19

Moncada S and Vane JR. Arachidonic acid metabolites and the interactions between platelets and blood vessel walls. N Engl J Med 1979; 300: 1142-7

Ricciotti E and Fitzgerald GA. Prostaglandins and inflammation. Arterioscler Thromb Vasc Biol 2011; 31(5): 986-1000

Cannon CP and Cannon PJ. COX-2 inhibitors and cardiovascular risk. Science 2012; 336(6087): 1386-7

Kaplan AP. Joseph K, Silverberg M. Pathways for bradykinin formation and inflammatory disease. Journal of Allergy and Clinical Immunology 2002; 109(2): 195-209

Golias Ch, Charalabopoulos A, Stagikas D. et al., The kinin system—bradykinin: Biological effects and clinical implications. Multiple role of the kinin system—bradykinin. Hippokratia 2007; 11(3): 124-8

Muller-Eberhard HJ. The membrane attack complex of complement. Ann Rev Immunol 1986; 4: 503-28

Landen NX, Li D, Stahle M. Transition from inflammation to proliferation: a critical step during wound healing. Cell Mol Life Sci, 73:3861-3885.

Dale DC, Boxer L, Liles WC. The phagocytes: neutrophils and monocytes. Blood 2008; 112: 935-45

Tang D, Kang R, Coyne CB et al., PAMPs and DAMPs: Signal 0s that spur autophagy and immunity. Immunol Rev 2012; 249(1): 158-75

Park BS and Lee JO. Recognition of lipopolysaccharide pattern by TLR4 complexes. Exp Mol Med 2013; 45(12): e66

Lawrence T. The nuclear factor NF-kB pathway in inflammation. Cold Spring Harb Perspect Biol 2009; 1(60): a001651

Guo S, Dipietro LA. Factor affecting wound healing. J Dent Res 2010; 89(3): 219-29

Gaffney L. Macrophages' role in tissue disease and regeneration. Results Probl Cell Differ 2017; 62: 245-71

Krystel-Whittemore M, Dileepan KN, Wood JG. Mast cell: A multi-functional master cell. Front Immunol 2016; 6: 620

Medzhitov R and Janeway C. Innate immunity. N Engl J Med 2000; 343: 338-44

Galli S, Nakae S, Tsai M. Mast cells in the development of adaptive immune responses. Nature Immunology 2005; 6: 135-42

Metcalfe DD, Baram D, Mekori YA. Mast cells. Physiological Reviews 1997; 77(4): 1033-79

Zipfel PF and Skerka C. Complement regulators and inhibitory proteins. Nature Reviews Immunology 2009; 9: 729-40

CHAPTER 5: Proliferative Phase

Anokhi Mehta & Devi Nampiaparampil

> **CHAPTER PREVIEW**
>
> In the proliferative phase, the body must break down the fibrin clot to make room for endothelial cells, epithelial cells, and fibroblasts to move in. Endothelial cells are part of the new blood vessels that are forming. Epithelial cells are part of the new wound surface (usually skin) that is forming. Fibroblasts will lay down early healing tissue called granulation tissue. In this chapter, we review these processes.

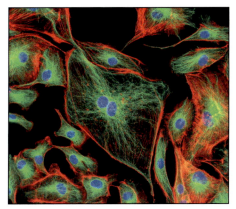

The proliferative phase starts approximately five days after an injury depending on the person's age and overall health. Although there is some overlap, this phase generally follows the inflammatory phase (Steed, 1997). It begins as the number of neutrophils in the wound decrease—from phagocytosis—and the numbers of macrophages and fibroblasts in the wound increase. This phase is sometimes referred to as "fibroplasia" (Steed, 1997). The focus in this stage is repairing the wound.

During the inflammatory phase, several mediators are released into the wound. These include C5a (a member of the complement system), a protein that can act as a molecular glue that is known as fibronectin, as well as growth factors. Growth factors are small proteins that bind to surface molecules found on cells, called receptors. When the growth factor and receptor on the cell surface join, a cascade of events inside the cell begins (Barrientos et al., 2008) that can facilitate healing.

Platelets release specific growth factors when there is an active wound. They release platelet-derived growth factor (PDGF), transforming growth factor-beta (TGF-beta), vascular endothelial growth factor (VEGF), and epidermal growth factor (EGF) (Barrientos et al., 2008). PDGF attracts neutrophils to the site to remove debris. TGF-beta helps transform monocytes to macrophages. Macrophages then release a variety of cytokines, or chemical messengers, including interleukin-1 (IL-1) and interleukin-6 (IL-6).

IL-1 can send various chemical messages. It can affect almost every type of cell in the body. It is highly inflammatory so there is a narrow margin between its beneficial and harmful effects (Dinarello, 1996). IL-6 is another highly inflammatory chemical messenger. It assists in the creation of C-reactive protein (CRP), another marker of inflammation. In the body as a whole, IL-6 increases the amount of glucose being produced, and then ultimately the amount of compensatory insulin produced (Pradhan et al., 2001).

The growth factors involved in wound healing include platelet-derived growth factor (PDGF), vascular endothelial growth factor (VEGF), basic fibroblast growth factor (b-FGF), insulin-like growth factor (IGF-1) and transforming growth factor (TGF-beta). All of them are involved in replenishing the extracellular space (Barrientos et al., 2008).

Some of these growth factors attract fibroblasts, which then release other cytokines, or chemical messengers, that promote both the formation of new tissue called granulation tissue, and the creation of new blood vessels in a process known as angiogenesis (Nguyen et al., 2011).

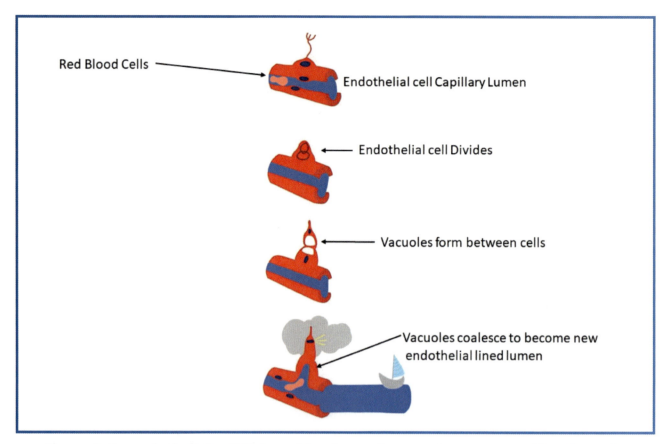

Figure 1: An endothelial cell lining a blood vessel generates a new capillary branch. That endothelial cell divides. Vacuoles form in each of those cells. When they connect, they form the lumen of the new capillary. This process repeats and repeats in a process known as angiogenesis-- or neovascularization.

VEGF, PDGF, and b-FGF are involved in creating new blood vessels. As they are created, they can bring more oxygen and nutrients to the area. This allows the cells, including fibroblasts (which we will come back to), to continue the work of wound healing.

Very simplified recap (simplified from Barrientos et al., 2008):

EGF: think E for epithelialization

VEGF: think V for vascularization

b-FGF: think F for fibroblasts; FGF stimulates them to make collagen (which we will discuss)

PDGF: think P for Proliferation of fibroblasts and P for production of extracellular matrix; PDGF can be applied to non-healing wounds to facilitate closure.

TGF-alpha: think A for Attracting keratinocytes to the wound

TGF-beta: no mnemonic for this one; it is involved in wound epithelialization and contraction; if a fetus sustains a wound, the fetus appears to decrease levels of this growth factor; this may be the reason fetal wounds don't form scars. Bone morphogenetic proteins are in this family. They are often used to facilitate healing after spinal fusions (Hustedt et al., 2014).

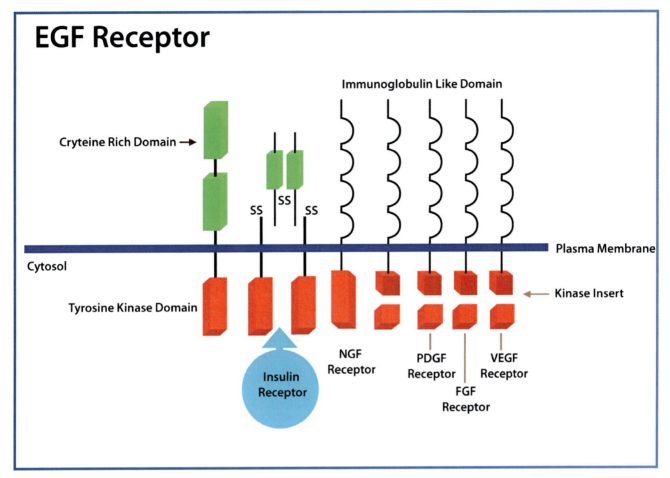

Figure 2: The horizontal gray line represents the cell membrane. Above that, we see the inside of the cell. Below it, we see the extracellular space, where growth factor binding sites are located.

New blood vessels must be formed to carry oxygen and nutrients to the wounded area. This process of creating blood vessels is called angiogenesis. The space su rounding the cells, called the extracellular space (a.k.a. extracellular matrix, interstitial space or third space) must be replenished with proteins and other materials to provide support to the local cells.

The formation of the fibrin clot was one of the main goals of the hemostasis phase. In the proliferative phase, the body must break down the fibrin clot to make room for endothelial cells, epithelial cells, and fibroblasts, among other cells, to move in (Navani et al., 2017). Endothelial cells are part of the new blood vessels that are forming. Epithelial cells are part of the new wound surface (usually skin) that is forming. Fibroblasts are going to lay down early healing tissues, or granulation tissues.

Fibroblasts have an important role in laying down the extracellular matrix. This is the structural support for the area-- the molecular scaffold, if you will- for cells. Initially, fibroblasts lay down a thin layer of scaffold, which is usually weaker than the layer that existed prior to the injury. This weaker layer is typically made of collagen type III. Although collagen type III is typically weaker than the pre-existing collagen, its main advantage is that it can be laid down quickly (Liu et al., 1995).

Collagen is a molecule that is found throughout the body: in the bones, joints, ligaments, tendons, blood vessels, skin, and even the eye. It is classified in different ways: according to the type (type I, II, III, IV, V, etc.) and according to the shape of the resulting structure it forms (ex. fibrillar vs. non-fibrillar) (Myllyharju et al., 2009).

Type I collagen is the most abundant form of collagen in the body. It is found in bones, tendons, blood vessel walls, skin, cornea, and in the endomysium that surrounds muscle fibers. Type II is found in hyaline cartilage, which comprises joints. Type III cartilage is a relatively weaker form of cartilage. It is usually found in the tissues that grow over a prior wound. It is also found in the uterus. Scar tissue is typically composed of a combination of type I and type III collagen. Type IV cartilage is found in the eye and in the capillaries. It is found in the glomeruli of the kidneys, for example. Type V is found mostly in the interstitial tissues. It can also be seen in the placenta. These are the five main types of collagen found in the body, although there are many others (Myllyharju et al., 2009).

Collagen can also be classified as fibrillar or non-fibrillar. The definition of "fibrillar" is small, slender fiber. Collagen molecules can be connected to each other like Legos. When certain types of collagen are stacked together, they form slender fibers, or fibrillar collagen structures. When other types of collagen are stacked together, they create a different shape, known as non-fibrillar collagen (Myllyharju et al., 2009).

One of the goals of the proliferative phase is wound closure. The wound must be covered to protect the organism from the surrounding environment. Collagen is being laid down in the wound in an orderly fashion. Another molecule, elastin, is being laid down in the wound in a disorderly fashion. Elastin forms random coils, which allow for stretch and recoil of the tissue in the wound (Steed, 1997). Meanwhile, new blood vessels are forming. Hypoxia stimulates the formation of blood vessels. It appears that as the oxygen level in the wound normalizes, the formation of new blood vessels slows down (Steed, 1997). Meanwhile, epithelial cells, found at the wound margins, begin to proliferate. These cells travel over the collagen to form a thickened surface.

The cells on the outer surface of the body are called epithelial cells. Most of these cells are skin cells. If the wound occurs on the corneal surface or on a mucosal membrane, for example, the type of epithelial cell may be something other than a skin cell. Keratinocytes, skin cells, travel to the surface of the wound to replenish the skin.

As practitioners of musculoskeletal medicine, we are often most concerned with impaired healing in injured muscles, tendons, ligaments, and joints. Together, these chapters discuss what should happen in normal healing.

References:

Steed DL. The role of growth factors in wound healing. Surgical Clinics of North America 1997; 77(3): 575-86

Barrientos S, Stojadinovic O, Golinko MS, et al., Growth factors and cytokines in wound healing. Wound Repair and Regeneration 2008; 16(5): 585-601

Dinarello CA. Biologic basis for interleukin-1 in disease. Blood 1996; 87(6): 2095-147

Pradhan AD, Manson JE, Rifai N. et al., C-reactive protein, interleukin 6, and risk of developing type 2 diabetes mellitus. JAMA 2001; 286(3): 327-34

Nguyen RT, Borg-Stein J, McInnis K. Applications of platelet-rich plasma in musculoskeletal and sports medicine: an evidence-based approach. PMR 2011: 3(3): 226-50

Hustedt JW and Blizzard DJ. The controversy surrounding bone morphogenetic proteins in the spine: A review of the current research 2014; 87(4): 549-61

Navani A, Li G, Chrysta J. Platelet rich plasma in musculoskeletal pathology: A necessary rescue or a lost cause? Pain Physician 2017; 20(3): E345-56

Liu SH, Yang RS, al-Shaikh R, et al., Collagen in tendon, ligament and bone healing: A current review. Clinical Orthopaedics and Related Research 1995; 318: 265-78

Myllyharju J and Kivirikko KI. Collagens and collagen-related diseases. Annals of Medicine 2001; 33(1): 7-21

CHAPTER 6 Maturation Phase

Arlene Lazaro

> **CHAPTER PREVIEW**
>
> This remodeling phase involves a delicate balance between constructing new tissue and breaking down old tissue. As the rate of new collagen formation decreases, the tensile strength of the wound increases. In this chapter, we review how this phase progresses in muscles, tendons, and ligaments.

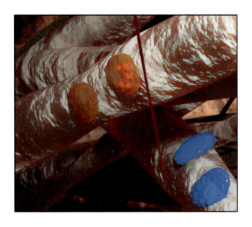

The final and longest phase of wound healing is the maturation, or remodeling phase. The goals of this phase are to produce collagen and lay down a scaffold in the extracellular space, allowing the new extracellular matrix to form, and to develop a scar (Beldon, 2010; Han, 2016).

Macrophages produce chemical signals, called cytokines, that attract cells called fibroblasts into the wound bed. These fibroblasts start producing collagen. The first type of collagen that is produced is type III collagen. This comprises about a third of the healing tissue, called granulation tissue. It is generally weaker than the pre-existing type of collagen. It does not increase the strength of the injured muscle, tendon, or ligament (Beldon, 2010; Janis et al., 2014).

The remodeling of collagen during the maturation phase is critically important in the healing of damaged tendons, ligaments, and muscles. As the collagen matures, it transforms into the stronger type I collagen. This is one of the sentinel events in the remodeling phase. In order for this to happen, an enzyme, a protein called collagenase, responsible for the breakdown of collagen, must get rid of the extra collagen while still allowing for new collagen to be made. Excess blood vessels also recede. The remodeling phase involves a delicate balance between constructing new tissue and breaking down old tissue (Gantwerker et al., 2012).

This collagen transformation continues for about 4 to 5 weeks. As the rate of new collagen formation decreases, the tensile strength of the wound increases (Han, 2014; Janis, 2016).

This is because the collagen molecules are forming bonds between themselves. They are linking their molecules together through a process called cross-linking. This cross-linking of collagen eventually produces solid, closely knit fibers. As the maturation phase progresses, more complex cross-linking occurs. This leads to greater strength and stability in the muscle. After approximately 3 months, depending on the circumstances, the wound can reach 80% of its original tensile strength. It will probably never reach 100% of its original tensile strength (Han, 2014; Janis, 2016).

The maturation phase varies depending on the musculoskeletal tissue type.

Skeletal Muscles:

In skeletal muscle (the muscles you can control voluntarily), mature muscle cells are called myotubes or myofibers. These myotubes or myofibers are organized into larger muscle fiber bundles. Along the margins of the fibers, muscle stem cells, called satellite cells, lie dormant. They are activated once there is an injury (Stocum et al., 2017).

CHAPTER 6 - MATURATION PHASE

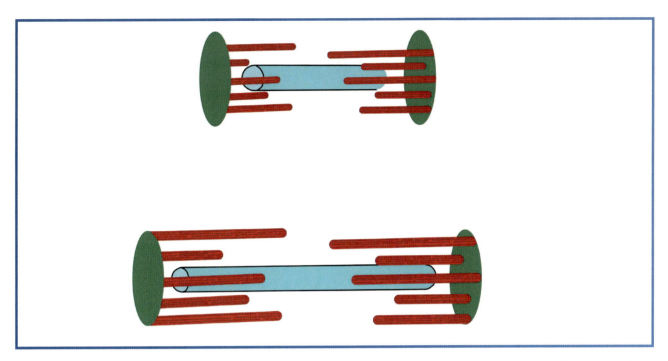

Figure 1: The sliding filament model of muscle contraction. The "thin" actin filaments (in red) and the "thick" myosin filaments (in blue) slide along each other. When they are close together, the muscle is contracting. When they are farther apart, the muscle is relaxed.

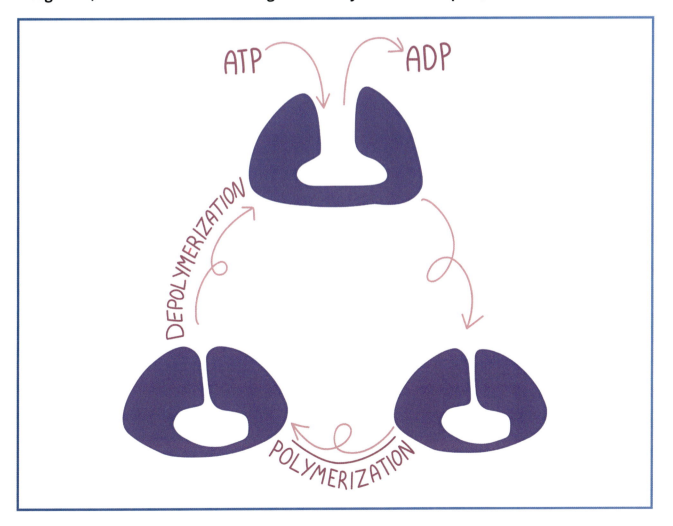

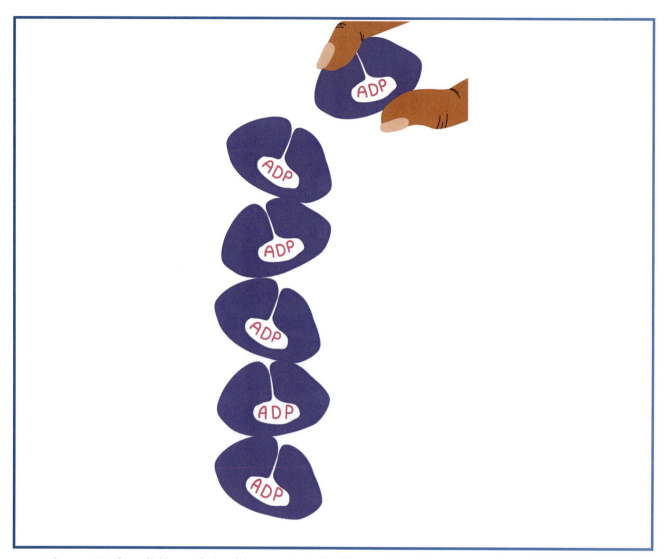

Figure 2: The sliding of the filaments is facilitated by the conversion of ATP to ADP. This conversion yields energy that powers the sliding of the filaments. The body stacks ADP as it is produced from the conversion of ATP to energy.

After an injury, the mature muscle cells die. This process is called necrosis. And the satellite cells transform into different types of cells called myogenic precursors. As wound healing progresses, these myogenic precursors become larger cells called myoblasts. Those myoblasts then fuse to become myotubes or myofibers. Ultimately, these cells grow into the injured region. While this process of transformation, also called cell differentiation, is occurring, other changes are occurring in the area (Juban et al., 2017).

In order for a muscle fiber to function effectively, it must connect to a nerve. The area where the two connect is called a neuromuscular junction. Not only will the nerve give the muscle directions. It will also nourish it. If a muscle does not receive signals from a nerve, it will ultimately shrink in a process called denervation atrophy. This area can then be replaced by scar tissue (Lennox, 1993).

As we discussed in earlier chapters, neutrophils and macrophages invade the area to engulf and remove (or phagocytose) dead myofiber cells. Fibroblasts rush into the area to lay down a collagen scaffold. Again, type III collagen is initially laid down and later replaced by type I collagen. As the myotubes grow between the collagen fibers, the size of the muscle fibers increases. This means that the number of collagen fibers laid down between the muscle fibers decreases (Lennox, 1993). When the body is repairing a muscle injury, there is a race between the myoblasts that are creating muscle fibers and the fibroblasts that are creating collagen.

Growth factors move in to stimulate new blood vessel formation. Then the macrophages themselves transform. They remove the neutrophils from the area. They also stimulate further growth and recovery of the muscle. The process of maturation, where the muscle tries to regain its former strength, takes several weeks to occur (Juban at al., 2017).

Muscles align in the direction of pull. If there is a muscle contraction, the muscle fibers will orient themselves parallel to the line of tension (Lennox, 1993).

It is possible that if the injured area returns to use or movement quickly, that will cause the muscle fibers to orient themselves more quickly. It may also cause more inflammation. If there is more inflammation, there will be more swelling in the area. That leads to more collagen being produced locally. This combination of events may enable the area to quickly gain tensile strength and return to its pre-injury status (Lennox, 1993).

The process of muscle regeneration appears to be the same regardless of the type of tissue injury: laceration (Novak et al., 2014), crush (Takagi et al., 2011), ischemia (Contreras-Shannon et al., 2006), exercise-induced muscle damage (Paulsen et al., 2002), or weight bearing after prolonged immobility (St. Pierre et al., 2004).

Tendons:

Tendons are tough fibrous bands that attach muscles to bones. They can have different shapes: cords, ribbons, or bands (Benjamin et al., 1995). Tendons are composed of various cells. Approximately 90% are tenocytes (mature tendon cells) or tenoblasts (immature tendon cells). The other 10% are cartilage cells called chondrocytes, joint fluid producing cells called synovial cells, and blood vessel related cells such as endothelial cells. This is because tendons share borders with cartilage, synovium and blood vessels (Sharma et al., 2005).

Under a microscope, tendon fibrils have a crumpled wrinkled appearance at rest. This is because they are slack at rest. They become taut during active muscle contraction (Ackerman, 2015). Compared to muscle, tendons have a lower metabolic rate. They lean towards more anaerobic processes than muscle. Because they use less energy than muscle, and because they do not rely on oxygen as much, tendons are able to carry greater weight for longer periods of time than muscle with less risk of dying. However, these same properties make them slower at healing from injuries (Williams, 1986).

Each tendon has a covering called an epitenon, which carries the blood supply and lymphatics to the tendon. When the epitenon extends into the tendon itself, it is called an endotenon. The epitenon is surrounded by a fibrous sheath called a paratenon. This paratenon is loose tissue comprising both type I and type III collagen, some elastic fibers composed of a substance called elastin, and synovial (or joint-fluid producing) cells. There are more of these synovial cells in the tendons in the hands and feet because those generally require more lubrication for movement (Jozsa et al., 1997).

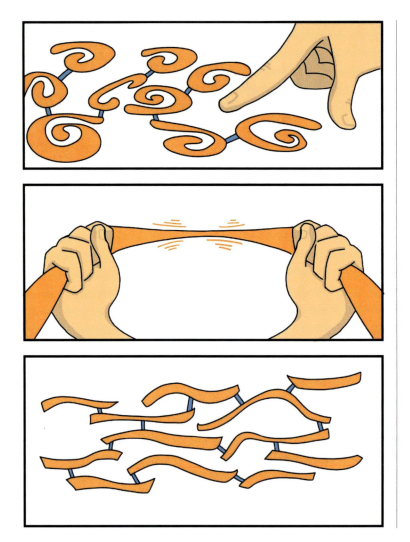

Figure 3: Elastin gives tendons the ability to stay slack at rest and taut with contractions

After a tendon injury, fibroblasts produce collagen. At first, the collagen fibers are disorganized. However, they still contribute to the overall strength of the tendon (Ackerman, 2015; Bown et al., 2016). As the tendon is contracted more often, through increased muscle loading, the contractions stimulate the fibroblasts to make more type I collagen, the stronger form of collagen. The contractions of the tendon cause the collagen to align with the long axis of the tendon (Ackerman, 2015; Riggin et al., 2015). This improves the ability of the tendon to carry more weight or to withstand more of a load (Ackerman, 2015). This process continues for approximately 4 weeks. The repaired tissue is still fibrous scar. It will probably never be as strong as it was prior to the initial injury (Stocum et al., 2012).

Many factors influence the rate and quality of tendon healing. One of the most important is the mechanical tension across the repair site. Mechanical tension affects the realignment of collagen fibers and ultimately tensile strength of the wound .This is why a patient's rehabilitation program iscritical. The protocol for loading a tendon after a regenerative injection may either improve or impair the outcome. More research is necessary to investigate which specific movement patterns or rehabilitation protocols are most likely to heal tendons.

Just a clarification of terms: tendinitis refers to inflammation around a tendon.Inflammation is more commonly seen with an acute injury or a tendon rupture. More chronic changes are seen in tendinopathy where the tendon turns from white to gray and thins out. Tendinopathy is a non-specific term that refers to overuse injury to the tendon. Some argue that technically the terms "tendinitis" and "tendinosis" should only be used after the tendon is evaluated under the microscope (Sharma et al., 2006).

Under the microscope, tendinosis has some common features. We can see disorganized thinned collagen, scattered blood vessels, a greater number of cells in general, and a greater number of glycosaminoglycans. Glycosaminoglycans are a type of protein that can attract water. Historically, the pain associated with tendinopathy has been attributed to inflammation. However, under the microscope, there doesn't appear to be a lot of inflammation going on with tendinopathy. This suggests there must be another reason that tendinopathies are painful (Khan et al., 1995).

The age-related decrease in tendon strength and power are thought to be related to decreases in collagen cross-linking (Bailey et al., 1984). It is possible that these changes can be reversed with resistance training (Reeves et al., 2003; Maganaris et al., 2004).

Ligaments:

Ligaments attach bone to bone, stabilize joints and guide them through their normal range of motion (Riggin et al., 2015). Like tendons, the collagen in ligaments has a crumpled, wrinkled appearance. This allows them to stretch slightly and stabilize the joint. If the collagen becomes more linear and more taut-- and less wrinkled, that increases the stiffness of the ligament, and therefore, the stiffness of the joint.

As with wounded muscles and tendons, during the proliferative phase, fibroblasts make type III collagen in injured ligaments. In ligaments in particular, the extracellular space is made up of randomly aligned collagen molecules. The collagen molecules are not as organized in ligaments as they are in muscles and tendons. The new collagen fibers that are formed in healing ligaments are narrower than the original uninjured collagen fibers. They are also cross-linked less effectively. As a result, the collagen fibers are not as tightly packed as they were originally. Therefore, the healed ligament is ultimately weaker than the prior uninjured ligament (Bown et al., 2016). In ligaments, tissue remodeling can go on for a year or longer after the initial injury (Woo et al., 2000).

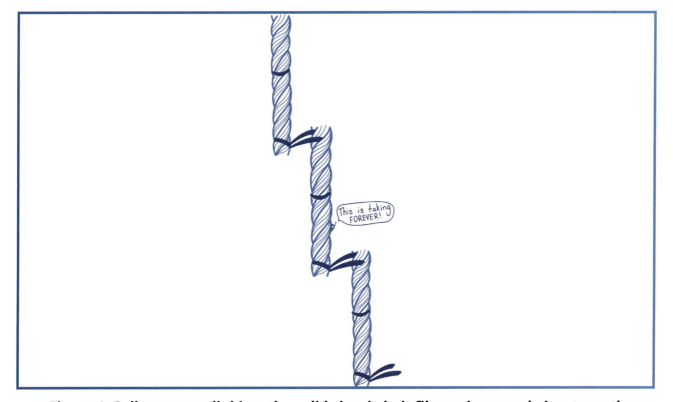

Figure 4: Collagen crosslinking; the solid closely knit fibers give muscle its strength and stability. There are intramolecular crosslinks (within each fiber) and intermolecular crosslinks (between each collagen fiber). The remodeling of these collagen fibers can take a year or longer.

Cortisone inhibits inflammation is by preventing lysosomes from releasing their digestive enzymes. Cortisone also prevents neutrophils from accumulating at the wound site and prevents the production of inflammatory cytokines, or chemical messengers (Kapetanos, 1982). They decrease collagen production (Scutt et al., 2006) and can even cause collagen fibers to die at the injection site (Wiggins et al., 1995). Ligaments injected with cortisone appear to be weaker when they heal (Nichols., 2005).

There is some evidence that prolotherapy injections, injections with a pro-inflammatory substance, increase the number of fibroblasts and the amount of growth factors in the local area (Hauser et al., 2011). Animal studies suggest that prolotherapy-injected ligaments may have a greater mass, thickness, and junction strength with bone (Lee et al., 2009) compared to ligaments that have healed through normal processes.

A note on your friendly neighborhood macrophage:

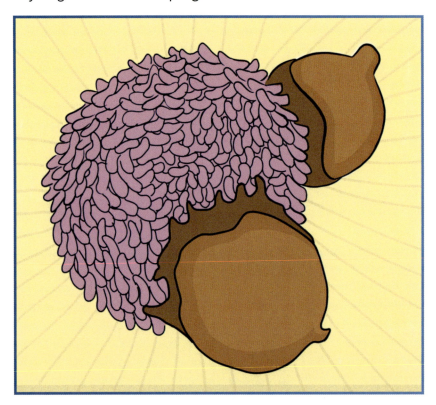

Figure 5: A macrophage (in purple) engulfing two dead cells (in brown)

The macrophage has a critical role to play in wound healing, particularly in muscle. An early study of muscle regeneration used a combination of anti-macrophage antibody serum and glucocorticoids (steroids) to minimize the participation of macrophages. As a result, there was a severe disruption in wound healing (Leibovich et al., 1975).

In diabetes, the macrophage's ability to transition from the pro-inflammatory M1 form to the pro-healing M2 form is affected. This may be one reason why diabetics have impaired wound healing (Koh et al., 2013).

References:

Beldon, Pauline. Basic science of wound healing. Surgery. 2010; 28(9): 409-412

Han, Seung-Kyu. Innovations and Advances in Wound Healing. Seoul, Korea: Springer, 2016: 26-28

Janis JE, Harrison B. Wound healing: part I. Basic science. Plast Reconstr Surg. 2014;133(2):199e-207e

Gantwerker EA, Hom DB. Skin: histology and physiology of wound healing. Clin Plast Surg. 2012;39(1):85-97

Stocum DL, Chapter 6: Regeneration of musculoskeletal tissues. Regenerative Biology and Medicine (2nd Edition). San Diego: Academic Press, 2012: 127-60

Juban G and Chazaud B. Metabolic regulation of macrophages during tissue repair: insights from skeletal muscle regeneration. FEBS Letters 2017; 591: 3007-21

Lennox C. Muscle injuries. In: McLatchie G, Lennox, CME, ed. The soft tissues: Trauma and sports injuries. Oxford; Boston: Butterworth-Heinemann; 1993:83-103

Novak ML, Weinheimer-Haus EM, Koh TJ. Macrophage activation and skeletal muscle healing following traumatic injury. J Pathol 2014; 232: 344-55

Takagi R, Fujita N, Arakawa T, Kawada S, et al., Influence of icing on muscle regeneration after crush injury to skeletal muscles in rats. J Appl Physiol 2011; 110:382-8

Contreras-Shannon V, Ochoa V, Reyes-Reyna O, et al., Fat accumulation with altered inflammation and regeneration in skeletal muscle of CCR2 -/- mice following ischemic injury. Am J Physiol Cell Physiol 2006; 292: C953-67

Paulsen G, Mikkelsen UR, Raastad T, et al., Leukocytes, cytokines and satellite cells: What role do they play in muscle damage and regeneration following eccentric exercise? Exerc Immunol Rev 2012; 18: 42-97

St. Pierre BA and Tidball JG. Differential response of macrophage subpopulations to soleus muscle reloading after rat hindlimb suspension. J. Appl Physiol 1994; 77: 290-7

Benjamin M and Ralphs J. Functional and developmental anatomy of tendons and ligaments. In: Gordon SL, Blair SJ, Fine LJ (eds) Repetitive Motion Disorders of the Upper Extremity. American Academy of Orthopedic Surgeons, Rosemont, USA 1995: 185-203

Sharma P and Maffulli N. Tendon injury and tendinopathy: healing and repair. J Bone Joint Surg Am 2005; 87: 187-202

Ackermann PW. Chapter 4- Tendinopathy I: Understanding Epidemiology, Pathology, Healing, and Treatment. In: Gomes, Manuela E., Reis, Rui L., Rodrigues, Marcia. Tendon regeneration: understanding tissue physiology and development to engineer functional substitutes. London: Elsevier, 2015: 113-147

Williams JG. Achilles tendon lesions in sport. Sports Med 1986; 3:114-35

Jozsa L and Kannus P. Human tendon: Anatomy, physiology and pathology. Human Kinetics, Champaign, USA 1997

Bown, MN, Shiple, BJ, Scarpone M. Regenerative Approaches to Tendon and Ligament Conditions. Phys Med Rehabil Clin N Am 27 2016: 941–984

Riggin CN, Morris TR, Soslowski LJ. Chapter 5- Tendinopathy II: Etiology, Pathology, and Healing of Tendon Injury and Disease. In: Gomes, Manuela E., Reis, Rui L., Rodrigues, Marcia. Tendon regeneration: understanding tissue physiology and development to engineer functional substitutes. London: Elsevier, 2015: 149-183

Sharma P and Maffulli N. Biology of tendon injury: Healing, modeling and remodeling. J Musculoskelet Neuronal Interact 2006; 6(2): 181-90

Khan KM, Cook JL, Bonar F, et al., Histopathology of common tendinopathies. Update and implications for clinical management. Sports Med 1999; 27: 393-408

Bailey AK, Robins SP, Balian G. Biological significance of the intermolecular crosslinks of collagen. Nature 1984; 251: 105-9

Reeves ND, Narici MV, Maganaris CN. Strength training alters the viscoelastic properties of tendons in elderly humans. Muscle Nerve 2003; 28: 74-81

Maganaris, Narici MV, Reeves ND. In vivo human tendon mechanical properties: Effect of resistance training in old age. J Musculoskelet Neuronal Interact 2004; 4: 204-8

Woo SLY, Debski RE, Zeminski J, et al., Injury and repair of ligaments and tendons. Annual Review of Biomedical Engineering 2000; 2: 83-119

Kapetanos G. The effect of the local corticosteroids on the healing and biomechanical properties of the partially injured tendon. Clinical Orthopedics 1982; 163: 170-9

Scutt N, Rolf CG, Scutt A. Glucocorticoids inhibit tenocyte proliferation and tendon progenitor cell recruitment. Journal of Orthopedic Research 2006; 24: 173-82

Wiggins ME, Fadale PD, Ehrlich MG, et al., Effects of local injection of corticosteroids on the healing of ligaments: A follow-up report. Journal of Bone and Joint Surgery 1995; 77A: 1682-91

Nichols AW. Complications associated with the use of corticosteroids in the treatment of athletic injuries. Clinical Journal of Sports Medicine 2005; 15: 370-5

Hauser RA and Dolan EE. Ligament injury and healing: An overview of current clinical concepts. Journal of Prolotherapy 2011; 3(4)

Lee JD, Lee DW, Jeong CW, et al., Effects of intra articular prolotherapy on sacroiliac joint pain. Korean Journal of Pain 2009; 229-33

Leibovich SJ, Ross R. The role of the macrophage in wound repair. A study with hydrocortisone and anti macrophage serum. Am J Pathol. 1975; 78:71–100

Koh T. DiPietro L. Inflammation and wound healing: The role of the macrophage. Expert Rev Mol Med 2013; 13: e23

CHAPTER 7 Platelet Rich Plasma

Puneet Ralhan, Mila Mogilevsky, Devi Nampiaparampil, Pradeep Albert & Alan Katz

CHAPTER PREVIEW

Platelet rich plasma (PRP) is a concentrated autologous mixture of blood plasma enriched with platelets, cytokines, and growth factors that are normally involved in the wound healing cascade. Injecting PRP is considered relatively safe and effective. It is generally supported by science. In this chapter, we will go over the different forms of PRP. We will also review PRP's use in the shoulder, elbow, hip and knee. We will specifically discuss PRP's effect on the tendons, ligaments, joints, tendons, fascia, bone and muscle.

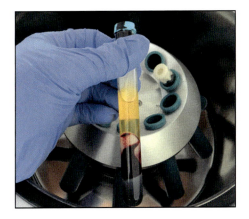

KEY FACTS THAT YOU SHOULD DOCUMENT ABOUT PRP:

Concentration
Erythrocyte-Rich vs. Erythrocyte-Poor
Activation in the body or in the kit
Leukocyte-Rich vs Leukocyte-Poor
Volume

Three consecutive intra-articular PRP injections in monthly intervals may improve clinical outcomes in patients with joint injuries or arthritis. (Cavazos et 2019). Dr. Albert and Dr. Nampiaparampil use this algorithm for tendon and soft tissue injections because they find that patients do better than with multiple injections compared to a single injection.

Platelets are non-nucleated discoid cell fragments derived from megakaryocytes in bone marrow that are about 2 microns in diameter. A platelet's life span is between 7 and 10 days (Pochini et al., 2016).

Platelets contain granules, which are storage reservoirs for bioactive proteins. There are alpha, delta and lambda granules. The alpha granules contain growth factors involved in chemotaxis (attracting other substances), mitogenesis (reproduction and growth), and cell differentiation(the specialization and maturation of cells). The delta granules contain agents involved in the clotting cascade, which stop bleeding. The lambda granules release lysosomal enzymes, which are proteins involved in cleaning up debris. These lysosomes break down lipids, proteins, and carbohydrates (Jurk et al., 2005).

There are normally 200,000 platelets/ uL in human blood. There is no universally accepted concentration of platelets in PRP, however we find a large range in the literature.

Whole blood contains 93% red blood cells, 6% platelets, and 1% white blood cells. With PRP, the goal is to reduce the red blood cell percentage to under 5% and to increase the platelet percentage to approximately 93% (Maffulli et al., 2016). The presence of both red and white blood cells can be controlled when preparing PRP to be used for different indications.

In most commercial kits, the PRP concentration achieved is 1.4 to 7 times higher than in the patient's baseline blood. Current consensus is that at least 1,000,000 platelets/ uL suspended in plasma are required for a therapeutic effect. Although there is no standard definition for PRP, this is a commonly used minimum platelet concentration.

CHAPTER 7 - PLATELET RICH PLASMA

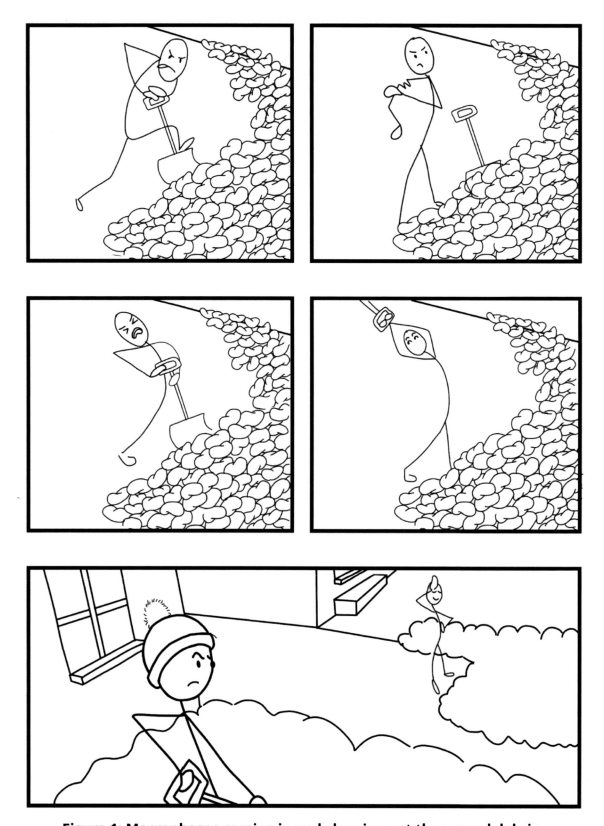

Figure 1: Macrophages coming in and cleaning out the wound debris

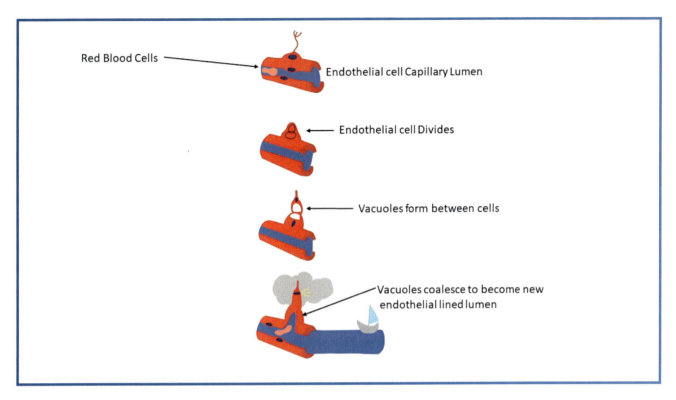

Figure 2: An endothelial cell lining a blood vessel generates a new capillary branch. That endothelial cell divides. Vacuoles form in each of those cells. When they connect, they form the lumen of the new capillary. This process repeats and repeats in a process known as angiogenesis or neovascularization.

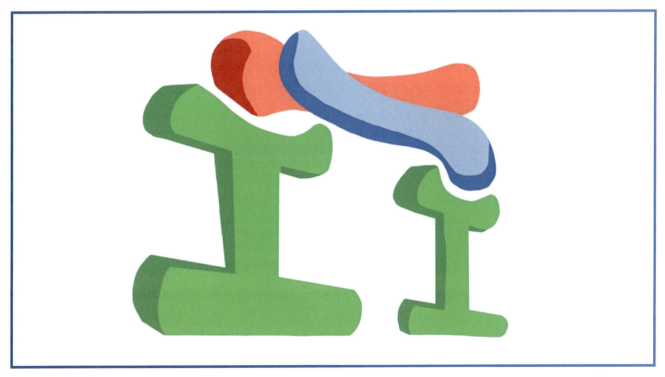

Figure 3: PDGF is a dimer that, because of its structure, acts as a scaffold for other substances involved in healing to bind and attach to. IGF-1 is also involved in building collagen. In addition, IGF-1 helps cells to grow and to mature and differentiate.

More platelets may not always be better. The jury is still out. In a study comparing 2 million to 5 million platelets/ uL on wound healing in intestinal anastomoses, the lower platelet concentration appeared to improve wound healing, whereas the higher concentration interfered with healing (Foster et al., 2009; Yamaguchi et al., 2010 Yoshida et al 2014).

The growth factors that platelets release include platelet-derived growth factor (PDGF), insulin-like growth factor (IGF-1), transforming growth factor (TGF-beta), vascular endothelial growth factor (VEGF), basic fibroblast growth factor (b-FGF), hepatocyte growth factor, and epidermal growth factor. These growth factors are each discussed in
detail in the Wound Healing section of this text, but let's go over them briefly here.

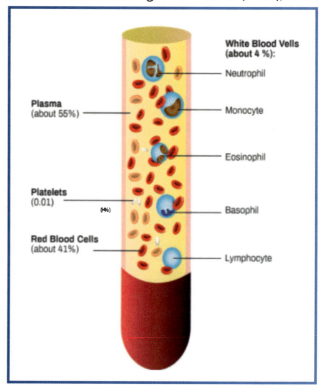

PDGF is involved in activating inflammatory cells, macrophages, to come in and to clean debris.

PDGF also stimulates new blood vessel growth in a process called angiogenesis. PDGF has a role in building collagen, a scaffold for new tissues, as well.

TGF-beta is a pro-inflammatory growth factor. It attracts cells to the wounded area, promotes the tightening or fibrosis of collagen strands, and helps bind substances to the collagen scaffold. It also stimulates new blood vessel growth to bring oxygen and nutrients to the area. TGF-beta prevents osteoclasts, cells that break down bone, from being formed.

VEGF promotes the growth of new blood vessels as well as the formation of granulation tissue, the new tissue that replaces the old wounded one.

Platelets release the contents of their granules when they get "activated." Approximately 70% of their growth factors are released within the first 10 minutes. All of the growth factors are released within an hour (Yun et al., 2016).

Platelets become activated when they contact collagen, thrombin, or the basement membrane of tissues. In PRP preparations, this happens when PRP is injected into the patient's body. Some kits allow you to activate platelets before they get injected. This early activation may lead to improved release of the growth factors from the platelets. However, the release may be premature, meaning that the damaged tissue may have less exposure to the growth factors (Yun et al., 2016). This author typically does not recommend early activation in orthobiologic use.

The types of growth factors found in PRP are variable. PRP contains growth factors that promote cartilage growth, such as TGF-beta 1, IGF-1, beta-FGF, and BMP-2. However, there can also be high levels of growth factors that inhibit cartilage growth. These factors include VEGF, PDGF, and EGF (Anitua et al., 2009).

Fibrin polymerization, determined by the ratio of fibrinogen to thrombin, plays a role in healing. Liquid PRP has soluble fibrinogen, which is the precursor to fibrin. If the thrombin concentration is high, there will be rapid polymerization. This creates a dense network that might slow down signals between cells and the mobility of cells. Slow polymerization might create a more flexible scaffold that could be more conducive to the spread of growth factors and cells involved in healing (Maffulli et al., 2016).

There are many commercially available kits for PRP processing. The four general categories of PRP preparations are: a) leukocyte-rich PRP (LR-PRP), leukocyte-poor PRP (leukocyte-poor PRP), leukocyte-rich with fibrin, and leukocyte poor with fibrin.

Single spin vs Double spin preparations exist. Single spin devices will produce a relatively low platelet concentration in the range of 1.4 to 3 times baseline. Double spin devices will typically produce a 5 to 7 times platelet concentration. Additionally, most single spin devices will produce only a leukocyte-poor product. Most dual spin devices allow for more user control of the final product.

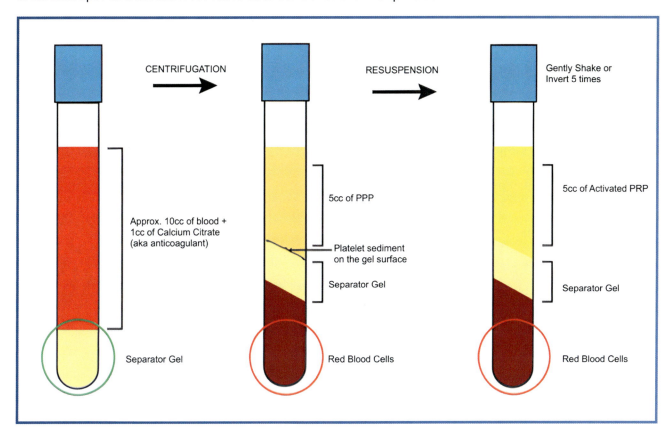

Leukocyte Rich vs Leukocyte-Poor

Leukocytes are white blood cells. When an organism has been wounded, neutrophils are the first type of white blood cell to arrive at the site of injury. Neutrophils are followed by monocytes, which release substances called matrix metalloproteinases (MMP-2, MMP-9, and MMP-13), which break down the debris between damaged cells and which allow cells promoting healing to migrate through the debris. These monocytes transform into macrophages, which can then engulf or encapsulate debris, necrotic tissue, and infectious organisms in a process called phagocytosis (Leick et al., 2014).

Leukocyte-rich PRP can increase inflammation. This can be beneficial in certain cases. On the other hand, white blood cells can also release toxic substances, such as reactive oxygen species and nitric oxide, which can be useful against bacteria, but can also impair wound healing. Therefore, it is not clear whether leukocyte-rich or leukocyte-poor preparations are more effective in healing. A recently published study demonstrated that intra-articular leukocyte-rich PRP or leukocyte-poor PRP injections produced similar clinical improvement in patients with symptomatic knee osteoarthritis. The presence of leukocytes did not significantly affect the clinical results of PRP injections (Di Martino et al., 2022)

Including leukocyte-rich preparations may help clinically in arthritis as well as in tendon injuries due to the positive effect of macrophage recruitment although there is no definitive consensus on this (Lana et al., 2019).

One study showed that-- in comparison to injections of 2 ml of leukocyte-poor PRP, injections of 2 ml of leukocyte-rich PRP showed a greater inflammatory response in the first 5 days after treatment. In a study of rabbit tendons, there was greater cellularity an+d greater vascularity within that time frame. The inflammation resolved by 14 days (Dragoo et al., 2012).

This inflammation may have a role in managing infectious disease. In a retrospective study of 1400 patients who underwent coronary artery bypass grafting (CABG), leukocyte-rich PRP appeared to decrease the incidence of chest wound infections and to decrease the incidence of chest and leg wound drainage (Khalafi et al., 2008).

PRP has been used in various forms including injectate, gel and spray. In the 1990s, platelet gel was used as an alternative to fibrin sealant to decrease bleeding during cardiac surgery (Everts et al., 2006). One meta-analysis combining data from 21 randomized controlled clinical trials as well as some non-randomized trials suggested that platelet gel was helpful in wound healing and wound closure. The wound area and volume decreased (Carter et al., 2011). Another study suggested that, for diabetic foot ulcers, PRP gel was more cost-effective than other therapies over a five-year period (Carter et al., 2003). In gel preparations, platelet-derived growth factors can become trapped in a fibrin glue (Araki et al, 2012).

For musculoskeletal applications most clinicians use the liquid form of PRP to inject intra-articularly as well to inject into areas of tendon injury. This is because most commercially available kits produce an injectate that clinicians administer via syringe non operatively. If using a gel or fibrin matrix it may be more advantageous to administer intraoperatively as it may be easier to adhere to the surgical site after repair.

PRP processing systems are considered medical devices. They have a 510(k) clearance under the Food & Drug Administration (the FDA). Essentially, the FDA approved a device that isolated platelet-rich plasma so that it could be mixed with bone graft materials in order to facilitate healing in bone surgeries, such as spinal fusions. Similar devices are used for processing PRP for off-label uses. These uses, including musculoskeletal wound healing, are left to the physician and patient's discretion.

As with all medical procedures, there are contraindications to consider, the biggest of which are severe thrombocytopenia, and infection at the site of proposed injection. Additionally one must consider recent use of steroids within 2 weeks, use of NSAIDS within 1 week, and patients that have active malignancies with hematogenous spread.

These four types of PRP are listed here below:
1. Leukocyte-rich PRP: has high levels of white blood cells and is in liquid form (anticoagulated)
2. Leukocyte-poor PRP: has low levels of white blood cells and is in liquid form (anticoagulated)
3. Platelet-Rich Fibrin (PRF) or Platelet-Rich Fibrin Matrix (PRFM): that has a low number of white blood cells
4. Platelet-Rich Fibrin (PRF) or Platelet-Rich Fibrin Matrix (PRFM): that has a high number of white blood cells.

In vitro and in vivo are two terms you will find when reading about scientific studies. In vivo means with or within a living organism. In vitro (in glass in Latin) is used to describe work performed outside of a living organism.

When the platelet is activated and becomes more solid, it can be "activated" by the following mechanisms:
1. With calcium inside a test tube (in vitro)
2. With thrombin inside a test tube (in vitro)
3. Inside the patient by collagen (in vivo); this is the most common method in musculoskeletal medicine.
4. PRP can also be activated mechanically by heating the sample or by mechanically damaging the platelet wall with a filter.

Dr. Albert recommends the following PRP classification system to standardize PRP.

Low or Standard Concentration	1X - 2X Platelet Concentration
Medium Concentration	2X - 5X Platelet Concentration
High Concentration	>5X Platelet Concentration

A PRP Kit that concentrates platelets 3X with an injectable volume of 10 ccs. Therefore, it would be documented as an injection of 10 ccs of medium concentration PRP.

A PRP Kit that concentrates platelets 1.4X with an injectable volume of 10 ccs. Therefore, it would be documented as an injection of 10 ccs of low or standard concentration PRP.

If you want to be more precise, you can consider the following criterion to document the presence or absence of RBCs and WBCs.

Generally speaking if the injectate is pink or red it's erythrocyte-positive; if its straw or yellow-colored, it's erythrocte-negative.

The kit manufacturer will decide whether the kit is leukocyte-poor or rich +/-.

Below are three examples that demonstrate Dr. Albert's PRP classification system:

Ex. A PRP kit that concentrates platelets by 3X with an injectable volume of 10 ccs that is straw or yellow-colored lacking WBC leukocyte-poor as stated by the manufacturer would be a classified as a double negative (negative for RBCs, and WBCs). Therefore, it would be documented as an Injection of 10 ccs of double negative medium concentration PRP.

Ex. A PRP kit that concentrates platelets by 1.4X with an injectable volume of 10 ccs that is pink-colored and is leukocyte-rich classified as a PRP injection with 10 CC of E+ leukocyte-rich low concentration PRP.

Ex. A PRP kit that concentrates platelets by 6X with 10 cc that is straw-colored and leukocyte poor would be classified as a PRP injection with 10 CC of E- leukocyte-poor high concentration PRP.

Remember that the higher concentration of PRP doesn't make the PRP better. There may be deleterious effects of high levels of PRP. This is a simple way to standardize PRP.

Clinical Studies:
At the time of publication there have been over 60 positive PRP randomized controlled trials where PRP was used in an orthopedic or musculoskeletal indication.

Shoulder

Tendon Injuries:
Tendons are dense connective tissues that connect muscles to bones. They receive less blood flow than muscle or bone, and are therefore harder to heal after injuries. Tendons are often subjected to large mechanical forces and therefore are susceptible to overuse injuries. Microscopically, these injured tendons show microtears, disrupted collagen fibers, calcification and debris, fat deposits, and disorganized new blood vessel growth. They have fewer total collagen strands compared to healthy tendons. They also show a greater ratio of Type III to Type I collagen strands. These changes alter the mechanical properties of the tendon and may also cause pain. These changes are collectively known as "tendinosis" (Maffulli et al., 2016).

Multiple studies have been published on the use of PRP for rotator cuff repair. In the lab, PRP induces the proliferation of tendon cells called tenocytes, and tendon stem/ progenitor cells, which are stem cells that can only mature into tendon cells. (Jo et al., 2012). Several studies have evaluated the use of PRP in the shoulder--for the treatment of rotator cuff tears. A meta-analysis of rotator cuff tears suggested PRP decreases the rate of recurrences among patients with small and medium rotator cuff tears, but not for large rotator cuff tears (Zhang et al., 2013). In a case report about a patient with a rotator cuff injury who underwent treatment with PRP gel rather than a tendon transposition, researchers observed complete tendon healing at 6 months (Maniscalco et al., 2008).

Elbow:
Many studies have demonstrated the superiority of PRP to corticosteroids or other therapies in terms of pain and function. A meta-analysis of randomized controlled trials found that local PRP injections were associated with superior outcomes for reducing pain and improving elbow joint function compared with local corticosteroids treatment for lateral epicondylitis at a follow-up of 6 months (Xu et al., 2019; Fitzpatrick

et al., 2017; Varshney et al., 2017; Martínez-Montiel et al., 2015).

Gautam et al 2015 reported PRP appeared to enable biological healing, whereas corticosteroid appeared to provide short-term, symptomatic relief but resulted in tendon degeneration.

Wrist:
In a prospective, randomized, blind, controlled, clinical trial of 33 patients, corticosteroids offer short-term relief of symptoms. PRP achieved 12 months of relief of early to moderate symptomatic trapeziometacarpal arthritis (Malaihas et al., 2018).

A randomized controlled trial of 150 patients in Egypt concluded that platelet-rich plasma could be an effective treatment of mild to moderate idiopathic carpal tunnel syndrome and superior to corticosteroid in improving pain, function, and distal sensory latency of the median nerve (Senna et al., 2019). A randomized controlled trial from China was published which demonstrated that PRP is a safe modality that effectively relieves pain and improves disability in the patients with carpal tunnel syndrome (Wu et al., 2017).

Dr. Albert uses 2cc of triple negative PRP (erythrocyte-poor, leukocyte-poor and non-activated) PRP for small joints.

Hip

Joint Injury:
PRP has an effect on growth factors involved in cartilage repair such as IGF-1, TGF-beta, and thrombospondin 1 (Xie et al., 2014).

In an observational study of 40 patients with unilateral hip osteoarthritis, three injections of PRP one week apart resulted in an approximately 30% decrease in pain at 6 months post-treatment (Sanchez et al., 2012). However, 11 out of 40 patients still required a metal resurfacing procedure.

A study of 20 patients with hip osteoarthritis treated with 3 intra-articular injections of PRP 2 weeks apart showed improvement at 1 year. However, there was a worsening of symptoms prior to the improvement (Battaglia et al., 2011).

The Orthopedic Institute in Bologna, Italy reported in the American Journal of Sports Medicine the results of ultrasound guided injections of PRP with and without Hyaluronic acid for hip osteoarthritis and did find significant clinical improvement.(Dallari et al., 2019).

Knee:
A systematic review in 2017 found that PRP is effective when treating Knee osteoarthritis. (Xing et al)
The Journal of Orthopaedic Surgery and Research also published a German manuscript in 2019 which studied 59 patients and concluded that there was a reduction of pain in knee osteoarthritis patients which was independent from the level of cartilage damage, with quantification by MRI. (Burchard et al., 2019).

Tendon Injuries:
A study utilizing three separate PRP injections, each 15 days apart, for the treatment of patellar tendinopathy showed significant improvement in pain, function, and quality of life with PRP (Kon et al., 2009).
In a prospective cohort study of patellar tendinopathy, PRP injections resulted in better clinical outcomes than focused extracorporeal shock therapy (Vetrano et al., 2013).

When the anterior cruciate ligament (ACL) tears and the patient elects to have a surgical repair, part of the patellar tendon is often taken by the surgeon and used to reconstruct the ligament. In a study of 27 patients who had ACL repairs, PRP was applied to the patellar ligament donor site in 12 of them. In this randomized controlled study, those patients had significantly better healing at the patellar tendon site at 6 months based on MRI. They also reported better postoperative pain control (Almeida et al., 2012).

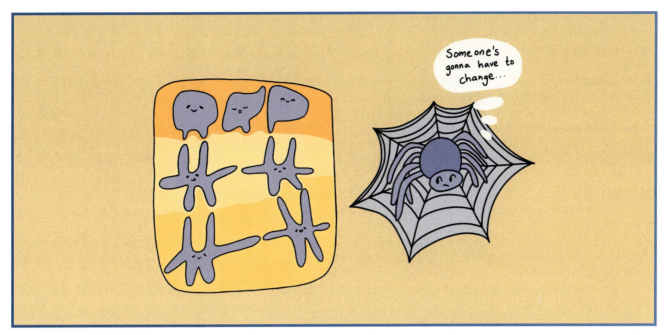

Figure 4: Growth factors acting like a spider with her web: attracting mesenchymal cells and then promoting them to change and differentiate into osteocytes to weave new bone. The osteocytes then get trapped in the bone they have weaved-- like a spider in her web.

Ligaments:
In a randomized controlled prospective study of 25 patients undergoing ACL repairs with tendon grafts, the ones who received platelet gel and leukocyte injections experienced better postoperative pain control and improved antero-posterior knee stability (Vogrin et al., 2010).

In another study, researchers evaluated how effectively autologous grafts took hold in ACL repairs. The patients who received PRP at the graft site had MRIs that showed the graft being incorporated more quickly than those who did not (Radice et al., 2010).

In a retrospective study of 100 patients who underwent ACL surgical repair, PRP appeared to improve postoperative pain. It also decreased the time necessary for the patients to resume normal activities (Sanchez et al., 2003).

Joint Injury:
Multiple studies show improvements in knee osteoarthritis symptoms with PRP (Spakova et al., 2012; Filardo et al., 2011; Sanchez et al., 2012). A randomized controlled double-blinded study compared PRP to saline for the treatment of knee osteoarthritis. Seventy eight patients (156 knees) were studied. At 6 months, the group that received PRP reported significantly better outcomes (Patel et al., 2013). In osteoarthritis, a disease of the cartilage, PRP injections appear to be more effective than saline and may even be more effective than hyaluronic acid (Dai et al., 2017; Shen et al., 2017).

A randomized controlled study of 120 patients with knee osteoarthritis showed better outcomes with four intra-articular injections of PRP vs. four intra-articular injections of hyaluronic acid at up to 24 weeks of follow-up (Cerza et al., 2012). Another randomized controlled study of 30 patients with knee osteoarthritis suggested that there was no difference between the PRP group and the hyaluronic acid group (Li et al., 2011).

A cross-sectional study of 30 patients with osteoarthritis who had received PRP vs. hyaluronic acid suggested that PRP yielded significant improvements in pain control (Sanchez et al., 2008). In a prospective study of 14 patients with osteoarthritis, three PRP injections within a four-week period resulted in significant pain relief (Sampson et al., 2010).

A case report of a 12 year-old soccer player suggested that PRP could heal a cartilage avulsion in the knee.

The patient resumed full sport activity at 18 weeks (Sanchez et al., 2003).

Foot And Ankle

Plantar fasciitis:
Several studies showed that PRP injections improved pain (Martinelli et al., 2012; Ragab et al., 2012; Aksahin et al., 2012). Randomized controlled studies have suggested that PRP is more effective than cortisone injections for the treatment of plantar fasciopathy (Monto et al., 2014; Omar et al., 2012).

PRP reduces pain in a double blinded control study in patients with plantar fasciitis. (Peerbooms et al 2019)

Bone Injuries:
Bone cells treated with PRP show an increase in alkaline phosphatase, a key enzyme in bone growth, in vivo.

A study was performed on patients that had PRP applied onto the bone and prosthetic surfaces, mixed into the graft, and packed into the joint. These patients had a higher fusion rate than expected based on the literature (Barrows et al., 2005). In another study comparing 66 patients to 114 historical controls, there was a decrease in the percentage of delayed unions and non-unions in the PRP-treated patients at 6 months (Coetzee et al., 2005).

Achilles tendon:
A positive response to PRP in combination with eccentric training was found in a randomized controlled trial of 60 patients in Denmark (Boesen et al., 2017).

Alsousou et al. demonstrated that a immunohistochemical response to topical PRP enhanced the maturity of the healing tendon tissues by promoting better collagen I deposition, decreased cellularity, less vascularity, and higher glycosaminoglycan content when compared with control samples.

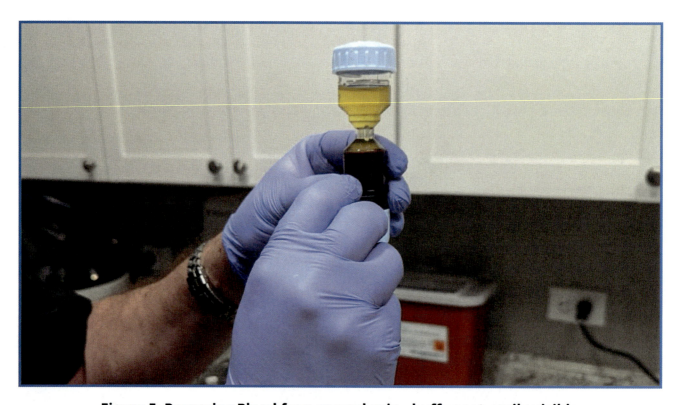

Figure 5: Preparing Blood for a second spin - buffy coat easily visible

Muscle Injuries:
There is debate about whether PRP could improve the healing of muscle tears. Post-traumatic hematomas resemble whole blood. Hematomas may slow healing. However, PRP may facilitate healing (Bobnov et al., 2013).

Combination Treatments with Stem Cells and PRP:
Some researchers and practitioners combine PRP with stem cell preparations. In one study, a mixture of PRP and bone marrow derived mesenchymal stem cells was injected into the injured tendons of dogs. These dogs experienced increased tensile strength in the injured tendons (Pandey et al., 2019).

Another randomized controlled trial of PRP combined with adipose-derived mesenchymal stem cells showed improvements in the organization of the collagen scaffold along with decreased inflammation (van Pham et al., 2013).

PRP in combination with tendon stem cell or progenitor cells may have a synergistic effect on Type I collagen production (Wang et al., 2017). PRP may increase the circulating levels of bone marrow derived stem cells and adipose-derived stem cells, which may be a secondary method for wound healing (Pandey et al., 2019). One study showed that stem cells mixed with platelet-rich plasma (PRP) was more effective at tendon healing than either substance alone (Rubio-Azpeitia et al, 2017).

However, in one study of injured sheep tendons, PRP in combination with peripheral blood derived mesenchymal stem cells did not show any improvements in tendon strength (Zhou et al., 2016).

Dr. Katz typically combines PRP injections with hyperbaric oxygen therapy, increasing the number of stem cells in circulation, while PRP attracts stem cells to the necessary areas.

Physicians who perform local cortisone injections often combine the cortisone with local anesthetic. However, evidence suggests that local anesthetics, including lidocaine and bupivacaine, can be toxic to cartilage cells. Therefore, most practitioners advise against mixing PRP preparations with local anesthetic (Maffulli et al., 2016).

There is evidence that anti-inflammatory drugs may interfere with muscle cell fusion, thereby hampering muscle healing (Shen et al., 2006). Therefore NSAIDs should be avoided when using PRP.

Limitations:
It is difficult to gauge and compare the safety and efficacy of PRP because there is no standard for comparison. Because we are using the patients' own blood, the risks of PRP appear to be very low. In terms of efficacy, there are several variables to consider. The current processing systems utilize different quantities and concentrations of platelets, growth factors, and leukocytes. In some cases, PRP is combined with other regenerative therapies. The timing of injections also varies. PRP is used for injuries with various expected wound healing times. Therefore, in some cases, we cannot be sure whether the PRP facilitated wound healing or if the wound healed spontaneously. We also cannot tell whether PRP improved the degree of healing in what would have been a non-healing injury.

ACUTE INJURY:
Most research in PRP focuses on treating chronic conditions. It is becoming clear that it may play a significant role in treating acute injury as well. Trunz recently reported in a trial of 55 athletes that when an injured hamstring had hematoma evacuation followed by PRP injection there was a return to play at 24 days rather than 32 days in the control group (Trunz et al., 2022).

Sample Dictation:
The procedure and potential complications were discussed with the patient. After written and verbal consent were obtained, the patient was placed in the seated position. A tourniquet was placed on the right arm and the area was surveyed for large palpable veins. The antecubital area was prepped and draped in the usual sterile fashion using alcohol. Using an 20G needle, approximately [ ] ccs of blood was drawn from the patient and transferred to a specially prepared PRP tube containing anticoagulants. After the needle was removed,

and a sterile bandage was placed over the entry site, the tube was vertically rotated back and forth five times.

The tube was placed in a centrifuge with an opposing counter-weight. After five minutes, the tube was removed and inspected. There was a visible gel, a buffy coat, and a golden liquid layer of PRP. The tube was vertically rotated back and forth five times. Afterwards, the PRP and buffy coat were gently extracted and transferred to a 10 cc syringe. The syringe was attached to a 22G 1.5" needle.

[Patient positioning as described above depending on the type of injection and approach]

The shoulder was prepped and draped in the usual sterile manner using three coats of betadine. The area of interest was identified using sonography. The area of interest was identified by the following landmarks: _____

With the probe held in place, a ½ a cc of 1% lidocaine was used to create a wheal at the entry site alongside the probe. The needle guidance software package was turned on. After a moment, with the probe held in place, the needle and syringe containing the PRP was advanced through the skin and the deeper tissues towards the target area. Under ultrasound guidance, the PRP was injected. The final image was recorded. The probe was moved, the needle was removed and a sterile gauze was held over the injection site with gentle pressure. A sterile bandage was applied. The patient was repositioned for comfort. The patient tolerated the procedure well with no apparent complications.

References:

Pochini AC, Antonioli E, Bucci DZ et al., Analysis of of cytokine profile and growth factors in platelet-rich plasma obtained by open systems and commercial columns. Einstein (Sao Paulo); 2016; 14(3): 391-7

Jurk K, Kehrel BE. Platelets: Physiology and biochemistry. Semin Thromb Hemost 2005; 31(4): 381-92

Maffulli N. Platelet rich plasma in musculoskeletal practice. 1st Ed. London: Springer-Verlag 2016

Foster TE, Puskas BL, Mandelbaum BR, et al., Platelet-rich plasma: from basic science to clinical applications. Am J Sports Med 2009; 37(11): 2259-72

Yamaguchi R, Terashima H, Yoneyama S, et al., Effects of platelet-rich plasma on intestinal anastomotic ealing in rats: PRP concentration is a key factor. J Surg Res 2010; 2

Yun SH, Sim EH, Goh RY, et al., Platelet activation: The mechanisms and potential biomarkers. Biomed Res Int 2016; 9060143

Anitua E, Sanchez M, Zalduendo MM, et al., Fibroblastic response to treatment with different preparations rich in growth factors. Cell Prolif 2009; 42(2): 162-70

Leick M, Azcutia V, Newton G, et al., Leukocyte recruitment in inflammation: Basic concepts and new mechanistic insights based on new models and microscopic imaging technologies. Cell Tissue Res 2014; 355(3): 647-56

Dragoo JL, Braun HJ, Durham JL, et al., Comparison of the acute inflammatory response of two commercial platelet-rich plasma systems in healthy rabbit tendons. Am J Sports Med 2012; 40(6): 1274-81

Khalafi RS, Bradford DW, Wilson MG. Topical application of autologous blood products during surgical closure following a coronary artery bypass graft. Eur J Cardiothoracic Surg 2008; 34(2): 360-4

Everts PA, Knape JTA, Weibrich G, et al., Platelet-Rich plasma and platelet gel: A review. J Extra Corpor Technol 2006; 38(2): 174-87

Carter MJ, Fylling CP, Parnell LKS. Use of platelet rich plasma gel on wound healing: A systematic review and meta-analysis. Eplasty 2011; 11: e38

Carter CA, Jolly DG, Worden CE, et al., Platelet-rich plasma gel promotes differentiation and regeneration during equine wound healing. Exp Mol Pathol 2003; 74(3): 244-55

Araki J, Jona M, Suga H, et al., Optimized preparation method of platelet-concentrated plasma (PCP) and non-coagulating platelet-derived factor concentrates (PFC): maximization of platelet concentration and removal of fibrinogen. Tissue Eng Part C Methods. 2012; 18(3): 176-85

Knighton DR, Ciresi KF, Fiegel VD, et al., Classification and treatment of chronic non-healing wounds: Successful treatment with autologous platelet-derived wound healing factors. Ann Surg 1986; 204(3): 322-30

Marx RE, Carlson ER, Eichstaedt RM, et al., Platelet-rich plasma: Growth factor enhancement for bone grafts. Oral Surg Oral Med Oral Pathol Oral RAdiol Endod 1998; 85(6): 638-46

Jo CH, Kim JE, Yoon KS, et al., Platelet-rich plasma stimulates cell proliferation and enhances matrix gene expression and synthesis in tenocytes from human rotator cuff tendons with degenerative tears. Am J Sports Med 2012; 40(5): 1035-45

Zhang Q, Ge H, Zhou J, Cheng B. Are platelet-rich products necessary during the arthroscopic repair of full-thickness rotator cuff tears: a meta-analysis. PLoS One. 2013;8(7), e69731

Maniscalo P, Gambera D, Lunati A, et al., The "Cascade" membrane: a new PRP device for tendpn ruptures. Description and case report on rotator cuff tendon. Acta Biomed. 2008;79(3):223-6.

Krogh TP, Fredberg U, Stengaard-Pedersen K, et al., Treatment of lateral epicondylitis with platelet-rich plasma, glucocorticoid, or saline: a randomized, double-blind, placebo-controlled trial. Am J Sports Med 2013; 41(3); 625-35

Creaney L, Wallace A, Curtis M, Connell D. Growth factor-based therapies provide additional benefit beyond physical therapy in resistant elbow tendinopathy: a prospective, single-blind, randomised trial of autologous blood injections. Br J

Sports Med. 2011;45(12):966-71.

Thanasas C, Papadimitriou G, Charalambidis C, et al., Platelet-rich plasma versus autologous whole blood for treatment of chronic lateral elbow epicondylitis: a randomized controlled clinical trial. Am J Sports Med. 2011;39(10):2130-4.

Peerbooms J, Sluimer J, Bruigin D, et al., Positive effect of an autologous platelet concentrate in lateral epicondylitis in a double-blind randomized controlled trail. Am J Sports Med. 2010; 38: 255-62.

Mishra A, Pavelko T. Treatment of chronic elbow tendinosis with buffered platelet-rich plasma. Am J Sports Med. 2006; 10:1-5.

Xie X, Zhang C, Tuan R. Biology of platelet-rich plasma and its clinical application in cartilage repair. Arthritis Res Ther 2014; 16(1): 204

Sanchez M, Anitua E, Fiz N, et al., Plasma rich in growth factors (PRGF-Endoret) in the treatment of symptomatic knee osteoarthritis: a randomized clinical trial. Arthroscopy. 2012;28:1070-8.

Battaglia M, Guaraldi F, Vannini F, et al., Platelet-rich plasma (PRP) intra-articular ultrasound-guided injections as a possible treatment for hip osteoarthritis: A pilot study. Clin Exp Rheumatol 2011; 29(4): 754

Kon E, Filardo G, Delcogliano M, et al., Platelet-rich plasma: new clinical application: a pilot study for treatment of jumper's knee. Injury.2009;40(6):598-603.

Vetrano M, Castorina A, Vulpiani MC, et al., Platelet-rich plasma verus focused shock waves in the treatment of jumper's knee in athletes. Am J Sports Med. 2013; 41(4):795-803

De Almeida AM, Demange MK, Sobrado MF, et al., Patellar tendon heLing with platelet-rich plasma: a prospective randomized controlled trial. Am J Sports Med. 2012;40(6): 1282-8.

Vogrin M, Rupreht A, Crnjac A, et al., The effect of platelet-derived growth factors on knee stability after anterior cruciate ligament reconstruction: a prospective randomized clinical study. Wien Klin Wochenschr. 2010; 122 Suppl 3:91-5.

Radice F, Yanez R, Gutierrez V, et al., Comparison of magnetic resonance imaging findings in anterior cruciate ligament grafts with and without autologous platelet-derived growth factors. Arthroscopy. 2010; 26(1):50-7.

Sanchez M, Azofra J, Anitua E, et al., Plasma rich in growth factors to treat an articular cartilage avulsion: A case report. Med Sci Sports Exerc 2003; 35(10): 1648-52

Frontera W, DeLisa J, Gans B, et al., Delisa's physical medicine and rehabilitation principles and practice. 5th Ed. Philadelphia: Lippincott Williams & Wilkins 2010

Spakova T, Rosocha J, Lacko M. Treatment of knee joint osteoarthritis with autologous platelet-rich plasma in comparison with hyaluronic acid. Am J Phys Med Rehabil. 2012; 91:411-7.

Filardo G, Kon E, Buda R, et al., Platelet-rich plasma intra-articular knee injections for the treatment of degenerative cartilage lesions and osteoarthritis. Knee Surg Sports Traumatol Arthosc. 2011; 19:528-35.

Vetrano M, Castorina A, Vulpiani MC, et al., Platelet-rich plasma verus focused shock waves in the treatment of jumper's knee in athletes. Am J Sports Med. 2013; 41(4):795-803

Dai WL, Zhou AG, Zhang H, et al., Efficacy of platelet-rich plasma in the treatment of knee osteoarthritis: A meta-analysis of randomized controlled trials. Arthroscopy 2017; 33(3): 659–670

Shen L, Yuan T, Chen S, et al., The temporal effect of platelet-rich plasma on pain and physical function in the treatment of knee osteoarthritis: systematic review and meta-analysis of randomized controlled trials. Journal of Orthopaedic Surgery and Research 2017; 12(1): 16

Cerza F, Carni S, Carcangiu A, et al., Comparison between hyaluronic acid and platelet-rich plasma, intra-articular infiltration in the treatment of gonarthrosis. Am J Sports Med 2012; 40(12): 2822-7

Li M, Zhang C, Ai Z, et al., Therapeutic effectiveness of intra-articular knee injection of platelet-rich plasma on knee articular cartilage degeneration. J Reparative Reconst Surg 2011; 25(10): 1192-6

Sanchez M, Anitua E, Azofra J, et al., Intra-articular injection of an autologous preparation rich in growth factors for the treatment of knee OA: a retrospective cohort study. Clin Exp Rheumatol. 2008;26(5):910-3.

Sampson S, Reed M, Silvers H, et al., Injection of platelet-rich plasma in patients with primary and secondary knee osteoarthritis: a pilot study. Am J Phys Med Rehabil. 2010;89(12):961-9.

Sanchez M, Azofra J, Anitua E, et al., Plasma rich in growth factors to treat an articular cartilage avulsion: a case report. Med Sci Sports Exerc. 2003;35(10):1648-52.

Schepull T, Kvist J, Norrman H. et al., Autologous platelets have no effect on the healing of human Achilles tendon ruptures: a randomized single-blind study. Am J Sports Med. 2011;39(1):38-47.

Owens Jr RF, Ginnetti J, Conti SF, et al., Clinical magnetic resonance imaging outcomes following platelet rich plasma injection for chronic midsubstance Achilles tendinopathy. Foot Ankle Int/ Am Orthop Foot Ankle Society Swiss Foot Ankle Soc 2011; 32(11): 1032-9

de Vos RJ, Weir A, van Schie HT, et al., Platelet-plasma injection for chronic Achilles tendinopathy: a randomized controlled trial. JAMA. 2010;303(2):144-9.

Sanchez M, Anitua E, Azofra J, et al., Comparison of surgically repaired Achilles tendon tears using platelet-rich fibrin matrices. Am J Sports Med. 2007;35(2):245-51.

Gaweda K, Tarczynska M, Krzyzanowski W. Treatment of Achilles tendinopathy with platelet-rich plasma. Int J Sports Med 2010; 31(8): 577-83

Delos D, Murawski C, Kennedy J. Platelet rich plasma for foot and ankle disorders in the athletic population. Tech Foot Ankle Surg 2011; 10:11-7

Monto RR. Platelet rich plasma treatment for chronic Achilles tendinosis. Foot Ankle Int/ Am Orthop Foot Ankle Soc Swiss Foot Ankle Soc 2012; 33(5): 379-85

Martinelli N, Marinozzi A, Carni S, et al., Platelet-rich plasma injections for chronic plantar fasciitis. Arch Orthop Trauma Surg 2012; 132(6): 781-5

Ragab EM, Orthman AM. Platelets rich plasma for treatment of chronic plantar fasciitis. Arch Orthop Trauma Surg 2012; 132(8): 1065-70

Aksahin E, Dogruyol D, Yuksei HY, et al., The comparison of the effect of corticosteroids and platelet-rich plasma (PRP) for the treatment of plantar fasciitis. Arch Orthop Trauma Surg 2012; 132(6): 781-5

Monto RR. Platelet-rich plasma efficacy versus corticosteroid injection treatment for chronic severe plantar fasciitis. Foot Ankle Int. 2014;35(4):313-8.

Omar ASIM, Ahmed AS, et al., Local injection of autologous platelet rich plasma and corticosteroid in treatment of laterl epicondylitis and plantar faciitis: randomized clinical trial. Egypt Rheumato. 2012;34:43-9

Kim E, Lee JH. Autologous platelet-rich verus dextrose prolotherapy for the treatment of chronic recalcitrant plantar fasciitis. PM & R J Injury Funct Rehabil. 2014; 6(2): 152-8.

Barrows CR, Pomeroy GC. Enhancement of syndesmotic fusion rates in total ankle arthroplasty with the use of autologous platelet concentrate. Fott Ankle Int/ Am Orthop Foot Ankle Soc Swiss Foot Ankle Soc 2005; 26(6): 458-61

Coetzee JC, Pomeroy GC, Watts JD, et al., The use of autologous concentrated growth factors to promote syndesmosis fusion in the AGility total ankle replacement. A preliminary study. Foot Ankle Int/ Am Orthop Foot Ankle Soc Swiss Foot Ankle Soc 2005; 26(10): 840-6

Boesen AP, Hansen R, Boesen MI et al., Effect of High-Volume Injection, Platelet-Rich Plasma, and Sham Treatment in Chronic Midportion Achilles Tendinopathy: A Randomized Double-Blinded Prospective Study. AM J Sports Med . 201, Jul; 45(9):2034-43

Bubnov R, Yevseenko V, Semeniv I, et al., Ultrasound-guided injections of platelet rich plasma for muscel injury in professional athletes. Comparative Study Med Ultrasound. 2013; 15: 101-5

Pandey S, Hickey DU, Drum M, et al., Platelet-rich plasma affects the proliferation of canine bone marrow-derived mesenchymal stromal cells in vitro. BMC Veterinary Research 2019; 269

Van Pham P, Bui KHT, Ngo DQ, et al., Activated platelet-rich plasma improved adipose-derived stem cell transplantation efficiency in injured articular cartilage. Stem Cell Res Ther 2013; 4(4): 9

Wang JHC, Nirmala X. Application of tendon stem/ progenitor cells and platelet-rich plasma to treat tendon injuries. Oper Tech Orthop 2016; 26(2): 68-7

Rubio-Azpeitia E, Sánchez P, Delgado D, Andia I. Adult Cells Combined With Platelet-Rich Plasma for Tendon Healing: Cell Source Options. Orthopaedic Journal of Sports Medicine. 2017;5(2):2325967117690846

Zhou Y and Wang JHC. PRP Treatment efficacy for tendinopathy: A review of basic science studies. Biomed Res Int 2016; 9103792

Shen W, Prisk V, Li Y et al., Inhibited skeletal muscle healing in cyclooxygenase-2 gene-deficient mice: the role of PGE2 and PGF2-alpha. J Appl Physiol 2006; 101(4): 1215-21

CHAPTER 8 Exosomes

Pradeep Albert, William Merritt & Vijay Vad

> **CHAPTER PREVIEW**
>
> Exosomes are extracellular vesicles extracted from a growth medium used for stem cell manufacturing; exosomes are being used more frequently in interventional musculoskeletal medicine.

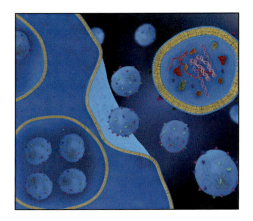

What are exosomes?

Exosomes are acellular substances produced by cells and used for communicating with other cells to make them do something (like multiply, grow or make other proteins). They are composed of proteins, peptides, growth factors, cytokines, cell signaling molecules, and extracellular vesicles.

What's a vesicle?

Vesicles are outward "blebbing" of the cell membrane consisting of the lipid bilayer, encapsulating mRNA, miRNA, or other proteins or peptides. It's a little packet of information for a cell, whether it's proteins, peptides, mRNA, or other signaling substances.

Why do cells excrete exosomes?

This is one of the ways that the cells communicate with each other. They will send extracellular vesicles to each other containing mRNA (messenger, RNA) sequences or miRNA (micro RNA) sequences. They will tell other cells to perform certain functions, activate, undergo morphological changes, and start secreting their own proteins. As far as stem cell exosomes are concerned, this can include instructions such as beginning healing, to regenerate tissue, and to perform other biological functions in the body.

How are exosomes made in a laboratory?

One can start with any cells. Since mesenchymal stem cells are precursor cells capable of transforming into any cell, most labs start with a mesenchymal stem cell line. Some scientists are using chondrocytes, fibroblasts, as well as other types of cell lines. The cells are cultured in a controlled laboratory setting. The broth that stem cells are grown in is extracted and filtered. This fluid is called exosomes. It is filled with acellular material that has cell signal molecules.

What does it mean to culture a cell? How do you grow a stem cell?

Stem cells are placed onto a plate or flask intended for growing cells. The cells start suspended in cell culture fluid. They adhere to the plastic and proliferate while bathed in micronutrients. By dividing, growing, and spreading across the plate. This is performed in an incubator that provides suitable conditions for cellular growth.

Similar to bacteria? In a Petri dish?

Yes. Many different cell types can be cultured, including stem cells, bacteria, fibroblasts, etc. And, as they are proliferating in culture, they're emitting proteins, peptides, cytokines, cell signaling molecules, and exosomes. They're telling each other to grow, to divide, to proliferate, and they do this by secreting these substances into the cell culture fluid. Cell culture fluid or cell media is rich in vitamins, amino acids, carbohydrates, and other substances that keep the cells nourished and healthy. And as previously mentioned, as the cells grow, they're also secreting proteins, growth factors, cytokines, and extracellular vesicles, into the fluid. As the cells start to reach confluence, there's not a lot of room for them to continue spreading out on the plate, the flasks are removed from the incubator, and the supernatant, which is the excess fluid covering the cells, is removed. This supernatant fluid has amino acids, peptides, proteins, growth factors, cytokines, and exosomes from the cells as they were cultured. By capturing these cell signaling molecules and extracellular vesicles, we can harness the power of the stem cell. We can capture all the signaling molecules, which is also what a stem cell excretes in your body during the healing process. Clinicians can then use this exosome fluid for regenerative medicine applications or as a way to capture some of the regenerative power of the stem cell without actually having to perform a cell transplant or cellular therapy on a patient.

How do you measure and isolate exosomes? Many labs claim that their exosomes are the best. How do you count them, and how do you determine the quality of their products?

There is no accepted standardization of exosome quality. There is no concrete answer for how to define what the best type of exosome product is, because exosomes and proteins are not currently standardized. The cell can respond in different ways to different stimuli. Adding a specific molecule to the cell culture broth can cause the stem cells to emit a different protein profile. In this way, it is possible for a unique secretome from a cell that's specific to a medical indication. The easiest way to characterize an exosome product is to identify how many extracellular vesicles (particles) there are in a product, identify how many different proteins/peptides there are, and identify the relative abundance of the proteins/peptides present. We perform an analytical technique called nanoparticle tracking analysis (NTA) to quantify extracellular vesicle concentration. It's a light scattering technique. Essentially, you're shooting a laser through a sample of the exosome product, then the laser bends and refracts around these microscopic extracellular vesicles that measure 30 nanometers to 150 nanometers. Through NTA, one can determine what sizes of exosomes there are in a given sample and how the exosome quantities are distributed over a given size range. Thus, we generate a curve of the number of exosome particles and their diameters. For the protein and peptide secretome, you can evaluate these with mass spectroscopy techniques – a kind of standard proteomics. We can also evaluate what's inside the extracellular vesicles using next-generation sequencing, which can break apart those extracellular vesicles and sequence the miRNA or mRNA in the exosome product.

What are miRNA and mRNA?

mRNA is messenger RNA, essentially a genetic sequence that the cell reads and tells the cell to do something like express a specific protein. miRNA (micro RNA) affects how proteins are expressed by interacting with mRNA. miRNA could bind to mRNA and mark it for destruction or save it for later. Higher levels of a particular miRNA could cause a specific protein to be under-expressed by suppressing the presence of a certain mRNA sequence. It's a complex system with a lot of potential in regenerative medicine. And so, with next-generation sequencing, we're able to sequence the genetic contents of the exosome product.

Is it fair to say that the better the stem cell or the cell line that you're growing, the better the exosomes?

The regenerative capability of the stem cell is well documented. That they're able to differentiate into many different cell types, they're able to secrete unique and potent protein profiles, and they're able to do things that other cells that have differentiated cannot. An exosome product from a non-stem cell product, like a fibroblast, doesn't mean it won't work. Perhaps a fibroblast-derived exosome product could be highly specific for a skin condition. But, it makes sense to target stem cells for most regenerative purposes.

There are internationally accepted definitions for the characteristics of a stem cell. A highly pure and potent source of stem cells is important. When creating exosome products, it is essential to try to have a high-quality pure mesenchymal stem cell line.

If you eventually take stem cells through enough passages – enough doublings – they lose certain cell surface markers used to characterize or define stem cells or reach a sort of planned senescence. They undergo apoptosis (cell death) or start to differentiate into other cell types. If you get greedy and culture the cells too far, you will be left with an impure stem cell culture. By limiting the number of passages that you're taking the cells through, you're increasing the chance that the stem cell product you have will remain pure. You're much more likely to have a product of consistent quality and efficacy.

As you multiply stem cells more and more, do they become less stem cell-ish? They lose some of their essential characteristics. If you extract these exosomes in the first four passes, you may have a better product than if you do it later.

If these products are acellular, is there still a risk of infection like HIV or hepatitis?

The risk is negligible if the product has proper testing and controls. We have to go to great lengths from a quality standpoint to ensure that. These stem cells typically come from birth tissue (placentas and umbilical cords), so we run maternal serological testing. To do this, we take blood samples from the mother and test them for known communicable viral agents such as HIV and West Nile virus and non-viral pathogens such as syphilis. The samples are tested for an entire suite of these infectious pathogens. As well as bacterial and fungal testing for microbial contamination of the actual cell culture line itself during handling. There are all sorts of ways of determining whether the cell line has been contaminated with bacterial fungus. We do send off representative samples from each batch for sterility testing. They're put into a growth media, and incubated, and you see if any bacteria or fungus grows over 14 days in prime conditions for bacterial or fungal growth. If nothing comes up, then you have a high level of confidence now that there's no bacterial contamination or fungal contamination in your cell line and exosome fluid and that the cells aren't potentially infected with communicative viral or adventitious agents from the donor. You can also do PCR and next-generation sequencing (NGS) on the samples. With NGS, you can look at all of the genetic data in the sample. From this data set, you can filter viral, bacterial, or fungal sequences to get an even higher level of assurance that there are no adventitious agents in the product. We run tests for pyrogens, the toxins the bacteria produce that can cause fever and inflammation when infused into or transfused into a body. We focus on ensuring that these products are as safe as possible and that they're not going to elicit any adverse event in the patient.

What is next-generation sequencing?

NGS is an analytical technique that evaluates the different genetic sequences in a given sample. It is a broad-panel-based approach to gene testing rather than things like PCR, that are looking for a single gene sequence.

What is the average number of particles that you expect to see in one cc of exosomes? Or does that vary?

It can vary. You want some level of standardization in your output. You would probably see anywhere between 1 billion and 15 billion. We get caught up in the numbers as a benchmark for comparing products, but a product may still be efficacious at 1 billion. Other highly concentrated products might have 100 billion exosomes in a dose. So you see a wide range of products. Does it mean it's better than another product? Not necessarily. People still see fantastic results with products that have a billion exosomes in a milliliter. Perhaps this is because those stem cells and their growth conditions were more focused on secreting growth factors and cytokines, which can do a lot of heavy lifting in the healing process. But it is fair and reasonable to want a product in the billions, as this is often a reported number in research and industry. Now, you would want to avoid having one of your batches have 1 billion in one and the next one have 15 billion. Given the same internal processes, you'd expect some standardization across your own batches. You'd want a level of reproducibility.

Can exosomes be stored at room temperature? Should they be frozen?

At ambient temperature, you make sure you're taking steps to prevent oxidation of the product of the proteins and the membranes of the exosomes. Storing it under cryopreservation, like in cryostorage, in theory, will increase the shelf life of the product just by reducing the potential for thermodynamic factors to affect protein integrity. You could potentially store it in liquid nitrogen for ten years or indefinitely. We have tested room-temperature products, we saw similar levels of proteins and exosomes after a two-year shelf-life test in some products. So it is possible that clinicians can store room-temperature products at ambient temperatures without protein degradation for up to two years.

Are people using ultrasound frequencies to elicit one type of exosome or another?

Light, sounds, and chemical additives can all affect stem cell signaling, providing different stimuli to the cells themselves as they're reproducing to get the cells to overexpress certain beneficial growth factors. There is much research needed on different ways to stimulate and/or stress the cells in culture to try to get them to overexpress certain proteins. Trying to figure out how to get the cells to behave slightly differently in culture to produce something unique that is patentable and provides a better clinical benefit is being explored by researchers worldwide.

What's the current FDA stand on exosomes? Are they allowed in the United States? Or are they completely illegal?

The FDA didn't regulate exosomes until recently; over the last few years, they've really come out strongly and clearly saying that you cannot market these exosomes as a way to treat or cure or prevent any diseases or conditions without FDA approval, which involves clinical trials and Biologics Licensing Application (BLA). However, there are specific indications that don't require FDA approval for exosomes to be marketed, topical applications for wound healing and aesthetics/cosmetics use are not currently excluded from FDA use as long as false claims are not made.

Are there any side effects from exosomes therapy?

There are no known adverse effects from exosome therapy , however since each formulation of exosomes is different, more research has to be performed. The biggest side effect in our opinion is promising cure that isn't possible, many are using exosomes without understanding what they are and how they work. Using bad quality exosomes may cause more problems than non treatment.

What clinical studies are there that prove that exosomes are beneficial?

Different formulations of exosomes are being studies, both human and plant exosomes are being studied in clinical trials. Many exciting and nascent studies are being pursued, with the cardiovascular system, and using dendritic exosomes to slow down tumor growth in cancer patients.

What are potential future therapies for exosomes?

If given intravenously, exosomes could play a role in cellular repair in acute events like myocardial infarctions, cerebrovascular accidents, or emphysema. They may play a role in reducing pain in chronic back pain and knee osteoarthritis, where local or regional exosome injections may significantly impact pain relief and potentially slow cartilage loss. Intrathecal injections may be helpful in patients that have neurodegenerative disorders. Whatever the future holds, it seems we are on the right track.

References:

Kalluri R and Lebleu VS (2020). Exosomes: Biology, Function, and Biomedical Applications. Volume 367, Issue 6478, Pages 1-12.

Muthu S, Bapat A, Jain R, Jeyaraman N, and Jeyaraman M (2021). Exosomal Therapy: A New Frontier in Regenerative Medicine. Volume 8, Issue 7, Pages 1-14.

The Endomembrane System and Proteins - Vesicles and Vacuoles (2022). Volume 4, Issue 11, Pages 1-10.

BioExplorer.net (2021). Explore Vesicles: Types and Their 9 Major Functions. Pages 1-8.

NIH Stem Cell Information Home Page (2021). In Stem Cell Information. Bethesda, MD: National Institutes of Health, U.S. Department of Health and Human Services.

Tiner S (2021). Beyond Stem Cells, Regenerative Medicine Finds Exosomes. Mayo Clinic News Network, July 22, Pages 1-3.

CHAPTER 9 Mesenchymal Stem Cells: An Introduction

Devi Nampiaparampil, Pradeep Albert & Laxmaiah Manchikanti

> **CHAPTER PREVIEW**
>
> In this chapter, we review the different types of stem cells: totipotent, pluripotent, multipotent and unipotent. We will also go over the mesenchymal family tree and how stem cells are being studied in bone, tendon, muscle, joint, ligament, meniscus, the spine, and even cancer.

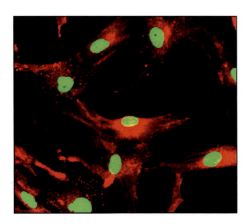

Stem cells can be categorized into four main groups; totipotent, pluripotent, multipotent, and unipotent. Totipotent stem cells are capable of forming all types of cells and have the potential to give rise to an entire organism, the placenta, as well as extra-embryonic cells. Pluripotent stem cells are embryologic in origin and capable of forming all embryonic germ layers. Multipotent stem cells arise from fetal or adult tissue and are less able to differentiate. Hematopoietic and mesenchymal stem cells falls into the "multipotent" category. Unipotent stem cells arise from adult tissue and can only differentiate into a single type of cell (Girlovanu et al., 2015).

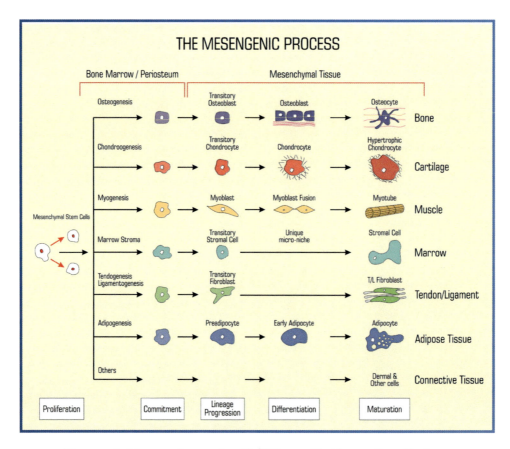

Figure 1: Mesenchymal cell differentiation a family tree

Although totipotent and pluripotent stem cells have the highest degree of differentiation potential-- and therefore regenerative or healing potential-- there are numerous ethical concerns that must be addressed before these cells can be studied effectively. There is one camp that believes these cells are isolated cells that can be studied for their regenerative potential in the same way as other treatment interventions. Others believe these cells represent human life. Therefore, manufacturing and manipulating them can be interpreted as another way of manipulating and potentially destroying human life (Girlovanu et al., 2015).

If you recall back to embryology, after the sperm meets the egg and conception occurs, the newly formed cell progresses to form three layers of cells: ectoderm (outer layer), mesoderm (middle layer), and endoderm (inner layer). The stem cells that descend from the mesoderm are referred to as mesenchymal stem cells. Mesenchymal stem cells are the stem cell precursors for bone, cartilage, muscle, tendon, ligament, adipocytes, connective tissue, dermis, and marrow stroma (Caplan, 1991). As research on bone marrow derived stem cells and cancer stem cells progressed, so did research on mesenchymal stem cells.

Dr. Arnold Caplan, for example, isolated mesenchymal stem cells from rat hind-limbs. He then influenced these stem cells to become either osteoblasts, cells that build bone, or chondroblasts, cells that build cartilage. He determined that these cells needed to be near blood vessels to form bone. They needed to be removed from blood vessels to form cartilage. He also determined what density of mesenchymal stem cells was more favorable for the formation of bone vs. cartilage (Caplan, 1991). Meanwhile, other scientists determined that, although human mesenchymal cells could form certain cell types around them, they retained their stem cell properties. Therefore, if they were moved to a different setting, they could still regenerate a different lineage of cells (Pittenger et al., 1999).

In one study, researchers isolated human mesenchymal stem cells and then injected them into the abdomens of 13-day old fetal mice in the uterus. Eight weeks after birth, those same mesenchymal stem cells were found in the bones, blood vessels, and heart of the mice. This suggests that mesenchymal stem cells isolated in a lab can be incorporated into an organism and can then differentiate (McBride et al., 2003).

This is substantiated in human studies as well. Normally, during pregnancy, some fetal cells cross the placenta and enter the mother's bloodstream. In one study, years after birth, the baby's cells were found in the mother's bone marrow (O'Donoghue et al., 2003; O'Donoghue et al., 2004). In another study, researchers found male cells incorporated into females' liver, lymph nodes, intestines, thyroid, and cervix. These women had previously had male pregnancies (Khosrotehrani et al., 2004).

There are differences between adult mesenchymal stem cells that can be harvested from an individual and then transplanted back into that individual-- either at a different time or different location-- and embryonic stem cells. Embryonic cells have proteins on the cell surface that might trigger an immune reaction if they are transplanted into a different recipient. In addition, embryonic stem cells can form into teratomas, tumors comprising various tissues: teeth, hair, muscle, bone, etc. (Campagnoli et al., 2001; Jones et al., 2012; Thurairajah et al., 2017).

Bone:
In normal fracture healing, bone morphogenic protein (BMP) and a growth factor called TGF-β help mesenchymal stem cells differentiate into chondrocytes (cartilage cells) and osteoblasts (bone-building cells); low levels of BMP cause the stem cells to turn instead into adipocytes (fat cells). Using a hydroxyapatite scaffold and this knowledge, a team of researchers was recently able to show that large bone defects could be repaired with the use of bone marrow-derived cells. Later studies showed how stem cells could be used to help fracture healing or to treat osteonecrosis (Zhang et al., 2019; Zhang et al., 2009).

Genetically-engineered bone marrow-derived mesenchymal stem cells have been used to treat mice with osteogenesis imperfecta (Pereira et al., 1998; Chamberlain et al., 2004).

In musculoskeletal medicine, bone marrow-derived mesenchymal stem cells have been studied in non-healing fractures with promising results (Granero-Molto et al., 2009).

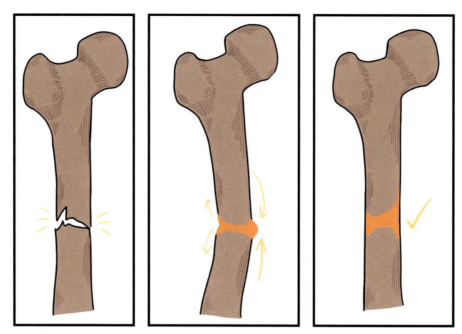

Figure 1: Bone healing typically occurs more readily on the compression side "the inside" of the fracture.

Tendon:
Stem cell therapy has also been proposed as a treatment option for tendinopathy. One small clinical study demonstrated healing of a complete rotator cuff tear using stem cells in conjunction with a surgical repair (Gomes et al, 2012). Another small study found that patients who received stem cells intraoperatively were twice as likely to have intact rotator cuffs ten years out (Hernigou et al, 2014).

Bone marrow-derived stem cells have also been transplanted to injured tendons with excellent results in the patellar tendon (Pascual-Garrido et al., 2012).

Bone marrow-derived and adipose-derived mesenchymal stem cells helped heal rotator cuff injuries in rabbit studies (Tornero-Esteban et al., 2015; Oh et al., 2014; Shen et al., 2012).

Muscle:
Adipose-derived mesenchymal stem cells have been injected into the soleus muscle of rats with an increase in the muscle tensile strength of the soleus. This may be because of their effects on the organization of muscle bundles (Tseng et al., 2008; Pecanha et al., 2012).

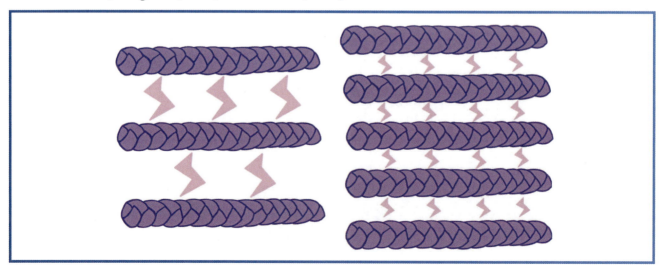

Figure 2: Contractile vs. parallel muscle bundles

Joint:
Recent systematic reviews have suggested improved pain relief and improved MRI findings in those treated with mesenchymal stem cells (Chahla et al., 2016; Gupta et al., 2012; Fellows et al., 2016).

In a horse cell model in the lab, a scaffold made with fibrin, facilitated the repair of a cartilage injury (Goodrich et al., 2016; Frisbie et al., 2015).

Mesenchymal stem cells have slowed down the progression of osteoarthritis in rabbits, mice, rats, guinea pigs, dogs, horses and sheep (Sierra et al., 2015).

Ligament:
In one animal study, mesenchymal stem cells increased the conversion of macrophages from the pro-inflammatory M1 form to the pro-healing M2 form in rat models of the Achilles tendon and of the medial collateral ligament of the knee. In both cases, the strength of the injured tendon and injured ligament returned almost to baseline (Chamberlain et al., 2017).

Meniscus:
One study suggested improved pain and meniscal height, as measured by MRI, with mesenchymal stem cells (Pak et al., 2017).

Putting bone marrow-derived mesenchymal stem cells on scaffolds has helped regenerate meniscus tissue in rabbits (Ding et al., 2015).

Spine:
In one preliminary study, allogeneic mesenchymal stem cells injected into a single lumbar intervertebral disc led to an improvement in pain symptoms in approximately 2/3 of the test group as compared to 1/3 of the control group (DePalma et al., 2014; Mascarinas et al., 2016).

In another study of five patients with chronic refractory low back pain, autologous bone marrow derived mesenchymal stem cells yielded improvements in pain, function and quality of life. There was no adverse events reported at between 4 to 6 years (Elabd et al., 2016).

Mesenchymal stem cells have been injected into the intervertebral discs in animal models. The transplanted cells slowed down the degeneration of the discs and appeared to improve disc regeneration (Crevenstein et al., 2004; Lee et al., 2006).

Cancer:
One potential problem is that mesenchymal stem cells may also be able to incorporate themselves into tumor cells (Djouad et al., 2003). One study showed that these donor cells found their way into a cancerous melanoma in the recipient and then facilitated its growth. In some cancer models, mesenchymal stem cells increased the incidence and the number of sites of cancer metastasis in the host (Li et al., 2018). Therefore, we must be cautious about injecting mesenchymal stem cells into humans. Interestingly, if the donor had cancer and the donor's cells were injected into a host, the host (the recipient of the cancer cells), did not develop cancer (Nardi et al., 2006).

Dr. Caplan hypothesized that, in the same way that hematopoietic cells could be used for autologous bone marrow transplants, perhaps mesenchymal cells could be collected from a patient and then returned to them when they needed them. For example, they could receive transplants of their own mesenchymal stem cells at a later date-- when they had osteoporosis (a weakening of the bone throughout the body) or osteoarthritis (a thinning of the cartilage throughout the body). FYI: the FDA does not allow for this type of procedure to be performed in the U.S.

Bone marrow-derived cells were first identified in Russia by Friedenstein in 1976 (Friedenstein et al., 1976).

Since that time, they became the main source of multipotent stem cells for medical procedures. However, there have been some barriers. First, in order to get them, patients must go through a bone marrow aspiration, which is an invasive and painful procedure that may or may not involve anesthesia and the risks of anesthesia (Berebichez-Fridman et al., 2017).

As the donor gets older, there are a variety of challenges. First, the bone marrow does not yield as many cells. The cells obtained do not last as long and their ability to differentiate (to mature into different cell types), decreases (Cheng et al., 2014).

Since mesenchymal stem cells are incorporated into cancers, scientists have considered the possibility of using mesenchymal stem cell transplants as a method of bringing anti-cancer medications and therapies directly into the cancer (Nardi et al., 2006).

And other scientists have looked at removing mesenchymal stem cells with a disease, genetically engineering them to correct the disease, and then returning the mesenchymal stem cells to the patient. The healthy stem cells could reconstitute the individual disease-free. This has been shown in osteogenesis imperfecta, a disease of collagen fibers that causes bone to be fragile (Pereira et al., 1998; Chamberlain et al., 2004). It is also being considered in hemophilia A (VanDamme et al., 2003). What if a person with hemophilia could incorporate mesenchymal stem cells that could make Factor VIII? (Remember the clotting cascade from our Hemostasis chapter)?

Bone marrow-derived stem cells are being studied in a variety of clinical conditions including hypertension, heart failure, asthma, systemic lupus erythematosus, and liver cirrhosis among others (Berebichez-Fridman R, et al., 2018).

CHAPTER 9 - MESENCHYMAL STEM CELLS

References:

Girlovanu M, Susman S, Soritau O, et al., Stem cells: Biological update and cell therapy progress. Clijul Medical 2015; 88(3): 265

Caplan AI. Mesenchymal stem cells. Journal of Orthopedic Research 1991; 9: 641-50

Pittenger MF, Mackay AM, Beck SC, et al., Multilineage potential of adult human mesenchymal stem cells. Science 1999; 284(5411): 143-7

McBride C, Gaupp D, Phinney DG. Quantifying levels of transplanted murine and human mesenchymal stem cells in vivo by real-time PCR. Cryotherapy 2003; 5: 7-18

O'Donoghue K, Coolani M, Chan J et al., Identification of fetal mesenchymal stem cells in maternal blood: Implications for non-invasive prenatal diagnosis. Mol Hum Reprod 2003; 9: 497-502

O'Donoghue K, Chan J, de la Fuente J, et al., Microchimerism in female bone marrow and bone decades after fetal mesenchymal stem-cell trafficking in pregnancy. Lancet 2004; 364: 179-82

Khosrotehrani K, Johnson KL, Cha DH, et al., Transfer of fetal cells with multilineage potential to maternal tissue JAMA 2004; 292: 75-80

Campagnoli C, Roberts IA, Kumar S, et al., Identification of mesenchymal stem/ progenitor cells in human first-trimester fetal blood, liver, and bone marrow. Blood 2001; 98(8): 2396 e402

Jones GN, Moschidou D, Puga-Iglesias TI, et al., Ontological differences in first compared to third trimester human fetal placental chorionic stem cells. PloS ONE 2012; 7(9): e43395

Thurairajah K, Broadhead M, and Balogh Z. Trauma and stem cells: Biology and potential therapeutic implications. International Journal of Molecular Sciences 2017; 18(3): 577

Zhang R, Li X, Liu Y, et al., Acceleration of bone regeneration in critical-size defect using BMP-9-loaded nHA/ Coll/ MWCNTs scaffolds seeded with bone marrow mesenchymal stem cells. BioMed Research International 2019; 7344957

Zhang ZY, Teoh SH, Chong MS, et al., Superior osteogenic capacity for bone tissue engineering of fetal compared with perinatal and adult mesenchymal stem cells. Stem Cells 2009; 27(1):126 e37
Pereira RF, O'hara MD, Laptev AV, et al., Marrow stromal cells as a source of progenitor cells for nonhematopoietic tissues in transgenic mice with a phenotype of osteogenesis imperfecta. Proc Natl Acad Sci USA 1998; 95: 1142-7

Chamberlain JR, Schwarze U, Wang PR et al., Gene targeting in stem cells from individuals with osteogenesis imperfecta. Science 2004; 303: 1198-201

Granero-Molto F, Weiss JA, Miga MI et al., Regenerative effects of transplanted mesenchymal stem cells in fracture healing. Tissue-Specific Stem Cells 2009; 27(8): 1887-98

Gomes JLE, da Silva RC, Silla LMR, et al., Conventional rotator cuff repair complemented by the aid of mononuclear autologous stem cells. Knee Surg Sports Traumatol Arthrosc 2012; 20(2): 373-7

Hernigou P, Flouzat Lachaniette CH, Delambre J, et al., Biologic augmentation of rotator cuff repair with mesenchymal stem cells during arthroscopy improves healing and prevents further tears: A case controlled study. Int Orthop 2014; 38(9): 1811-8

Pascual-Garrido C, Rolon A, Makino A. Treatment of chronic patellar tendinopathy with autologous bone marrow stem cells: A 5-year follow-up. Stem Cells Int 2012; 953510

Tornero-Esteban P., Hoyas J. A., Villafuertes E., et al., Efficacy of supraspinatus tendon repair using mesenchymal stem cells along with a collagen I scaffold. Journal of Orthopaedic Surgery and Research. 2015; 10(124): 1–7

Oh J. H., Chung S. W., Kim S. H., Chung J. Y., Kim J. Y. 2013 Neer award: effect of the adipose-derived stem cell for the improvement of fatty degeneration and rotator cuff healing in rabbit model. Journal of Shoulder and Elbow Surgery. 2014; 23(4): 445–455

Shen W., Chen J., Yin Z., et al., Allogenous tendon stem/progenitor cells in silk scaffold for functional shoulder repair. Cell Transplantation. 2012; 21(5): 943–958

Tseng S. S., Lee M. A., Reddi A. H. Nonunions and potential of stem cells in fracture-healing. The Journal of Bone & Joint Surgery. 2008;90 (Supplement 1):92–98

Peçanha R., De Lima L., Ribeiro M. B., et al., Adipose-derived stem-cell treatment of skeletal muscle injury. The Journal of Bone & Joint Surgery. 2012; 94-A(7): 609–617

Chahla J, et al., Concentrated Bone Marrow Aspirate for the Treatment of Chondral Injuries and Osteoarthritis of the Knee: A Systematic Review of Outcomes. Orthop J Sports Med. 2016 Jan 13;4(1):2325967115625481.

Gupta PK, Das AK, Chullikana A, Majumdar AS. Mesenchymal stem cells for cartilage repair in osteoarthritis. Stem Cell Research & Therapy. 2012;3(4):25

Fellows CR, Matta C, Zakany R, Khan IM, Mobasheri A. Adipose, Bone Marrow and Synovial Joint-Derived Mesenchymal Stem Cells for Cartilage Repair. Frontiers in Genetics. 2016;7:213

Goodrich L. R., Chen A. C., Werpy N. M., et al., Addition of mesenchymal stem cells to autologous platelet-enhanced fibrin scaffolds in chondral defects. The Journal of Bone & Joint Surgery. 2016; 98(1): 23–3

Frisbie D. D., McCarthy H. E., Archer C. W., Barrett M. F., McIlwraith C. W. Evaluation of articular cartilage progenitor cells for the repair of articular defects in an equine model. The Journal of Bone & Joint Surgery. 2015; 97(6): 484–493

Sierra R., Wyles C., Houdek M., Behfar A. Mesenchymal stem cell therapy for osteoarthritis: current perspectives. Stem Cells Cloning. 2015; 8(Supplement 1): 117–124

Chamberlain EE, Saether E, Aktas E, et al., Mesenchymal stem cell therapy on tendon/ ligament healing. J Cytokine Biol 2017; 2(1)

Pak J, Lee JH, Park KS, Jeon JH, Lee SH. Potential use of mesenchymal stem cells in human meniscal repair: current insights. Open Access Journal of Sports Medicine. 2017;8:33-38

Ding Z, Huang H. Mesenchymal stem cells in rabbit meniscus and bone marrow exhibit a similar feature but a heterogenous multi-differentiation potential: Superiority of meniscus as a cell source for meniscus repair. BMC Musculoskelet Disord 2015; 16:65

DePalma MJ, Gasper JJ. Cellular Supplementation Technologies for Painful Spine Disorders. PM&R. 2015.7:S19-S25

Mascarinas A, Harrison J, Boachie-Adjei K, Lutz G. Phys Med Rehabil Clin N Am. Regenerative Treatments for Spinal Conditions. 2016 Nov;27(4):1003-1017.

Elabd C, Centeno CJ, Schultz JR, Lutz G, et al., Intra-discal injection of autologous, hypoxic cultured bone marrow-derived mesenchymal stem cells in five patients with chronic lower back pain: a long-term safety and feasibility study. Elabd et al., J Transl Med. 2016;14:253:1-9.

Crevensten G., Walsh A. J., Ananthakrishnan D., et al., Intervertebral disc cell therapy for regeneration: mesenchymal stem cell implantation in rat intervertebral discs. Annals of Biomedical Engineering. 2004; 32(3): 430–434

Lee E. H., Hui J. H. P. The potential of stem cells in orthopaedic surgery. Journal of Bone and Joint Surgery. 2006; 88(7): 841–851

Djouad F, Plence P, Bony C, et al., Immunosuppressive effect of mesenchymal stem cells favors tumor growth in allogeneic animals. Blood 2003; 102: 3837-844

Li JH, Fan WS, Wang MM, et al., Effects of mesenchymal stem cells on solid tumor metastasis in experimental cancer models: A systematic review and meta-analysis. J Transl Med 2018; 16(1): 113

Nardi NB and da Silva ML. Mesenchymal stem cells: Isolation, in vitro expansion and characterization. Handb Exp Pharmacol 2006; 174: 249-82

Friedenstein AJ. Precursor cells of mechanocytes. Int Rev Cytol 1976;47:327–59

Berebichez-Fridman R, Gómez-García R, Granados-Montiel J, et al., The holy grail of orthopedic surgery: Mesenchymal stem cells - Their current uses and potential applications. Stem Cells Int 2017

Cheng HY, Ghetu N, Wallace CG, et al., The impact of mesenchymal stem cell source on proliferation, differentiation, immunomodulation and therapeutic efficacy. J Stem Cell Res Ther 2014;4:237

Van Damme A, Chuah MK, Dell'accio F, et al., Bone marrow mesenchymal cells for haemophilia A gene therapy using retroviral vectors with modified long-terminal repeats. Haemophilia 2003; 9(1): 94-103

Berebichez-Fridman R and Montero-Olvera PR. Sources and clinical applications of mesenchymal stem cells: State of the art review. Sultan Qaboos Univ Med J 2018; 18(3); e264-77

CHAPTER 10: Bone Marrow Aspirate Concentrate

Craig Chappell, Pradeep Albert, Alan Katz, Patrick Cleary & Richard Chang

> **CHAPTER PREVIEW**
>
> Bone marrow-derived mesenchymal cells secrete growth factors and decrease inflammation. They are most commonly harvested from the iliac crest. We describe a sample procedural technique here.

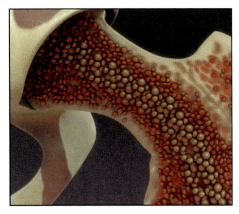

The main benefits of using bone marrow concentrate (BMAC) as an OrthoBiologic treatment include:
1. The ability to specifically target injured areas with minimal side effects.
2. The ability to increase the chances of successful healing by increasing the number and quality of stem cells present in the patient's tissue.

It's best to collect marrow from multiple sites rather than a single location to increase the odds of finding enough STEM cells. Once harvested, the bone marrow aspirate is concentrated by centrifuge. The red blood cells, white blood cells, platelets, and immature precursor cells are removed. The best concentration of BMAC to use is controversial and will vary dependent on the age of the patient. Younger patients will require less concentrated BMAC than those older than 50.

The Total Nucleated Cell Count (TNCC) required for autologous BMAC ranges from 500,000 cells/ml for children and young adults to 1 million cells/ml for those over the age of 50 (Hernigou et al., 2017).

The volume of aspirate can vary from 60 to 120 CC of marrow aspirate depending on patient size and application. To maximize stem cell collection, 10 ccs or less is taken at each pass to optimize stem cell yield.

BMAC success is best when ultrasound or fluoroscopy is used. Blind injections are discouraged (Centeno et al., 2017). Some people find BMAC therapy to be painful, but most people tolerate it well. Most people experience mild pain during the procedure, which lasts for about an hour. Some people also experience swelling and redness at the extraction site, but these symptoms typically subside within a few days.

Patient selection is extremely important when deciding to offer BMAC to a patient. Patients with mild to moderate disease respond best to BMAC therapy. Patients with severe diseases may not respond as well.

CLINICAL STUDIES:

Multiple studies show that bone marrow derived mesenchymal stem cells migrate and engraft with various musculoskeletal tissues, especially at the site of injury. There, they undergo tissue-specific differentiation (Caplan, 2005).

Bone marrow derived mesenchymal stem cells seem to be as effective as chondrocytes for articular cartilage repair in improving symptoms in patients. These stem cells have additional advantages in that they require less surgery and they generally cost less.

CHAPTER 10 - BONE MARROW DERIVED STEM CELLS

QUICK FACTS:

What's in the Bone Marrow?
Medicinal Signaling Cells formerly known as Adult Mesenchymal Stem Cells - Cells that are derived from mesodermal cells
Hematopoietic Stem Cells - Cells are important in producing the components of blood
Endothelial Progenitor cells - Progenitor cells facilitate vascular neogenesis
Pericytes - Cells that surround blood vessels
There are retinue of other cells that help in healing

Relative Contraindications
Prednisone or corticosteroids for 4 weeks prior to therapy
NSAID use for 1 week prior to therapy
Inabilty to perform procedure secondary to patient limitations or body habitus
Patients Age >60 have fewer stem cells and this may reduce the efficacy of treatment

Indications for using BMAC	Absolute Contraindications for Injecting BMAC in the outpatient setting.
Arthritis	Severe Anemia
Tendon Injury	Active local or systemic bacterial Infection
Muscle Injury	Active hematologic or metastatic neoplasm
Ligament Injury	Bleeding diathesis or anticogulant therapy that cannot be stopped for procedure
Avascular necrosis	Myelofibrosis

Multiple studies show that chondro-genetically-induced mesenchymal stem cells can transiently form fibrocartilaginous tissue, terminally differentiated calcifying cartilage, or osteophytes, all of which can be problematic depending on the type of tissue defect that they are being used to correct (Koga, 2007).

Bone marrow derived mesenchymal stem cells had a greater expression of Type I collagen compared to skin fibroblasts and tenocytes and a high ratio of Type I to Type III collagen, suggesting strong mechanical properties (Li, 2019).

One study compared bone marrow derived mesenchymal stem cells to placebo in the treatment of calvarial defects in dogs. The defects treated with BMAC formed bone faster and more extensively than those without.

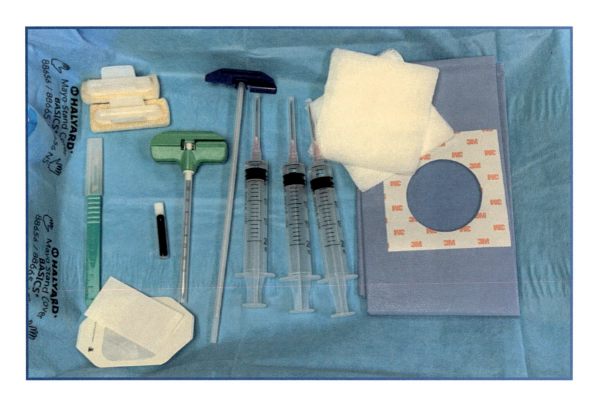

Supplies Needed to Aspirate Bone Marrow:

- 10 cc of 1% Lidocaine
- Jamshidi Needle or similar bone marrow aspiration kit
- 10 cc of Heparin (1,000 U/ml)
- 10 cc Syringes for aspiration
- Sterile Fenstrated Drape
- #11 blade scalpel
- 27 gauge ½ inch needle
- 20 gauge 3 - 4 3/4 inch spinal needle depending on size of patient
- BMAC Kits with centrifuge and 200 Micron Filters
- Ultrasound with Curvilinear Probe or Fluoroscopy

- Conscious sedation if clinically warranted

CHAPTER 10 - BONE MARROW DERIVED STEM CELLS

Medicinal signaling cells (MSC), formerly referred to as mesenchymal stem cells, are immunomodulatory and potentially can migrate to injured tissue (Caplan et al., 2010). The term "Mesenchymal Stem Cell" began in 1991 based on a belief that what happened in vitro would also occur in vivo. This turned out not to be the case (Caplan et al., 1991). Newer information lets us know that MSCs are secretory and produce an extensive array of cytokines and growth factors, prompting the new name, "Medicinal Signaling Cell." MSCs act as a sort of drug store at sites of injury (Caplan et al., 2010). MSCs also participate in the recruitment of other cells needed in tissue repair. They promote survival of existing cell repair, secrete growth factors, modulate the local environment and decrease inflammation. They can be obtained from bone marrow, referred to as bone marrow aspirate concentrate.

BMAC is most commonly harvested from the iliac crest. Like platelet-rich plasma, BMAC is generated by density-gradient centrifugation to remove red blood cells and plasma. Centrifugation increases MSC concentration and produces high levels of interleukin-1 receptor antagonists, which may function as an anti-inflammatory.

In a study conducted in 2014, the ilium was divided into six 4cm sectors, anterior to posterior, to determine the safest sectors to obtain bone marrow (Hernigou, 2014). It was shown that most breaches through the ilium were in sectors 1, 4, and 5. Sector 6 had the thickest transverse distance between the inner and outer cortex and the fewest overall breaches. One possible danger in obtaining bone marrow in sector six would include injury to the sciatic nerve or gluteal vessels secondary to a breach into the greater sciatic notch at depths greater than 6 cm. In the author's opinion, if practitioners desire to participate in bone marrow aspiration, they should start in sector 6 with guidance.

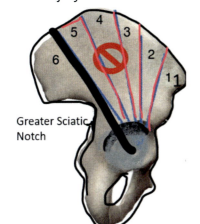

With the patient in the prone position, start by palpating the most prominent portion of the posterior sacroiliac spine (PSIS) and make a mark with a surgical marker corresponding to sector 6.

Then confirm with ultrasound. Dr. Chappell prefers a low-frequency curvilinear probe for deeper and broader visualization.

Confirm the mark over the PSIS and revise the mark if needed.

Then slide the probe laterally over the ilium so the probe is parallel with the ilium in a line from the anterior superior iliac spine (ASIS) to the PSIS so that the ilium can be visualized through the gluteal musculature.

Then slide the probe using a short-axis linear slide caudad until the greater sciatic notch is seen. Confirm the greater sciatic notch by using a doppler to visualize the gluteal vessels.

Once the greater sciatic notch is confirmed, slide the probe cephalad until the notch is no longer visualized.

In this position, angle the posterior portion on the probe to line up with your mark on the PSIS and draw a line. Anything on or cephalad to this line will fall in sector six and be safe to perform a bone marrow aspiration.

Next, sterilely prep the area and apply a sterile drape with a fenestration large enough to allow for the use of a sterilely covered ultrasound probe. Next, deliver an anesthetic with ultrasound guidance to the skin, subcutaneous tissue, and periosteum. Dr. Chappell generally uses 5-10 cc 1% lidocaine to anesthetize the periosteum.

The procedure is much more tolerable if the periosteum is thoroughly blocked. In Dr. Chappell's opinion, delivering an anesthetic is the most crucial step as this is when you can confirm the trajectory of your needle and the trocar once introduced.

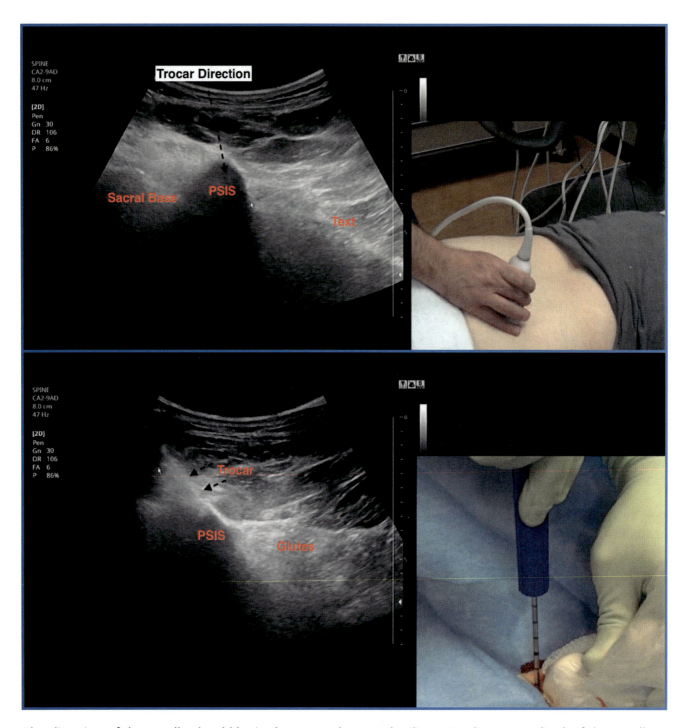

The direction of the needle should be in the same plane as the ilium. Readjust accordingly if the needle is even slightly out of plane.

Once the target and trajectory are confirmed, place an #11 blade through the skin wheel previously made during anesthetic placement. The width of the #11 blade is sufficient, and the incision does not need to be extended.

All syringes and the trocar should be heparinized before the procedure and the anticoagulant of choice is added to each syringe.

Then introduce the trocar with ultrasound guidance making sure to land the tip of the trocar on the middle of the PSIS. If needed, confirmation can be made by walking the trocar off the PSIS medially and laterally until it is confirmed in the center.

Then seat the trocar with firm pressure. Now advance the trocar through the cortex by manually rotating the handle of the trocar clockwise and counterclockwise with continued downward pressure directed into the PSIS, making sure not to change the angle of the trocar to avoid skiving off the ilium into the glute laterally or worse, medially onto the sacrum and potentially into a posterior sacral foramen.

Continue to advance, keeping an eye on the depth markers on the trocar and monitoring for a loss of resistance. Dr. Chappell prefers the manual technique vs. drill or hammer as he's found that some patients get a little nervous with the drill, and there appear to be more complaints of pain several days following the procedure with the use of a hammer.

Once the cortex is accessed, remove the trocar stylet and aspirate marrow to ensure successful cortex access per your device protocol.

Protocols differ based on the device you have decided to use. Many people believe that regardless of the system used, it appears to result in higher yields of desired cells by using small syringes (10ml) and creating strong negative pressure at multiple levels (Bohr et al., 2018).

This is accomplished by pulling small volumes of bone marrow at 1 level, then placing a blunt in the trocar and advancing 0.5-1cm, withdrawing the blunt and aspirating a small volume of bone marrow, and repeating the process until the trocar is advanced 3-5cm into the PSIS. If more bone marrow is required, one could go to the contralateral side and do the same thing or back the trocar out to the cortex and reangle in the direction of sector 5 and repeat the process.

Once the desired amount of bone marrow is obtained the trocar is withdrawn and the wound can be dressed with steristips and sterile dressing. Dr. Chappell generally has the patient flip to a supine position and put body weight pressure on the wound while the BMAC is processing per specific product protocol.

In one study, 1–4cc of bone marrow was aspirated with a 10cc syringe resulting in optimal harvesting. Filling a 10cc syringe to 10-20% of the total syringe volume resulted in higher MSC concentrations (Hernigou et al., 2005).

In other studies, there were no significant differences in the number of MSCs obtained in a single site, multiple depth harvest versus a multiple site single depth harvests. However, there was significantly more pain following the procedure in the multiple-site harvest.

SAMPLE

Please see Consent forms and Post procedure Care Provided by Dr. Craig Chappell. Please consult your local laws and use this as a guideline only.

POST PROCEDURE CARE: STEM CELL BMAC / ADIPOSE

Day of Procedure:
- Rest and avoid strenuous activities for the remainder of the day.
- Do not drive a car for the remainder of the day.
- If a dressing or ace wrap was applied after your procedure, you will need to keep that on for 2 hours. Then, you may remove it and just cover the site with a band-aid if needed.
- You may take Tylenol or pain medication as prescribed.

Days 2-5:
- You may experience an increase in pain and soreness for 2-5 days after your procedure.
- You may take Tylenol or pain medication as prescribed.
- Do not take any anti-inflammatory medication (i.e. Ibuprofen, Motrin, Aleve, or Naprosyn) for at least 5 days following the procedure.
- Try to abstain from icing but if you need to you may ice for no longer than 10 minutes every 2 hours as needed for pain and swelling using a barrier between the skin and ice. Numbness is too cold.
- The clear waterproof bandage should remain over the bone marrow aspiration site for 3 days.
- Aside from showering, avoid swimming or water activities for 3 days.
- It is normal to experience some soreness at both the aspiration site and the injection site. Please contact the office if redness, swelling, or warmness to touch occurs at either site.

Up to Day 14:
- You may experience a "roller coaster" syndrome where you feel great one day and then feel pain again for no apparent reason. This is normal in the healing process.
- The initial inflammatory phase lasts 7 days and the second phase can last up to 14 days.

Follow-Up Care:
- We will call to check on your healing 3-6 weeks following your procedure.
- If at any time during the 6 week healing phase, you have concerns that cannot be addressed over the phone, please schedule an appointment to be seen in the office.
- If your treatment plan includes multiple treatment sessions, please be sure to schedule your next procedure(s) as advised.

Additional Instructions (follow any checked boxes):
- Non-weight bearing:
    - Non-weight bearing for _____ days/weeks, then partial weight bearing on the _____ day/week.
    - No weight restriction on the _____ day/week.
- Activity Restrictions:
    - No lifting over _____ lbs for _____ days/weeks
    - No running for _____ days/weeks
    - No squatting or weight bearing exercises for _____ days/weeks
    - No above head activities/exercises for _____ days/weeks
    - No strenuous stretching of the area for _____ days/weeks
    - Follow exercise instructions provided
- Brace Wearing:
    - Wear brace during waking hours for _____ days/weeks
    - Wear brace during physical activity _____ days/weeks

Please note that your DME benefits might vary from your medical benefits. It is important to contact your insurance and understand your coverage for your brace

CONSENT TO BONE MARROW ASPIRATE CONCENTRATE (BMAC) AND/OR ADIPOSE WITH PRP

I, _____, hereby authorize Dr. Chappell and his assistants to perform bone marrow aspiration and stem cell injections using bone marrow aspirate and/or adipose with PRP on _____.

If any unforeseen condition arises in the course of the procedure calling for, in the physician's judgment, additional or different procedures/techniques from those I have consented to, I further request and authorize him to perform any other procedure/technique he deems necessary and advisable.

The nature and purpose of the procedure, possible alternative methods of treatment and the possibility of complications have been fully explained to me. I acknowledge that no guarantee or assurance has been made as to the results that may be obtained.

I understand the alternatives to PRP injections are:
- Surgical Intervention
- Other regenerative injections such as Prolotherapy or PRP
- Steroid Injections
- Osteopathic manipulation for temporary pain relief
- Acupuncture
- Bracing, splint and/or sacral belt
- Do nothing

I consent to the drawing of the blood as well as administration of local anesthetic agents to be applied by or under the direction of Dr. Chappell and to the use of such anesthetics, as he may deem advisable. The nature and purpose of the anesthesia, possible alternative methods of its administration, the risks involved, and the possibility of complications have been fully explained to me. I acknowledge that no guarantee or assurances have been made as to the results that may be obtained.

Possible risks may include however are not limited to:
- Immediate pain in the injection site lasting 3-4 days or more
- Stiffness in the injected joint
- Bruising
- Headache with back injections
- Allergic reaction to the solution
- Injury to the nerve/muscle
- Spinal cord injury during back injections
- Temporary or permanent nerve paralysis
- No effect from the treatment
- Pneumothorax (collapsed lung) when injecting near the lungs
- Death from complications of the treatment
- Itching at the injection sites
- Nausea/vomiting
- Dizziness or fainting
- Swelling after injections
- Bleeding
- Lumps/bumps will usually subside within 2 weeks from injection

I authorize this medical facility or members of its staff to retain, preserve and use for scientific or teaching purposes, or dispose of at their convenience and in their sole discretion, any specimens or tissues removed from my body, and I waive any interest I may have or have had in such specimens or tissues.

Please initial:

_____I certify that I have read and fully understand the above consent to the procedure.

_____That the explanations therein referred to were made as needed.

_____All my questions have been addressed by the physician.

_____That all blanks or statements requiring insertion or completion were filled in before I signed.

_____   _____
Patient/Guardian   Date

_____   _____
Witness   Physician Signature

References:

Hernigou P., and Beaujean, F. Bone marrow concentrate: A review of the current status and controversies. BioMed Research International 2017; 1-13.

Centeno C. J., Al-Sayegh H., Bashir J., and Goodyear, S. A dose response analysis of a specific bone marrow concentrate treatment protocol for knee osteoarthritis. BMC Musculoskeletal Disorders 2015; 16(1): 1-8.

Caplan A. I. Review: mesenchymal stem cells: cell-based reconstructive therapy in orthopedics. Tissue Engineering 2005; 11(7-8): 1198-1211.

Koga H., Muneta T., Ju YJ., Nagase T., Nimura A., Mochizuki T., and Sekiya I. Synovial stem cells are regionally specified according to local microenvironments after implantation for cartilage regeneration. Stem Cells 2007; 25(3):689-96.

Li Y., Chen S. K., Li L., Qin L., Wang X. L., and Wu J. L. Comparative characterization of mesenchymal stem cells from human bone marrow and adipose tissue for bone tissue engineering. Stem Cell Research & Therapy 2019; 10(1):206.

Shi Y., Zheng Y., Qu X., Gong T., Yang Y., Li W., Chen L., Wang J., Zhang X., and Fan Q. Bone marrow mesenchymal stem cell-derived exosomes facilitate bone marrow regeneration by regulating the biologic functions of recipient cells and activating the PI3K/Akt pathway in dogs with calvarial defects. Journal of Cellular Biochemistry 2019; 120(10):16916-16928.

Caplan A. I. What's in a name? Tissue Eng Part A 2010; 16(8):2415-7.

Caplan A. I. Mesenchymal stem cells. Journal of Orthopaedic Research 1991; 9(5): 641-650.

Hernigou J., Alves A., Homma Y., Guissou I., and Hernigou, P. Anatomy of the ilium for bone marrow aspiration: map of sectors and implication for safe trocar placement. International Orthopaedics (SICOT) 2014; 38(12): 2585-2590.

Bohr S., Patel S. J., Flick L. M. The influence of aspiration technique and syringe volume on the yield and quality of human mesenchymal stem cells from bone marrow aspirates. Journal of Orthopaedic Research 2018; 36(9):2427-2435.

Hernigou P., and Beaujean F. Percutaneous autologous bone-marrow grafting for nonunions: Influence of the number and concentration of progenitor cells. The Journal of Bone and Joint Surgery 2005; 87(7): 1430-1437.

CHAPTER 11 Adipose Derived Stem Cells

Norr Santz

CHAPTER PREVIEW

In this chapter, we discuss all the different types of adipose tissue: white, which is involved in appetite regulation; brown, which is involved in energy regulation in newborns; mechanical, which pads vulnerable structures; bone marrow, which acts as a reservoir for chemical messengers; and mammary, which provides nutrients. Then we discuss in detail the different types of mesenchymal stem cells found in adipose tissue and how to harvest them.

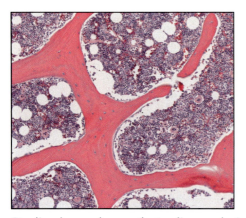

Assuming that our goal is to harvest as many functional mesenchymal stem cells as possible from an adult, in the safest most effective manner, we have different options. We can obtain these cells from the blood, the bone marrow, and the adipose, or fatty, tissue. Comparing those three options, the blood is the safest route, but has the lowest yield of stem cells. The bone marrow is a little less safe. Harvesting stem cells from the bone marrow involves a painful invasive procedure. Therefore, many doctors prefer to harvest stem cells from the patient's adipose tissue. Fatty tissue contains an abundance of stem cells—particularly the mesenchymal stem cells we are interested in. There can be some pain involved in harvesting them, but the procedure is usually less painful than a bone marrow aspiration (Kolaparthy et al., 2015). Studies have shown that adipose-derived mesenchymal stem cells can then differentiate into multiple cell lineages: adipocytes, osteocytes, and chondrocytes (Zuk et al., 2002).

Let's rewind a bit and talk about fat. As a human embryo develops, the cells form three layers: the ectoderm (or outer layer), the mesoderm (or middle layer), and the endoderm (or inner layer). Fat comes from the middle layer, the mesoderm. Fat cells, or adipocytes, first appear in the fetus during the second trimester. As they mature, the cells become rounded almost like grapes. They can have one lobe (unilobular) or multiple (multilobular). These lobules are separated by connective tissue borders. In order to get enough oxygen and nutrients for growth, these adipose-derived mesenchymal stem cells release a variety of growth factors. These include vascular endothelial growth factor (VEGF), transforming growth factor-beta (TGF-beta), and hepatocyte growth factors (Sbarbati et al., 2010).

As the fetus grows, five different types of adipose tissue form. We have brown fat and white fat, which are used for energy, mechanical adipose, which is used for padding, bone marrow adipose, which acts as a reservoir, and mammary adipose, which is used for nutrients. Let's go through each one individually.

Brown adipose or brown fat is found in the fetus and newborn. It is used for energy—it generates heat. It is found in the vital organs: the heart, aorta, and kidneys. It is also in the reproductive organs. It disappears as the individual gets older.

White adipose tissue, the most common form of fat in an adult, is also used for energy. White fat releases different hormones involved in appetite because they help determine how much food or energy we think we need. They are also involved in energy expenditure or how much energy you burn to maintain a certain weight. And they are involved in inflammation. Leptin, resistin, and adiponectin are the names of a few of these hormones. They travel through the bloodstream to communicate with the brain, liver, muscle, immune cells, and other fat cells (Kwon et al., 2013).

The term "mechanical adipose" refers to fat pads. We have fat pads in the face to support certain structures. We also have fat pads to protect vulnerable areas. Examples are the heel fat pads or metatarsal fat pads,

CHAPTER 11 - ADIPOSE DERIVED STEM CELLS

which protect the feet since they are constantly hitting the ground and ripe for injury (Kolaparthy et al., 2015).

Bone marrow adipose tissue is the yellow fat that we find in marrow. It is a reservoir of chemical messengers that regulate both bone growth and blood development.

There is also mammary adipose tissue, which is found in both males and females. Female breast tissue is composed of adipose tissue and glandular tissue and contains both lobules and milk ducts. Mammary adipose tissue provides nutrients and energy to babies through lactation (Kolaparthy et al., 2015). It also contains lymphatic vessels, blood vessels, lymph nodes, fibrous connective tissue and ligaments (National Cancer Institute, 2019).

This chapter focuses on mesenchymal stem cells found in the adipose tissue. These cells have different names: adipose-derived stem cells (ASCs), stromal vascular fraction, and processed lipoaspirates (PLAs). The intermediary cells between mesenchymal stem cells and adipocytes may be referred to as preadipocytes, lipoblasts, and pericytes (Bunnell et al., 2008).

Human body fat comprises mature adipocytes, preadipocytes, mesenchymal stem cells, fibroblasts, endothelial cells, immune cells, and other progenitors. The highest yield of mesenchymal stem cells comes from the abdomen, thigh, arm, and breast (Kolaparthy et al., 2015). Plastic surgeons can perform liposuctions and remove almost 3 liters of fat at a time, which translates to about 100 ml of "usable" fat. However, most practitioners of regenerative medicine use interventional techniques for fat harvesting. If you are using a needle to percutaneously aspirate fat ("lipoaspirate"), with local anesthetic and conscious sedation, your best bet might be the abdomen. There is less risk of injury to neurovascular bundles than in other areas. For the same volume of bone marrow and lipoaspirate, lipoaspirate often yields more mesenchymal stem cells and is technically easier than bone marrow aspirate (Illouz et al., 2011).

Once the fat has been collected, it must be washed and prepared in order to separate out the mesenchymal stem cells from the other cells including hematopoietic stem cells (Priya et al., 2014). This separation process can be performed in different ways. When researchers first tried to isolate mesenchymal stem cells, they used to mince the fat by hand.

Now different methods are used including filtration (separation based on particle size) and by centrifugation (separation based on density). An enzyme that can digest and break down the fat, called lipase, is often used as well (Klar et al., 2017).

With the advent of liposuction, clinicians inserted large-bore cannulas into the fat and injected and engorged the fat with solutions containing mixtures of saline, local anesthetic, and/ or epinephrine. This mixture of fat and other substances was then suctioned back through cannulas. The resulting aspirate contained finely minced fragments that could then be separated out further. Another method of obtaining fat aspirate is to perform ultrasound-assisted liposuction. The number of stem cells obtained is less than with liposuction (Bunnell et al., 2008). Despite the mechanical trauma involved in liposuction, the mesenchymal cells still appear to work normally.

In order to differentiate the mesenchymal stem cells from the hematopoietic stem cells, clinicians often use identifying markers on the cell surface. These include CD31 or platelet endothelial cell adhesion molecules, for example, which are found on the cell surfaces of endothelial precursors or progenitors (Weyand et al., 2013). Different immunologic techniques can be used to separate out these cells.

Because of the large amounts of fats and oils involved, the process of cell harvesting can be time-consuming and tedious. Many practitioners use a "bag within a bag" approach. They connect the suction catheter to a bag that acts as a sieve. Some tissue drips out and is removed. The fat that remains in the sieve can be washed and prepared afterwards. Another method involves transferring fat to a rotating centrifuge while collagenase digests the tissue. This allows larger amounts of fat to be processed at any given time (Gimble et al., 2007).

There are variations with respect to the optimal harvesting and processing of adipose-derived mesenchymal stem cells. There are also debates about the optimal number of cells to inject as well as how to steer the cells to the area of injury.

Adipose-derived mesenchymal stem cells repair and regenerate tissues in different ways. First, stem cells may release chemical messages, called cytokines, as well as growth factors that promote recovery. When nearby cells receive these chemical messages, they are also recruited to mature into the needed cell types (Bouhassira et al., 2015).

Second, these stem cells may release antioxidants into areas of injury. These antioxidants neutralize the actions of free radicals, uncharged molecules, that cause significant damage to living tissues. Some of these free radicals are produced by neutrophils, white blood cells that are more active during the inflammatory phase of wound healing (Bouhassira et al., 2015).

Third, adipose-derived mesenchymal stem cells are active in healing the extracellular matrix, the space between cells outside of blood vessels. They can promote the growth of fibroblasts that create a collagen scaffold and keratinocytes that build new layers of skin. This can reduce tissue scarring. They can also promote the growth of new blood vessels for healing (Hyldig et al., 2017).

Adipose-derived mesenchymal stem cells can also improve neurologic deficits after stroke and spinal cord injuries. It appears they decrease the pro-inflammatory immune response and they also promote nerve repair. In rats with occlusions of their middle cerebral arteries, intravenous injections of adipose-derived mesenchymal stem cells decreased the size of the area of brain injury. It also decreased the number of apoptotic neurons (Zhao et al., 2017). These are neurons that the body programs to commit suicide after an injury.

Because adipose-derived mesenchymal stem cells can differentiate into chondrocytes, and because they have immunosuppressant qualities, they may be an effective therapy for osteoarthritis. In one animal study, adipose-derived mesenchymal stem cells were injected subcutaneously into mice. Afterwards, the rate of osteophyte and fibrous tissue formation decreased (Tang et al., 2017).

In one human study, adipose tissue was aspirated from the patellar fat pads or infrapatellar fat pads surrounding the patients' knees. Then it was injected back into the knee joints of the same patients. The patients reported improved pain and function afterwards (Tang et al., 2017).

Adipose-derived mesenchymal stem cells may also have a role in the treatment of rheumatoid arthritis. There are higher amounts of inflammatory substances like TNF-alpha, interleukin 6 (IL-6), and interleukin 1-beta (IL-1-beta) in rheumatoid arthritis. Human adipose-derived mesenchymal stem cells were injected into models of mice with rheumatoid arthritis. They decreased the production of these inflammatory chemical messengers (Zhang et al., 2017).

In the chronic wound environment, adipose-derived mesenchymal stem cells may be able to curtail the inflammatory phase and promote the transition from the proliferative to the maturation phase. They do this by changing the chemical messages that white blood cells (T-cells and B-cells) send out. They also promote macrophages to change from the inflammatory M1 form to the anti-inflammatory M2 form. Adipose-derived mesenchymal stem cells may also promote new blood vessels to grow, carrying oxygen and nutrients, and they improve the function of fibroblasts, which create collagen (Hyldig et al., 2017).

CHAPTER 11 - ADIPOSE DERIVED STEM CELLS

References:

Kolaparthy LK, Sanivarapu S, Moogla S, et al., Adipose tissue: Adequate, accessible regenerative material. Int J Stem Cells 2015; 8(2): 121-7

Zuk P, Zhu M, Ashijan P, et al., Human adipose tissue is a source of multipotent stem cells. Mol Biol Cell 2002; 13(12): 4279-95

Sbarbati A, Accorsi D, Benati D, et al., Subcutaneous adipose tissue classification. Eur J Histochem 2010; 54(4): e48

Kwon H and Pessin JE. Adipokines mediate inflammation and insulin resistance. Front Endocrinol (Lausanne) 2013; 4: 71

National Cancer Institute. Breast Anatomy [Accessed on April 13, 2019] https://www.nationalbreastcancer.org/breast-anatomy

Bunnell BA, Flaat M, Gagliardi C, et al., Adipose-derived stem cells: Isolation, expansion, and differentiation. Methods 2008; 45(2): 115-20

Illouz YG and Sterodimas A, eds. Adipose stem cells and regenerative medicine. Springer Science & Business Medial 2011

Priya N, Sarcar S, Majumdar AS, et al., Explant culture: a simple, reproducible, efficient and economic technique for isolation of mesenchymal stromal cells from human adipose tissue and aspirate. Tissue Engineering and Regenerative Medicine 2014; 8(9): 706-16

Klar AS, Zimoch J, and Biedermann T. Skin tissue engineering: Application of adipose-derived stem cells. Biomed Res Int 2017

Weyand B, Dominici M, Hass R, et al., Mesenchymal stem cells: Basics and clinical application II. Springer-Verlag Berlin Heidelberg 2013

Gimble JM, Katz AJ, and Bunnell BA. Adipose-derived stem cells for regenerative medicine. Circ Res 2007; 100: 1249-60

Bouhassira EE. The SAGE encyclopedia of stem cell research. Los Angeles, CA: SAGE Publications 2015; [Accessed on April 13, 2019]

Hyldig K, Riis S, Pennisi CP, et al., Implications of extracellular matrix production by adipose tissue-derived stem cells for development of wound healing therapies. Int J Mol Sci 2017; 18(6): 1167

Zhao K, Li R, Gu C, et al., Intravenous administration of adipose-derived stem cell protein extracts improves neurological deficits in a rat model of stroke. Stem Cells Intl 2017

Tang Y, Pan Z, Zou Y, et al., A comparative assessment of adipose-derived stem cells from subcutaneous and visceral fat as a potential cell source for knee osteoarthritis treatment. J Cell Mol Med 2017; 20(10): 1-10

Zhang L, Wang XY, Zhou PJ, et al., Use of immune modulation by human adipose-derived mesenchymal stem cells to treat experimental arthritis in mice. Am J Transl Res 2017; 9(5): 2595-607

CHAPTER 12: Fetal Stem Cells

Bhavi Patel & Devi Nampiaparampil

> **CHAPTER PREVIEW**
>
> Mesenchymal stem cells are found in the fetus can be in supportive tissues such as the amniotic fluid that protects the fetus; the placenta that nourishes the fetus; the umbilical cord blood and tissues connecting the fetal and maternal circulation; and in the Wharton's jelly, the substance that covers the umbilical arteries and vein. Manufacturing and manipulating fetal stem cells is illegal in the United States.

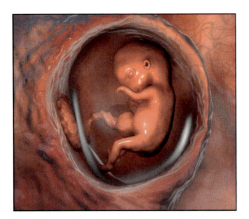

Stem cells can be categorized into four main groups; totipotent, pluripotent, multipotent, and unipotent. Totipotent stem cells form all types of cells and have the potential to give rise to an entire organism, the placenta, as well as extra-embryonic cells. Pluripotent stem cells are embryologic in origin and capable of forming all embryonic germ layers. Multipotent stem cells arise from fetal or adult tissue and are less able to differentiate. Hematopoietic and mesenchymal stem cells fall into the "multipotent" category. Unipotent stem cells arise from adult tissue and can only differentiate into a single type of cell (Girlovanu et al., 2015).

Although totipotent and pluripotent stem cells have the highest degree of differentiation potential-- and therefore regenerative or healing potential-- there are numerous ethical concerns that must be addressed before these cells can be studied effectively. There is one camp that believes these cells are isolated cells that can be studied for their regenerative potential in the same way as other treatment interventions. Others believe these cells represent human life. Therefore, manufacturing and manipulating them can be interpreted as another way of manipulating and potentially destroying human life (Girlovanu et al., 2015).

There are various types of stem cells: embryonic stem cells, fetal stem cells, adult stem cells and induced pluripotent stem cells. After conception, the fertilized egg divides into an inner cell mass, called a blastocyst, and an outer cell mass. The blastocyst will become the fetus. The outer cell mass will develop into the placenta and supporting structures. The inner cell mass is composed of embryonic stem cells. These have the largest differentiation potential. For that reason, there is an ethical debate about using these cells for research (DeLong et al., 2016). Fetal stem cells are obtained from the differentiating growing fetus.

Adult stem cells can be harvested from different areas of the body. The bone marrow, adipose tissue, and peripheral blood are the areas clinicians commonly use. Adult stem cells can also be found in cardiac muscle, the skin, articular cartilage, the gingiva, and even menstrual blood (Rodrigues et al., 2016).

Induced pluripotent stem cells are somatic cells that have been engineered and reprogrammed to retain the ability to differentiate into all three germ layers (Antoniadou et al., 2016).

The first human embryonic stem cell line was created in 1998. Since that time, the techniques that can be used to isolate and expand human embryonic stem cells have advanced significantly. In in vitro fertilization, an egg and a sperm are joined to achieve conception. That one cell is typically allowed to grow for 3 to 8 days until it develops into a blastocyst of approximately eight cells. Often, one of those eight cells is sent for genetic biopsy. This can either be preimplantation genetic screening (PGS) for chromosomal abnormalities or preimplantation genetic diagnosis (PGD) for specific genetically transmitted diseases. That one cell can be removed from the blastocyst without harm. Then, when the results of the PGS or PGD come back, the parent can decide whether or not to proceed with implanting the blastocyst into the uterus (Rodin et al., 2014; Rodin et al., 2014).

CHAPTER 12 - FETAL STEM CELLS

Scientists have figured out related techniques to remove one cell, one human embryonic stem cell, from the blastocyst to develop a cell line without harming the embryo. They can also use the biopsied single cell to develop a cell line. Nevertheless, the debate continues about whether or not it is acceptable to manipulate human life in this manner (Rodin et al., 2014; Rodin et al., 2014).

These human embryonic stem cells can be developed into full cell lines in the lab itself—without using animal models to grow them (Rodin et al., 2016).

Animal models are used to determine both the functionality of these cells and the safety of their use. These cells have been transplanted into animals to regenerate and repair organs and tissues derived from all three of the embryonic cell layers. However, the more times that the cells divide or reproduce, the more likely they are to accumulate genetic mutations. As a result, they are more likely to transform into a cancer after being transplanted (Narva et al., 2010, Amps et al., 2011).

There are certain markers or identifiers on the cell surface that can identify these cells as pluripotent stem cells. Some of these markers are named Oct-4, Sox-2 and Nanog. At present, there is no method to quickly isolate the cells with these markers. Instead, approximately 1 million cells from a cell lineage are often subcutaneously injected into mice to determine whether a teratoma will form. If so, then the population of cells, the cell line, must be derived from a human embryonic stem cell (Wesselschmidt RL, 2011; Gertow K et al., 2007).

Once these cells are identified, they can be removed from any population of cells that would be used for human trials. They can be removed by various methods including sorting cells by centrifuge (Tang et al., 2011), using stem cell inhibitors (Ben-David et al., 2013), using cytotoxic (or deadly) antibodies (Choo et al., 2008), or promoting a process of cell suicide, also known as apoptosis (Di Stasi et al., 2011).

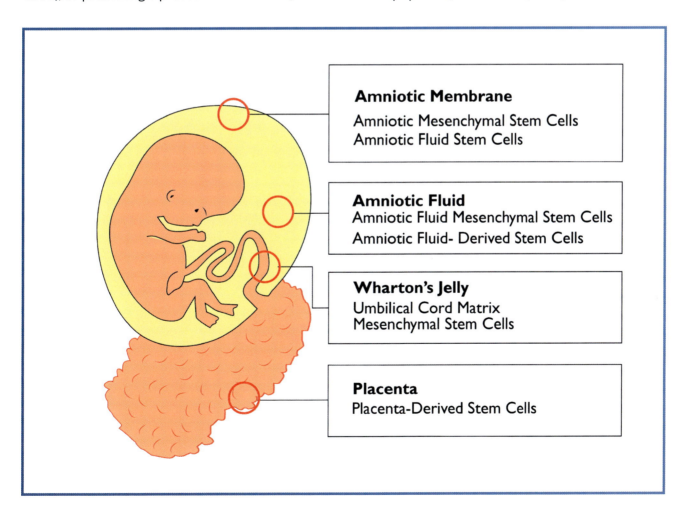

At present, safety trials—safety, not efficacy trials-- are in progress for the use of these cells in two conditions: spinal cord injuries and age-related macular degeneration that causes blindness. Thus far, they appear to be safe (Schwartz et al., 2012; Seiger, 1989; Piltti et al., 2013; Schwartz et al., 2015).

Injury precipitates stem cell activation. The stem cells migrate to the site of injury and differentiate into the cells required for healing the damaged tissue. Depending on the type of injury, the stem cells' quantity and quality can be affected. This can lead to poor tissue regeneration.

There are several types of stem cells associated with fetal tissue. Fetal stem cells can be obtained from the fetus itself. Fetal stem cells can also potentially be collected from the tissues that support the fetus: the amnion and amniotic fluid that protect and bathe the fetus, the placenta that nourishes the fetus, the umbilical cord blood and tissues that connect the fetal circulation with maternal circulation, and Wharton's jelly the substance inside the umbilical cord that covers the umbilical cord arteries and vein.
In terms of the prevalence of mesenchymal stem cells (Gotherstrom et al., 2016)—

Fetal bone marrow: 1/ 400 cells with a nucleus is a mesenchymal stem cell
Newborn bone marrow: 1/ 10,000 cells with a nucleus is a mesenchymal stem cell
Adult bone marrow: 1/ 250,000 cells with a nucleus is a mesenchymal stem cell

Fetal mesenchymal stem cells may play a greater role in hematopoiesis than adult stem cells. Fetal stem cells appear to travel with hematopoietic stem cells to facilitate their creation of red blood cells, white blood cells and platelets (Van den Heuvel RL, et al., 1987).

Compared to adult mesenchymal stem cells, fetal stem cells divide more rapidly. They divide every 30 hours rather than every 80 hours. One theory of aging relates to telomere shortening with each division. Because fetal stem cells have longer telomeres, they appear to age more slowly (Guillot et al., 2007; Gotherstrom et al., 2003; Gotherstrom et al., 2005). Both fetal mesenchymal and adult mesenchymal stem cells form elongated spindle shapes as they grow. Fetal stem cells form colonies. Adult stem cells do too, but the number decreases with age.

Mesenchymal stem cells obtained in the first trimester have a doubling time of thirty hours when compared to adult mesenchymal stem cells which have a doubling time of eighty hours. In the lab, they have achieved approximately 28 doublings in fifty days while adult mesenchymal stem cells have only been able to double about 7 times in the same period. Fetal mesenchymal stem cells are capable of expanding approximately 70 times before showing signs of senescing while adult mesenchymal stem cells are capable of expanding about 15-40 times (Heo et al., 2016).

Compared to human embryonic stem cells, mesenchymal stem cells do not appear to form tumors (Bernardo et al., 2007; Prockop et al., 2010; von Bahr et al., 2012).

In 2002, the first fetal mesenchymal cell transplant was performed in humans to treat osteogenesis imperfecta type III. This is a disease where collagen is formed abnormally. As a result, the patient's bones were frail and broke easily. The transplant appeared to slow down her rate of fractures. When she received additional transplants of mesenchymal stem cells, the rate of fractures slowed even further (Gotherstrom et al., 2016; Le Blanc et al., 2005; Gotherstrom et al., 2014)

Both hematopoietic and mesenchymal stem cells can be harvested from the umbilical cord blood and tissues. Hematopoietic stem cells can mature into red blood cells, white blood cells and platelets. Mesenchymal stem cells can mature into muscle, tendon, cartilage, bone, and adipose tissue. Both types of stem cells travel to the area of injury and then differentiate into the types of cells necessary for the injury to heal. They can stimulate other progenitor or precursor cells to reproduce and mature, promote the growth of new blood vessels to the area, prevent a form of cell suicide known as apoptosis, reduce inflammation and minimize scarring (Antoniadou et al., 2016).

Stem cells applied directly to the site of injury may improve healing. The optimal form, preparation, dose, and frequency of mesenchymal stem cell treatment still has to be defined. Moreover, we are still learning how mesenchymal stem cells can migrate to—and stay in—the correct location, differentiate into the correct cell type, and survive post-transplant. We are also still identifying factors that may stimulate undifferentiated cells to form cancerous cells.

By the mid-thirties, the human skeleton has reached maturity or adulthood. However, it still goes through changes. It undergoes bone formation and bone loss, replenishing itself in whole every two to ten years depending on the individual's age. The rate of bone formation and bone loss are about even during the thirties. After that age, bone loss can exceed bone formation, particularly during menopause. These individuals are more at risk for fracture.

As a person ages, responsive mesenchymal stem cells decrease in number. Their function remains intact. Therefore, injecting or applying mesenchymal stem cells to fracture sites might speed up healing by increasing the number of cells available for regeneration.

Cartilage is composed of chondrocytes (cartilage cells) and extracellular matrix, which comprises molecules such as proteoglycans and glycosaminoglycans like hyaluronic acid and chondroitin sulfate. Hyaluronic acid attracts cells to injured areas to facilitate wound healing (Voinchet et al., 2006). Chondroitin sulfate appears to be anti-inflammatory. It also stimulates the production of more proteoglycans and hyaluronic acid (Iovu et al., 2008).

Because cartilage does not contain blood vessels, it is slow to heal. Cartilage is predisposed to degenerative conditions such as osteoarthritis. There are theories that suggest that older cartilage cells release chemicals, called catabolic cytokines, and proteins known as matrix-degrading enzymes, which can decrease the number of cells available for regeneration and repair. A molecule called ADAMTS5 causes stem cells to differentiate into fibroblasts rather than into chondrocytes (cartilage cells). This molecule is thought to be involved in the breakdown of cartilage because mice lacking ADAMT25 do not develop osteoarthritis (Glasson et al., 2005).

References:

Girlovanu M, Susman S, Soritau O, et al., Stem cells: Biological update and cell therapy progress. Clijul Medical 2015; 88(3): 265

DeLong JM. The current state of stem cell therapies in sports medicine. Operative Techniques in Orthopedics 2016; 124-34

Rodrigues MC, Lippert T, Nguyen H, et al., Menstrual blood-derived stem cells: In vitro and in vivo characterization of functional effects. Adv Exp Med Biol 2016; 951: 111-21

Antoniadou E and David AL. Placental stem cells. Best Practice & Research Clinical Obstetrics and Gynaecology 2016; 31: 13 e29

Rodin S, Antonsson L, Niaudet C, et al., Clonal culturing of human embryonic stem cells on laminin-521/ E-cadherin matrix in defined and xeno-free environment. Nat Commun 2014; 5:3195

Rodin S, Antonsson L, Hovatta O, et al., Monolayer culturing and cloning of human pluripotent stem cells on laminin-521 based matrices under xeno-free and chemically defined conditions. Nat Protoc 2014; 9: 2354 e68

Rodin S, Stenfelt S, Antonssen L. Human embryonic stem cells. Best Practice & Research Clinical Obstetrics and Gynaecology 2016; 2e12

Narva E, Autio R, Rakhonen N, et al., High-resolution DNA analysis of human embryonic stem cell lines reveals culture-induced copy number changes and loss of heterozygosity. Nat Biotechnol 2010; 28: 371e7

Amps K, Andrews PW, Anyfantis G, et al., Screening ethnically diverse human embryonic stem cells identifies a chromosome 20 minimal amplicon conferring growth advantage. Nat Biotechnol 2011; 29(12): 1132-44

Wesselschmidt RL. The teratoma assay: an in vivo assessment of pluripotency. Methods Mol Biol 2011; 767: 231e41

Gertow K, Przyborski S, Loring JF, et al., Isolation of human embryonic stem cell-derived teratomas for assessment of pluripotency. Curr Protoc Stem Cell Biol 2007; Chapter 1: Unit 1B4

Tang C, Lee AS, Volkmer JP, et al., An antibody against SSEA-5 glycan on human pluripotent stem cells enables removal of teratoma-forming cells. Nat Biotechnol 2011; 29: 829e34

Ben-David U, Gan QF, Golan-Lev T, et al., Selective elimination of human pluripotent stem cells by an oleate synthesis inhibitor discovered in a high-throughput screen. Cell Stem Cell 2013; 12: 167e79

Choo AB, Tan HL, Ang SN, et al., Selection against undifferentiated human embryonic stem cells by a cytotoxic antibody recognizing pdocalyxin-like protein-1. Stem Cells 2008; 26: 1454e63

Di Stasi A, Tey SK, Dotti G, et al., Inducible apoptosis as a safety switch for adoptive cell therapy. N Engl J Med 2011; 365: 1673e83

Schwartz SD, Hubschman JP, Heilwell G, et al., Embryonic stem cell trials for macular degeneration: a preliminary report. Lancet 2012; 379:713 e20

Seiger A. Collection and use of fetal central nervous system tissue. Fetal Ther 1989; 4 (Suppl 1): 104 e7

Piltti KM, Salazar DL, Uchida N, et al., Safety of human neural stem cell transplantation in chronic spinal cord injury. Stem Cells Transl Med 2013: 2:961 e74

Schwartz SD, Regillo CD, Lam BL, et al., Human embryonic stem cell-derived retinal pigment epithelium in patients with age-related macular degeneration and Stargardt's macular dystrophy: follow-up of two open-label phase ½ studies. Lancet 2015; 385:509 e16

Gotherstrom C. Human foetal mesenchymal stem cells. Best Practice & Research Clinical Obstetrics and Gynaecology 2016; 31: 82e87

Van den Heuvel RL, Versele SR, Schoeters GE at al. Stromal stem cells (CFU-f) in yolk sac, liver, spleen and bone marrow of pre- and postnatal mice. Br J Haematol 1987; 66(1): 15 e20

Guillot PV, Gotherstrom C, Chan J, et al., Human first-trimester fetal MSC express pluripotency markers and grow faster and have longer telomeres than adult MSC. Stem Cells 2007; 25(3) 646 e54

Gotherstrom C, Ringden O, Westgren O, et al., Immunomodulatory effects of human foetal liver-derived mesenchymal stem cells. Bone Marrow Transplant 2003; 32(3):265 e72

Gotherstrom C, West A, Liden J, et al., Difference in gene expression between human fetal liver and adult bone marrow mesenchymal stem cells. Haematologica 2005;90(8): 1017 e26

Heo JS, Choi Y, K HS, et al., Comparison of molecular profiles of human mesenchymal stem cells derived from bone marrow, umbilical cord blood, placenta and adipose tissue. International 2016; 37(1): 115-25

Bernardo ME, Zaffaroni N, Novara F, et al., Human bone marrow derived mesenchymal stem cells do not undergo transformation after long-term in vitro culture and do not exhibit telomere maintenance mechanisms. Cancer Res 2007; 67(19):9142 e9

Prockop DJ, Brenner M, Fibbe WE, et al., Defining the risks of mesenchymal stromal cell therapy. Cytotherapy 2010;12(5): 576 e8

von Bahr L, Batsis I, Moll G, et al., Analysis of tissues following mesenchymal stromal cell therapy in humans indicates limited long-term engraftment and no ectopic tissue formation. Stem Cells 2012; 30(7):1575 e8

Le Blanc K, Gotherstrom C, Ringden O, et al., Fetal mesenchymal stem-cell engraftment in bone after in utero transplantation in a patient with severe osteogenesis imperfecta. Transplantation 2005; 79(11): 1607-14

Gotherstrom C, Westgren M, Shaw SW, et al., Pre- and postnatal transplantation of fetal mesenchymal stem cells in osteogenesis imperfecta: a two-center experience. Stem Cells Transl Med 2014; 3(2):255 e64

Antoniadou E and David AL. Placental stem cells. Best Practice & Research Clinical Obstetrics and Gynaecology 2016; 31: 13 e29

Voinchet V, Vasseur P, Kern J. Efficacy and safety of hyaluronic acid in the management of acute wounds. Am J Clin Dermatol 2006; 7(6):353-7

Iovu M, Dumais G, du Souich P. Anti-inflammatory activity of chondroitin sulfate. Osteoarthritis Cartilage 2008; 16 Suppl 3: S14-8

Glasson SS, Askew R, Sheppard B, et al., Deletion of active ADAMTS5 prevents cartilage degradation in a murine model of osteoarthritis. Nature 2005; 434(7033): 644-8

CHAPTER 13 Stem Cells in Amniotic Fluid, Placenta and Wharton's Jelly

Brian Pekkerman & Devi Nampiaparampil

> **CHAPTER PREVIEW**
>
> Amniotic fluid protects and cushions the fetus. It also insulates the fetus and provides nutrients and growth factors. Placental tissues, which have contributions from both the fetus and the mother, have the ability to repair and regenerate tissues. Wharton's jelly has similarities to cartilage. In this chapter, we discuss the roles of each of these substances in regenerative medicine.

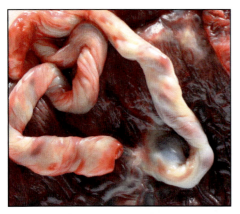

Amniotic Fluid:
During pregnancy, the amniotic fluid surrounds the fetus and serves as a protective liquid barrier. It also provides nourishment (Underwood et al., 2005). The amniotic fluid is made up of water, cells and chemicals. The cells, which include mesenchymal stem cells, are typically shed by the fetus (Polgar et al., 1989). Amniotic fluid also contains other stem cell types that can go on to form liver cell, nerve cell, and other cell lines (Roubelakis et al., 2007).

Amniotic fluid consists of proteins, carbohydrates, lipids, phospholipids, electrolytes, and waste products like urea. It usually appears during the second week of gestation (Hamid et al., 2017). The amniotic fluid cells can be separated into: amniocytes (~60%), epithelioid (~33%), and fibroblastic type (~5%) (Hamid et al., 2017). Only 1% of all amniotic fluid derived stem cells show pluripotent characteristics. The rest of the stem cells are committed to specific germ lines. They can only mature into cells from their specific primary germ layer (Da Sacco et al., 2010).

Amniotic fluid has several functions. It protects and cushions the fetus and umbilical cord from trauma and also provides cushioning to allow fetal movements. It thermoregulates and insulates the fetus. The amniotic fluid provides nutrients and growth factors to the fetus. It also defends the fetus from infection (Hamid et al., 2017).

During the first half of pregnancy, amniotic fluid is formed by the passive movement of water from the fetus. Sodium and chloride are also actively transported between the fetus's skin and the amniotic membrane (Hamid et al., 2017).

In the lab, amniotic fluid stem cells were able to build bone. Scaffolds containing amniotic fluid stem cells have been implanted subcutaneously into mice. Eight weeks later, x-rays suggested bone formation (Loukogeorgakis et al., 2016).

There is evidence that amniotic fluid stem cells can regenerate nerves. Rat models with sciatic nerve crush injuries experienced better foot movement as well as improved nerve conduction velocities and muscle action potentials after the administration of amniotic fluid stem cells (Loukogeorgakis et al., 2016).

In certain medical conditions-- when the baby has chromosomal abnormalities or gastrointestinal malformations, for example—the fetus may be surrounded by more amniotic fluid than usual. This is called polyhydramnios. In those cases, clinicians can remove some amniotic fluid in a procedure called amnioreduction. This procedure is typically performed in the second or third trimester to prevent premature labor (Dickinson et al., 2014).

Amniocentesis is a procedure used to diagnose chromosomal abnormalities and infections. It is performed by aspirating amniotic fluid from the womb around the fetus. Because some of the cells from the fetus are contained in the amniotic fluid, it is possible to test those cells for genetic abnormalities in the lab. The procedure is usually performed between weeks 15-16 of gestation because earlier aspirations are associated with an increased risk of miscarriage (The Canadian Early and Mid-Trimester Amniocentesis Trial Group, 1998).

Amniotic fluid can be collected during the second trimester via amniocentesis, during the third trimester via amnioreduction, and at birth via c-section. Most often, the cells captured at birth are from umbilical cord blood and the placenta (Loukogeorgakis et al., 2017). The amniotic fluid changes as pregnancy progresses. The amniotic fluid stem cells that are collected in the first trimester appear to be more primitive and share more in common with embryonic fetal stem cells than cells collected later in pregnancy (Schiavo et al., 2015; Moschidou et al., 2012).

In animal models, amniotic fluid derived mesenchymal cells can heal and repair bone, cartilage and muscle injuries (Fuchs et al., 2005; Kunisaki et al., 2006; Kunisaki et al., 2006; Steigman et al., 2005). In animal models, amniotic fluid stem cells do not form tumors—even when they are injected into immunocompromised mice (Coppi et al., 2007).

There is a difference between amniotic fluid derived stem cells (AFSCs) and amniotic fluid derived mesenchymal stem cells (AF-MSCs). Amniotic fluid derived stem cells express markers associated with pluripotent cells. That means they could potentially mature into cells derived from any of the three primary germ layers. Amniotic fluid derived mesenchymal stem cells, on the other hand, can only mature into cells derived from one of the primary germ layers: the mesoderm.

Placenta:

Going back to human embryology, the blastocyst grows into a trophoblast. When the trophoblast pierces the uterine endometrium and burrows a hole, the placenta starts to form. As the embryo develops, the yolk sac and amniotic cavity form.

Placental tissue has contributions from both the fetus and the mother. Therefore, mesenchymal cells obtained from the placenta can have different properties. If they are from the fetus, they have a greater ability to regenerate and repair tissues. If they are from the mother, they have less regenerative potential (Zhu et al., 2014). Placental mesenchymal cells obtained earlier in gestation are more likely to be primitive and pluripotent than placental mesenchymal cells obtained during labor and delivery (Sung et al., 2010; Poloni et al., 2012; Park et al., 2013).

Compared to adult bone marrow derived mesenchymal stem cells, placental mesenchymal stem cells appear to have more growth potential. They also have a greater ability to control inflammation (Ziaei et al., 2017).

Placental mesenchymal stem cells and fetal bone marrow-derived stem cells appear to be able to form bone tissue equally effectively (Shafiee et al., 2017).

In the lab and in animal studies, placental mesenchymal stem cells could produce muscle myofibers (Park et al., 2011).

Placental mesenchymal stem cells are used to treat non-healing wounds, particularly in epidermolysis bullosa, a condition that causes the skin to blister and peel off in layers (Nevala-Plagemann et al., 2015).

Placental mesenchymal stem cells can also be used to treat graft-vs.-host disease. Graft-vs.-host disease occurs when donor tissue—transplanted tissue—attacks the recipient. This can happen with bone marrow transplants. Placental mesenchymal stem cells have treated graft-vs.-host disease in patients who were not responding to immunosuppression with steroids. With placental mesenchymal stem cells, the survival rates improved to greater than 70% as opposed to under 10% (Ringden et al., 2015).

There are certain cell markers or identifiers that can be found on pluripotent stem cells, primitive stem cells that can form any cell type derived from the three embryonic cell layers. One of these identifiers is called

Oct-4. This cell identifier has come up on certain placental stem cells, suggesting that pluripotent stem cells can be harvested from the placenta. However, to our knowledge, no tumors or cancers have formed from placental stem cell transplants (Fong et al., 2007; Fariha et al., 2010).

Placental mesenchymal stem cells are being used in clinical studies of neurologic diseases. In Parkinson's Disease, a condition where the brain loses its ability to produce a chemical called dopamine, injections of processed placental stem cells into mice improved the affected nerve cells ability to produce dopamine (Park et al., 2012).

Placental-based mesenchymal stem cell therapies are also being evaluated for the treatment of multiple sclerosis, a neurodegenerative condition that can affect the brain and spinal cord. Injections of placental stem cells into the brains of mice appeared to slow down the progression of the disease (Fisher-Shoval et al., 2012).

Research is also ongoing regarding the use of placental stem cells for the treatment of traumatic brain injuries (Chen et al., 2009).

There have been attempts to set up a public biobank for donated placental products. However, there have been challenges. A bill called the Stem Cell Research Enactment Act was vetoed by President George W. Bush (Congress, 2007). In the past decade, private companies have entered the market allowing parents to pay to store their child's placental products. Nevertheless, there is a wide variability in how familiar hospital staff are with biobanking protocols (Antoniadou et al., 2016).

Wharton's Jelly:

The stem cells found in Wharton's jelly are high in hyaluronic acid and glycosaminoglycans. Compared to other types of stem cells, they may have more similarities to cartilage. Therefore, they may be better for repairing cartilage. In the lab, when grown in cell culture media, mesenchymal stem cells derived from Wharton's jelly were more effective than those derived from bone marrow at differentiating into cartilage cells (Richardson et al., 2016).

Mesenchymal stem cells have also been harvested from Wharton's jelly. These cells have been used in animal studies of traumatic brain injury, stroke, Parkinson's Disease, Huntington's Disease, and multiple sclerosis (Joerger-Messerli et al., 2016).

In one human study, a 5 year-old child with cerebral palsy received multiple transfusions of Wharton's jelly derived mesenchymal stem cells from her sister. In that one case, her speech and gait improved (Wang et al., 2013).

Medical conditions that arise during pregnancy might affect the mesenchymal stem cells in the Wharton's jelly. In women who had preeclampsia, a greater number of the Wharton's jelly derived mesenchymal stem cells were further along in the pathway to becoming nerve cells (Joerger-Messerli et al., 2015).

References:

Underwood MA, Gilbert WM, and Sherman MP. Amniotic fluid: Not just fetal urine anymore. J Perinatol 2005; 25: 341– 348

Polgar, K, Adany, R, Abel, G et al., Characterization of rapidly adhering amniotic fluid cells by combined immunofluorescence and phagocytosis assays. Am J Hum Genet 1989; 45: 786– 792

Roubelakis, MG, Pappa, KI, Bitsika, V et al., Molecular and proteomic characterization of human mesenchymal stem cells derived from amniotic fluid: Comparison to bone marrow mesenchymal stem cells. Stem Cells Dev 2007; 16: 931– 952

Hamid A, Joharry M, Mun-Fun H, et al., Highly potent stem cells from full-term amniotic fluid: A realistic perspective. Reproductive Biology 2017: 9-18

Da Sacco S, Sedrakyan S, Boldrin F, et al., Human amniotic fluid as a potential new source of organ precursor cells for future regenerative medicine applications. J Urol 2010; 183(3); 1193-200

Loukogeorgakis SP, De Coppi P. Stem cells from amniotic fluid—potential for regenerative medicine. Best Pract Res Clin Obstet Gynaecol 2016; 31: 45-57

Dickinson JE, Tijoe YY, Jude E, et al., Amnioreduction in the management of polyhydramnios complicating singleton pregnancies. American Journal of Obstetrics and Gynecology 2014; 211(4): 434 e1- 434 e7

The Canadian Early and Mid-Trimester Amniocentesis Trial Group. Randomised trial to assess safety and fetal outcome of early and midtrimester amniocentesis. Lancet 1998; 351(9098): 242-7

Loukogeorgakis SP, Coppi P. Concise review: Amniotic fluid stem cells: The known, the unknown, and potential regenerative medicine applications. Stem Cells 2017; 35(7): 1663-73

Schiavo AA, Franzin C, Albiero M et al., Endothelial properties of third-trimester amniotic fluid stem cells cultured in hypoxia. Stem Cells Res Ther 2015; 6: 209

Moschidou D, Mukherjee S, Blundell M, et al., Human mid-trimester amniotic fluid stem cells cultured under embryonic stem cell conditions with valproic acid acquire pluripotent characteristics. Stem Cells Dev 2012; 22: 444-58

Fuchs JR, Kaviani A, Oh JT, et al., Diaphragmatic reconstruction with autologous tendon engineered from mesenchymal amniocytes. J Pediatr Surg 2004; 39: 834-8

Kunisaki SM, Fuchs JR, Kaviani A, et al., Diaphragmatic repair through fetal tissue engineering: A comparison between mesenchymal amniocyte- and myoblast-based constructs. J Pediatr Surg 2006; 41: 34-39

Kunisaki SM, Freedman DA, Fauza DO. Fetal tracheal reconstruction with cartilaginous grafts engineered from mesenchymal amniocytes. J Pediatr Surg 2006; 41: 675-82

Steigman SA, Ahmed A, Shanti RM, et al., Sternal repair with bone grafts engineered from amniotic mesenchymal stem cells. J Pediatr Surg 2009; 44: 1120-6

Coppi, P, Bartsch, G, Siddiqui, MM et al., Isolation of amniotic stem cell lines with potential for therapy. Nat Biotechnol 2007; 25: 100– 106

Zhu Y, Yang Y, Zhang Y, et al., Placental mesenchymal stem cells of fetal and maternal origins demonstrate different therapeutic potentials. Stem Cell Res Ther 2014; 5:48

Sung HJ, Hong SC, Yoo JH, et al., Stemness evaluation of mesenchymal stem cells from placentas according to developmental stage: comparison to those from adult bone marrow. J Korean Med Sci 2010; 25:1418 e26

Poloni A, Maurizi G, Serrani F, et al., Human AB serum for generation of mesenchymal stem cells from human chorionic villi: comparison with other source and other media including platelet lysate. Cell Prolif 2012; 45:66 e75

Park S, Koh SE, Hur CY, et al., Comparison of human first and third trimester placental mesenchymal stem cell. Cell Biol Int 2013; 37:242 e9

Ziaei M, Zhang J, Patel D, et al., Umbilical cord stem cells in the treatment of corneal disease. Survey of Opthalmology 201; 62(6): 803-15

Shafiee A, Baldwin JG, Patel J, et al., Fetal bone marrow-derived mesenchymal stem/ stromal cells enhance humanization and bone formation of BMP7 loaded scaffolds. Biotechnol J 2017; 12(12)

Park TS, Gavina M, Chen C-W, et al., Placental perivascular cells for human muscle regeneration. Stem Cells Dev 2011; 20:451 e63

Nevala-Plagemann C, Lee C, Tolar J. Placenta-based therapies for the treatment of epidermolysis bullosa. Cytotherapy 2015; 17:786 e95

Ringden O, Solders M, Erkers T, et al., Placenta-derived decidual stromal cells for graft-versus-host disease, hemorrhaging, and toxicity after allogeneic hematopoietic stem cell transplantation. Biol Blood Marrow Transplant 2015; 21: S149

Fong CY, Richards M, Manasi N, et al., Comparative growth behaviour and characterization of stem cells from human Wharton's jelly. Reprod Biomed Online 2007; 15:708 e18

Fariha M-MN, Chua K-H, Tan G-C, et al., Human chorion-derived stem cells: changes in stem cell properties during serial passage. Cytotherapy 2011; 13:582 e93

Park S, Kim E, Koh SE, et al., Dopaminergic differentiation of neural progenitors derived from placental mesenchymal stem cells in the brains of Parkinson's disease model rats and alleviation of asymmetric rotational behavior. Brain Res 2012; 1466:158 e66

Fisher-Shoval Y, Barhum Y, Sadan O, et al., Transplantation of placenta-derived mesenchymal stem cells in the EAE mouse model of MS. J Mol Neurosci 2012; 48:176 e84

Chen Z, Tortella FC, Dave JR, et al., Human amnion-derived multipotent progenitor cell treatment alleviates traumatic brain injury-induced axonal degeneration. J Neurotrauma 2009; 26:1987 e97

Congress US. Congressional record, V. 153, PT. 12, June 18, 2007 to June 26, 2007. US Congress. 2007

Antoniadou E and David AL. Placental stem cells. Best Practice & Research Clinical Obstetrics and Gynaecology 2016; 31: 13 e29

Richardson SM, Kalamegam G, Pushparaj PN, et al., Mesenchymal stem cells in regenerative medicine: Focus on articular cartilage and intervertebral disc regeneration. Methods 2016; 99: 69-80

Joerger-Messerli MS, Marx C, Oppliger B, et al., Mesenchymal stem cells from Wharton's jelly and amniotic fluid. Best Practice & Research Clinical Obstetrics and Gynaecology 2016; 31: 30 e44

Wang L, Ji H, Zhou J, et al., Therapeutic potential of umbilical cord mesenchymal stromal cells transplantation for cerebral palsy: a case report. Case Rep Transplant 2013

Joerger-Messerli M, Bruhlmann E, Bessire A, et al., Preeclampsia enhances neuroglial marker expression in umbilical cord Wharton's jelly-derived mesenchymal stem cells. J Matern Fetal Neona 2015; 2015; 28:464 e9

CHAPTER 14: Stem Cells: History & Foundation

Patrick Cleary & Richard Chang

> **CHAPTER PREVIEW**
>
> World War II served as a catalyst for tissue transplantation research. Researchers made advances in skin grafting to treat burns and in ABO blood typing to perform safe and effective blood transfusions. Meanwhile, Hiroshima and Nagasaki taught the world that high-dose radiation can cause marrow failure and death. In this chapter, we explain how historical events led to the underpinnings of regenerative medicine.

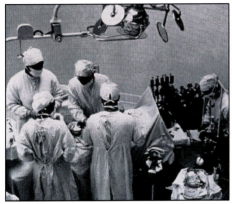

Controversy surrounds stem cell treatment in regenerative medicine. But stem cell treatment is not a new concept. In fact, stem cell transplants are done everyday to treat leukemia, lymphoma, multiple myeloma, and aplastic anemia. In 1990, E. Donnall Thomas and Joseph Murray, won Nobel Prizes for their transformative work on stem cells, HLA-typing, and transplantation (www.nobelprize.org). In musculoskeletal medicine, we are focusing on mesenchymal stem cells, the precursors to bone, cartilage, and muscle cells. In the Nobel Prize winning work, the investigators concentrated on hematopoietic stem cells. We will discuss their work here since they laid the foundation for the work that stem cell researchers are undertaking today (de la Morena et al., 2011).

Stem cells are cells that can change their form and function. Depending on the situation, they can become specialized cells, such as nerve, muscle, or blood cells.

Stem cells can be categorized into four main groups; totipotent, pluripotent, multipotent, and unipotent. Totipotent stem cells form all types of cells and have the potential to give rise to an entire organism, the placenta, as well as extra-embryonic cells. Pluripotent stem cells are embryologic in origin and capable of forming all embryonic germ layers. Multipotent stem cells arise from fetal or adult tissue and are less able to differentiate. Hematopoietic and mesenchymal stem cells fall into the "multipotent" category. Unipotent stem cells arise from adult tissue and can only differentiate into a single type of cell (Girlovanu et al., 2015).

One source of human stem cells is the human embryo. Approximately three to five days after fertilization, the human embryo is a ball of stem cells known as a blastocyst. These cells, known as pluripotent stem cells, can become any kind of cell needed in the body. They can also form more stem cells. These cells are known as embryonic stem cells. These cells can be obtained from fetuses that have been aborted. Because abortion is extremely controversial, the United States does not allow these cells to be used clinically.

Adults also have stem cells. The bone marrow contains hematopoietic stem cells. These stem cells can transform into three different lines of blood cells: red blood cells, white blood cells and platelets.

Once the red blood cells, white blood cells, and platelets mature, they leave the bone marrow to enter the blood. A small number of hematopoietic stem cells also enter the blood. They are known as peripheral blood stem cells. The number of hematopoietic stem cells circulating in the blood can be increased with certain medications such as granulocyte colony stimulating factor (G-CSF) (Panopoulos et al., 2008).

In certain types of blood cancer, such as leukemia, chemotherapy may be used to kill rapidly growing cancer cells. The problem is that the patient's healing stem cells are also killed in the process. Bone marrow transplants, an FDA-approved form of treatment for certain blood and lymph cancers, involves capturing hematopoietic stem cells from a patient before chemotherapy and then returning those stem cells to the patient afterwards. Those stem cells can reconstitute the red blood cells, white blood cells and platelets that the patient needs to survive (Sagar et al., 2007; Blogowski et al., 2016; Moore et al., 2017).

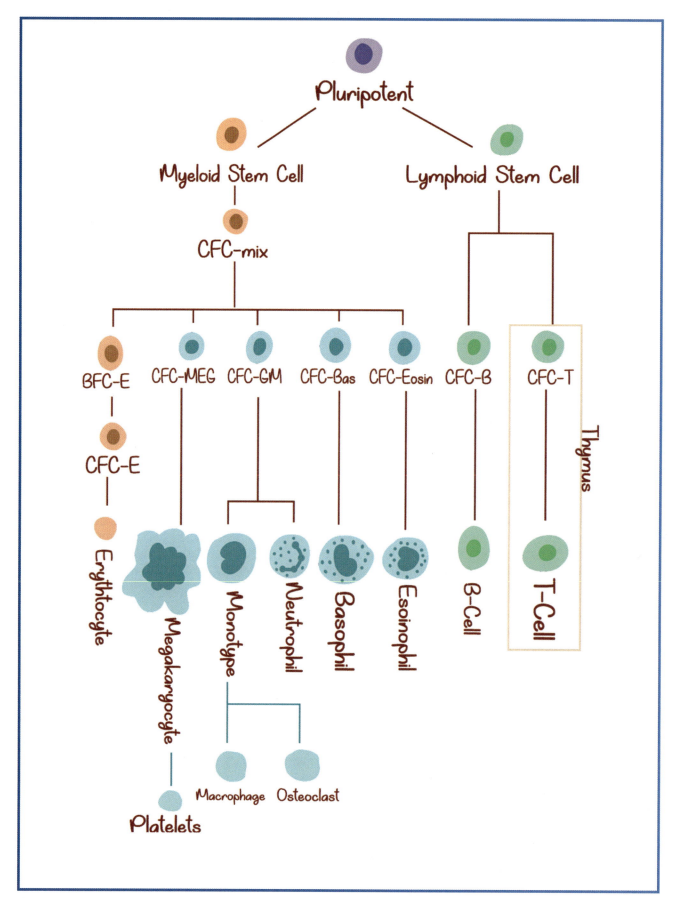

Figure 1: The hematopoietic family tree

Hematopoietic Stem Cell Transplants

In the history of medicine, stem cells transplants are a relatively new phenomenon. The research on stem cell transplants began just 80 years ago. In 1939, a patient received intravenous bone marrow from his brother as a treatment for his aplastic anemia (Forkner, 1938). There were several historical events that contributed to bone marrow transplantation becoming an accepted treatment option for certain forms of leukemia and lymphoma.

World War II served as a catalyst for tissue transplantation research. Researchers made advances in skin grafting to treat burns and ABO blood typing to perform safe and effective blood transfusions. Meanwhile, Hiroshima and Nagasaki taught the world that high-dose radiation can cause marrow failure and death. In 1949, researchers found that shielding certain areas of the body could allow an organism to survive high doses of radiation. Specifically, researchers found that shielding the spleen, part of the liver, the head or the hind leg could be life-saving when it came to full-body irradiation. Two years later, they found that injecting spleen or marrow cells could also protect against radiation (Thomas, 1999). These investigators deduced that there was something in these areas of the body that allowed the mice to regenerate or repair the damage caused by the radiation.

Later work showed mice who had received bone marrow infusions could repopulate their bone marrow and produce new blood cells. The successful animal studies spurred researchers to try human trials. The first bone marrow infusion was performed in France by George Mathe for leukemia. The patients appeared to go into remission from leukemia. However, they all died—either from infection or from what we now understand to be graft-vs.-host disease. This is where the transplanted donor cells attack the host or recipient cells. Around the same time in the United States-- again before graft vs. host disease was understood.

E. Donnall Thomas performed a bone marrow transplant for patients with leukemia. He emphasized that the transplanted marrow was free of pathogens, with the implication that that should minimize the patients' risks of dying from infection (Thomas et al., 1975). The transplant was considered a success because the patients were in remission from cancer. However, all of the patients still died.

What happened in these early experiments is that transplanted marrow cells caused a harmful, even fatal, immune response. Because the donor and recipient marrow were not compatible, two things could happen. The host could attack the donor cells. This would result in a "rejection" of the transplant. Or the donor cells (the graft cells) could attack the host. This is referred to as graft-vs.-host disease (Armitage et al., 1994).

In 1956, researchers found that leukemia in mice could be treated by radiation followed by infusion of normal bone marrow; when this was tried in humans, however, only those patients who received marrow from an identical twin survived (Bortin, 1970). This provided clues about HLA-matching. Research performed in dogs demonstrated that compatible human leukocyte antigen (HLA) was the key to performing safe bone marrow transplants (Thomas, 1999).

In the late 1960's, doctors in Seattle recruited patients suffering from either aplastic anemia or end-stage leukemia. In aplastic anemia, the bone marrow has failed completely and is no longer producing red blood cells, white blood cells or platelets. In end-stage leukemia, the cancer cells in the bone marrow have overtaken the normal cells. Both conditions are deadly. The patients' siblings donated their bone marrow for transplantation into these patients. The HLA typing from the siblings was similar. They were HLA-matched or HLA-compatible. Approximately 15% of those patients lived for more than a year, which was considered a success at that time. Of the patients who survived, about 50% survived for over 20 years (Thomas, 1999).

When a sibling, or any other individual, gives a person their bone marrow, it is referred to as an allogeneic transplant. The donor bone marrow is different from the recipient bone marrow. When a person donates their own bone marrow to themselves, this is referred to as an autologous transplant. If there is something inherent—something about the diseased bone marrow itself-- that predisposes it to developing cancer or aplastic anemia, we can infer that someone else's bone marrow may not have that intrinsic problem. Someone else's bone marrow (except for maybe an identical twin) may be more resistant to cancer. It was this theory that drove the increase in allogeneic transplants (Armitage et al., 1994).

The problem with allogeneic transplants is that the donor cells may not recognize the recipient cells. Therefore, they can attack. In order to receive a transplant, and to decrease the likelihood of this attack, called graft-vs.-host disease, the person undergoing the transplant must take medications that suppress the immune system. These medications will affect both the donor and the recipient immune systems. Therefore, they increase the risk that the person will die of an infection. Infection is the most common cause of death after an allogeneic transplant (Singh et al., 2016).

Hematopoietic stem cells for transplant may be harvested from the bone marrow, the peripheral blood, or from the umbilical cord blood at the time of birth. For clarification, a "bone marrow transplant" is the same as a "(hematopoietic) stem cell transplant;" the only difference is the source of the cells.

In 1988, a worldwide bone marrow donor registry was created (Henig, 2014). Over 80,000 transplants have been performed. With advances in research and technology, both allogeneic and autologous stem cell transplants have become safer and more prevalent in the treatment of leukemia, lymphoma, multiple myeloma, and aplastic anemia.

What About Other Cancers?

Although stem cell transplant has been used to treat a variety of blood cell cancers, it is not currently indicated for the treatment of most solid tumors (Karadurmus et al., 2016).

Current research suggests that most solid tumors, and some refractory forms of leukemia and lymphoma, do not respond to treatment (Dawood et al., 2014). One theory for why they are unresponsive to treatment is the existence of cancer stem cells. These cells are thought to be similar to adult stem cells, in that they can self-renew, or divide into any kind of tissue. However, unlike adult stem cells, cancer stem cells cannot slow down their growth. Therefore, unlike normal stem cells, cancer stem cells can cause cancer when transplanted. A small number of cancer stem cells may be responsible for the development of breast cancer and lung cancer (Dawood et al., 2014).

Our current treatment options, which include surgery, chemotherapy and radiation, generally target cancer cells. They do not capture all the cancer stem cells. Therefore, for tumors where a cancer stem cell exists and is left in place, the cancer stem cell can regenerate a tumor back to its original size. These cancer stem cells can then enter the bloodstream and spread to other sites through a process called metastasis. Cancer stem cells also may lack the chemical markers that most chemotherapy drugs target. This further complicates treatment (Dawood et al, 2014). Studies continue about how we can use stem cells to target cancer.

References:

The Nobel Prize Organization. The Nobel Prize in physiology or medicine 1990: Press Release; 1990 [cited April 4, 2019] Accessed at: https://www.nobelprize.org/prizes/medicine/1990/press-release/

de la Morena MT and Gatti RA. A history of bone marrow transplantation. Hematology/ Oncology Clinics of North America 2011; 25(1): 1-15

Girlovanu M, Susman S, Soritau O, et al., Stem cells: Biological update and cell therapy progress. Clijul Medical 2015; 88(3): 265

Panopoulos AD and Watowich SS. Granulocyte colony-stimulating factor: Molecular mechanisms of action during steady state and "emergency" hematopoiesis. Cytokine 2008; 42(3): 277-88

Sagar J, Chaib B, Sales K, et al., Role of stem cells in cancer therapy and cancer stem cells: a review. Cancer Cell International. 2007; 7(1): 9

Błogowski W, Bodnarczuk T, and Staandrzyńska T. Concise Review: Pancreatic Cancer and Bone Marrow-Derived Stem Cells. Stem Cells Translational Medicine 2016; 5: 938–945

Moore TM, Ikeda AK. Bone Marrow Transplantation: Background, Basic Information, Indications for Transplantation. http://emedicine.medscape.com/article/1014514-overview#a1. Published January 20, 2017. Accessed April 23, 2017

Forkner CE. Leukemia and allied disorders. New York: Macmillan, 1938

Thomas ED. A history of haemopoietic cell transplantation. British Journal of Haematology. 1999;105:330–339

Thomas ED, Storb R, Clift RA, et al., Bone Marrow Transplantation. N Engl J Med 1975; 292: 832-843

Armitage J. Bone marrow transplantation. New Eng J Med 1994; 330: 827-38

Bortin MM. A compendium of reported human bone marrow transplants. Transplantation 1970; 9(6): 571-871970

Singh A and McGuirk JP. Allogeneic stem cell transplantation: A historical and scientific overview. Cancer Research 2016; 76(22): 6445-51

Henig I, Zuckerman T. Hematopoietic Stem Cell Transplantation - 50 Years of Evolution and Future Perspectives. Rambam Maimonides Med J 2014; 5(4)

Karadurmus N, Sahin U, Basgoz BB, et al., Review of allogeneic hematopoietic stem cell transplantation with reduced intensity conditioning in solid tumors excluding breast cancer. World J Transplant 2016; 6(4): 675-81

Dawood S, Austin L, Cristofanilli M. Cancer Stem Cells: Implications for Cancer Therapy. Oncology (Williston Park) 2014; 28(12): 1101-7, 1110

CHAPTER 15: Stem Cells and Cancer

Sohan Nagrani

> **CHAPTER PREVIEW**
>
> Not all cancer cells are created equal. Cancers appear to follow a hierarchical model with the cancer cell at the top of the hierarchy and the cells it created-- of varying levels of maturity, appearance, and differentiation-- surrounding it. Therefore, the cancer stem cell model has similarities to normal stem cells responsible for the production and differentiation of normal healthy tissues.

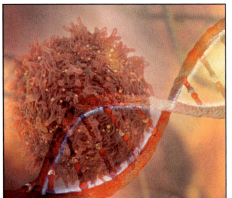

Stem cells are cells that can regenerate themselves. It's not just that they can proliferate-- they can reproduce other stem cells to ensure that the organism can always reconstitute itself. In that sense, stem cells are immortal until they choose to mature and differentiate themselves into specific cell types. There is some evidence that stem cells are at risk to become cancerous because they live for so long. They have more time to accumulate mutations. They need to live for as long as the entire organism (Reya et al., 2001). The cancer stem cell model is a relatively modern theory in medicine. There are two main reasons why we are including a chapter on cancer stem cells in this text.

First, to help themselves grow and multiply, cancer stem cells appear to hijack the normal wound healing pathways. Cancer stem cells activate the clotting cascade described in our hemostasis chapter, produce inflammatory chemical messengers, called cytokines, as described in our inflammatory phase chapter, increase (cancer) cell proliferation as explained in our proliferative phase chapter, and then stimulate the differentiation of tumor cells as discussed in our maturation phase chapter (Tanno et al., 2011; Arwert et al., 2012). To paraphrase the pathologist Harold Dvorak, tumors are wounds that do not heal (Dvorak, 1986).

Second, stem cells are of almost universal interest in medicine—not just musculoskeletal medicine. Hematologists and oncologists are actively searching for methods to destroy aberrant stem cells (cancer stem cells) and to enhance the function of normal stem cells that can heal and regenerate tissues. That means practitioners in musculoskeletal medicine may want to stay on top of developments in other areas of medicine. We can't silo ourselves if we want to advance our own understanding of regenerative medicine.

Early cancer research suggested that there was some variability in how effectively cancer cells could grow and spread. Not all cancer cells were equal. We are not sure how this passed the Institutional Review Board... but in one study, researchers took 20 young and healthy prisoners from the Ohio State Penitentiary and injected each of them subcutaneously with either normal cells or with cancer cells from 9 different cancer cell lines. The two prisoners injected with normal cells had no significant response. The 18 prisoners who had been injected with 2-3 million cancer cells had a significant localized immune response. The responses were successful. None of those prisoners developed cancer (Itoh et al., 1963). This sparked two different ideas. First, there was something about the cancer cells that identified them as cancerous. This is why the prisoners' immune systems were able to recognize the cells and wall them off. Second, not all cancer cells are equally powerful. The cancer cell clones injected into these prisoners might be front-line "soldiers." However, there might be a more powerful cancer driver, a cancer stem cell, that was missing from these cell lines.

The first cancer stem cells were found in leukemia. Every cell has a variety of identifiers on its cell surface. Think facial recognition. In leukemia, certain cells have identifiers called CD34 and CD38. When researchers isolated leukemic cells with these markers and injected them into mice, the mice developed leukemia. The more cells that were transplanted, the more likely the mice were to develop leukemia. This suggested that

CD34 and CD38 might be identifiers for cancer stem cells (Arnold et al., 2015). Researchers also noted that those cells cycled through cell division (or cell reproduction) more slowly than normal cells (Kreso et al., 2014).

In the early 2000s, the first cancer stem cells were isolated from breast cancer (Kreso et al., 2014; Arnold et al., 2015). These cells carried the cell surface identifiers, CD44 and CD24 (Grandics et al., 2006; Gonda et al., 2009). These cells appeared to be different from other cells in the cancer (Kreso et al., 2014), suggesting the cancer stem cell model was not unique to leukemia. Cancer stem cells could play a role in solid tumors (tumors formed from a tissue other than blood or lymphatic fluid).

After this discovery, cancer stem cells were found in brain, head and neck, pancreatic, lung, prostate, and colon cancers. These cancers appear to follow a hierarchical model with the cancer cell at the top of the hierarchy and cells it created—of varying levels of maturity, appearance, and differentiation—surrounding it. Therefore, the cancer stem cell model has similarities to normal stem cells responsible for the production and differentiation of normal healthy tissues (Kreso et al., 2014).

Our immune system comprises a variety of immune cells. Among the white blood cells, there are cells called lymphocytes. Within that group, there are B- cells and T- cells that travel around in the blood and protect us from threats. There are some cell surface markers found both on our normal immune T-cells and on cancer cells (Grandics et al., 2006).

For example, the identifier, or antigen, CD45, is normally found on T-cells (Altin et al., 1997). But it is also found in leukemia, lymphoma, seminoma, rhabdomyosarcoma, and several neuroendocrine carcinomas.

The CD57 antigen is found on our body's normal T cells and natural killer cells (Kared et al., 2016). (Natural killer cells are our immune cells that specifically attack cancers and viruses). However, they are also found on cancer cell surfaces in small cell lung cancer, astrocytoma, neuroblastoma, retinoblastoma, and carcinoid tumors (Kreso et al., 2014).

The CTLA-4 antigen, or identifier, is also found on both normal T-cells on cells found in gastric epithelial cell carcinomas (Grandics et al., 2006; Rowshanravan et al., 2018). These findings suggest cancer stem cells may develop from our own immune system's T cells.

Some scientists argue that infections stimulate the development of the cancer stem cell (Grandics et al., 2006). An infection initiates an immune response. White blood cells are activated. These cells produce chemical messengers and growth factors that fight the infection and promote tissue healing. The identifiers, called surface antigens, interact with the body's normal immune cells. Some of these immune cells, known as B- and T- cells, clear the infection.

Some bacteria, viruses, and cancers can elude these immune cells. A bacteria, virus or cancer cell may have surface antigens that look like the body's normal cell surface antigens. If the body mistakenly thinks those pathogens are normal, the pathogen can grow. It can invade blood vessels and travel throughout the body.

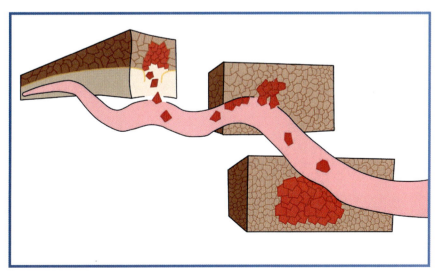

Figure 2: Cancer metastasizing through the blood

To hedge against this danger, our bodies develop "autoimmune" self-attacking T cells. These autoimmune cells may be a necessary evil. These self-destructive cells will attack camouflaged pathogens. It is possible that rogue autoimmune T cells may give rise to cancer stem cells (Grandics et al., 2006).

Cancers often develop in areas of prior injury or inflammation. The presence of inflammatory chemical messengers in these areas of chronic inflammation may be related to the development of cancer. In multiple myeloma and gastric cancer, an inflammatory chemical messenger called tumor necrosis factor (TNF-alpha), is present in high quantities. TNF-alpha creates inflammation by producing reactive oxygen species (a.k.a. free radicals). Normally, TNF-alpha is actively involved in the maturation phase of wound healing. Therefore, it seems to have a role both in wound healing and in cancer development (Gonda et al., 2005).

There are other chemical messengers that are involved both in wound healing and in cancer development. We discussed interleukin-1 in the chapter on the proliferative phase of wound healing. There are two genes for IL-1: IL-1-alpha and IL-1-beta. Both TNF-alpha and interleukin 1-beta cause machinery within individual cells to become active. This machinery has different names. They are generally referred to as transcription factors. Specifically, they are called hypoxia-inducible factors. These hypoxia-inducible factors are particularly active in stem cells. They cause the stem cells to build proteins that facilitate the cell's own reproduction, thereby promoting the proliferation of cells involved in healing (Krizhanovsky et al., 2008).

Interleukin-6 (IL-6) is another inflammatory chemical messenger that is active in the proliferative phase. It plays a role in cancers such as multiple myeloma, non-Hodgkin's lymphoma, and hepatocellular carcinoma. IL-6 stimulates immune B-cells and T-cells. The purpose of this in wound healing is probably to prevent the wound from getting infected. But in chronic inflammation or cancer, IL-6 may have a different role. (Krizhanovsky et al., 2008).

Mesenchymal stem cells are a type of stem cell within the body. These are cells that can transform into bone, cartilage and muscle. Stem cells within a wound release cytokines, or chemical messengers, to attract mesenchymal stem cells (Korbling et al., 2003). Like cancer stem cells, mesenchymal stem cells promote proliferation and cell maturation in tumors.

Both mesenchymal stem cells and cancer stem cells produce factors that protect them from the normal programmed self-destruction known as apoptosis (Dittmer et al., 2014). These factors also stimulate the formation of new blood vessels, which can either bring oxygen and nutrients to a healing wound or to a growing cancer (Dittmer et al., 2014). This allows for both wound healing and cancer progression (Eming et al., 2014; Sandanha et al., 2015).

In summary, the local environment established by cancer stem cells is similar to that of normal stem cells (Arnold et al., 2015). Stem cells play a critical role in both tissue repair and cancer development. Normal stem cells facilitate wound healing. Cancer stem cells may produce a microenvironment supporting its own healing. However, cancer stem cells promote dysfunctional processes that cause the abnormal growth and progression of tumors (Reya at al., 2001).

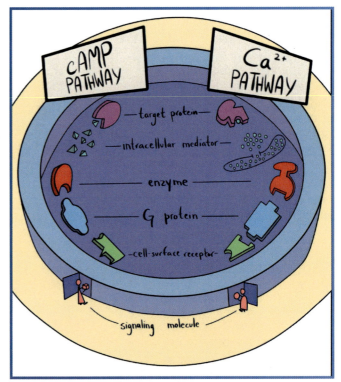

Figure 3: The cancer stem cell uses growth factors to trigger cellular processes that advance its own growth

References:

Reya T, Morrison SJ, Clarke MF, et al., Stem cells, cancer and cancer stem cells. Nature 2001; 414(1): 105-111

Dvorak HF. Tumors: wounds that do not heal. Similarities between tumor stroma generation and wound healing. N Engl J Med. 1986 Dec 25; 315(26): 1650-9

Tanno T, Matsui W. Development and maintenance of cancer stem cells under chronic inflammation. J Nippon Med Sch. 2011; 78(3):138-45

Arwert EN, Hoste E, Watt FM. Epithelial stem cells, wound healing and cancer. Nat Rev Cancer. 2012 Feb 24; 12(3):170-80

Itoh T and Southam CM. Isoantibodies to human cancer cells in healthy recipients of cancer homotransplants. J Immunol 1963; 91(4): 469-83

Arnold KM, Opdenaker LM, Flynn D, Sims-Mourtada J. Wound healing and cancer stem cells: inflammation as a driver of treatment resistance in breast cancer. Cancer Growth Metastasis. 2015 Jan 29; 8:1-13

Kreso A; Dick JE. Evolution of the cancer stem cell model. Cell Stem Cell 2014; 14(3): 275-91

Grandics P. The cancer stem cell: evidence for its origin as an injured autoreactive T cell. Mol Cancer. 2006 Feb 14; 5:6

Gonda TA, Tu S, Wang TC. Chronic inflammation, the tumor microenvironment and carcinogenesis. Cell Cycle. 2009 Jul 1; 8(13):2005-13

Altin JG and Sloan EK. The role of CD45 and CD45-associated molecules in T cell activation. Immunol Cell Biol 1997; 75(5): 430-45

Kared, Martelli S, Ng TP, et al., CD57 in human natural killer cells and T-lymphocytes. Cancer Immunol Immunother 2016; 65(4): 441-52

Rowshanravan B, Halliday N, Sansom DM. CTLA-4: A moving target in immunotherapy. Blood 2018; 131(1): 58-67

Kørbling M, Estrov Z. Adult stem cells for tissue repair – a new therapeutic concept? N Engl J Med. 2003; 349(6):570-82

Dittmer J, Leyh B. Paracrine effects of stem cells in wound healing and cancer progression (review). In J Oncol. 2014; 44(6):1789-98

Eming SA, Martin P, Tomic-Canic M. Wound repair and regeneration: mechanisms, signaling, and translation. Sci Transl Med. 2014; 6(265):265sr6

Saldanha SN, Royston KJ, Udayakumar N, Tollefsbol TO. Epigenetic regulation of epidermal stem cell biomarkers and their role in wound healing. Int J Mol Sci. 2015; 17(1)

Krizhanovsky V, Xue W, Zender L, et al., Implications of cellular senescence in tissue damage response, tumor suppression, and stem cell biology. Cold Spring Harb Symp Quant Biol. 2008; 73:513-22

CHAPTER 16: Hyperbaric Oxygen

Alan Katz & Devi Nampiaparampil

> **CHAPTER PREVIEW**
>
> How does hyperbaric oxygen therapy work? It increases the amount of oxygen carried in the blood stream, stimulates the growth of new blood vessels, reduces inflammation and swelling, strengthens the immune system, and stimulates the release of stem cells. At increased atmospheric pressures, levels of interleukin 1 (IL-1), interleukin 6 (IL-6), and tumor necrosis factor alpha (TNF-alpha) decrease. There is evidence that hyperbaric oxygen may have as potent an anti-inflammatory effect as dexamethasone. Hyperbaric therapy can also promote collagen deposition and osteoblast proliferation.

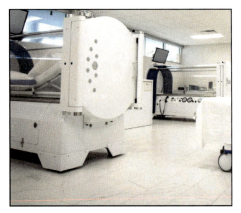

Hyperbaric oxygen therapy exposes patients to 100% oxygen at pressures greater than atmospheric pressure to decrease inflammation and enhance the proliferative phase of wound healing (Sutherland et al., 2016). What does this mean? If you stood outside at sea level, you would be exposed to 1 atmosphere of pressure. If you were 33 feet underwater, you would be exposed to 2 atmospheres of pressure. Hyperbaric therapy typically exposes patients to 1-2 atmospheres of pressure. This type of oxygen exposure increases the oxygen pressure in the lungs, and in turn, increases the amount of oxygen in the blood (Jain et al., 1999). This allows the body to carry more oxygen to injured ischemic tissues, which are not receiving enough oxygen. As the oxygenation in the tissues increases, the development of new blood vessels in the tissues is stimulated. Improved oxygenation also improves the function of the white blood cells in the area (Thom et al., 2011).

The history of hyperbaric therapy ties into other notable scientific discoveries. Hyperbaric therapy was first documented in 1662 by the British clergyman, Nathaniel Henshaw, to treat respiratory and digestive ailments. He used a system of bellows to control the atmospheric pressure in a chamber that he called "the domicilium." (Henshaw, 1664).

In 1774, the British-American, Joseph Priestley, characterized air as a mixture of substances, including a highly reactive gas that the French chemist, Antoine Lavoisier, later named "oxygen." (A Swedish apothecary,

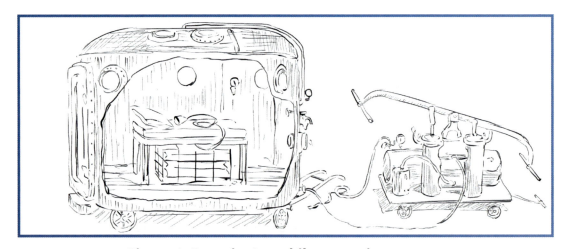

Figure 1: Fontaine's mobile operating room

Carl Wilhelm Scheele, had identified the same gas the year prior, but Priestley published his discovery first). Priestley noted that oxygen might have some wound healing properties. Incidentally, Priestley also invented carbonated water and created the first rubber eraser while drafting his papers (American Chemical Society, 2019).

In 1877, the French surgeon, Rene Fontaine (who created the Fontaine classification system for peripheral arterial disease and claudication), started using hyperbaric oxygen clinically. He developed the first mobile operating room that used hyperbaric oxygen (Fontaine et al., 1954).

The neurologist, James Leonard Corning, built the first hyperbaric chamber in the United States, in New York, to treat central nervous system disorders (Williams et al., 1885). Corning had achieved fame for performing the first epidural injection with a local anesthetic—in this case, cocaine—and successfully numbing the patient to painful stimuli (Gorelick et al., 1987).

In the 1880s and 1890s, the U.S. undertook several great engineering projects including the construction of the Brooklyn Bridge, connecting Manhattan to Brooklyn, and the Hudson Tunnel (a.k.a. Holland Tunnel), connecting Manhattan to New Jersey. Some of the casualties of these engineering feats were the construction workers who developed decompression sickness, later named Caisson Disease. If you take an open box, flip it over and push it quickly through river water into the ground below where you partially bury and anchor it, there's a good chance there will be some air in the now sealed container. This is how a caisson operates. A caisson is a large watertight container used for construction on bridges, piers, and ships. The workers stay inside while they work. If the workers leave the caisson and swim upward out of the water, the rapid atmospheric pressure change can cause gases dissolved in their blood to come out of solution. This can cause damage to the ears, sinuses, and lungs. It causes severe pain and can be deadly (Knight, 1977).

How does this happen? Remember Henry's Law of solubility from high school Chemistry. Assuming a constant temperature, the volume of gas dissolved in a liquid or tissue is proportional to the partial pressure of the gas in contact with the liquid or tissue. Think of what happens when you open a closed (pressurized) can of soda. The pressure in the can decreases. There's a release of bubbles. That is what happens when the deep sea construction workers rose to the surface of the water. The pressure decreased and the gases that were in solution in their blood came out of solution and formed bubbles.

In 1917, Bernhard and Heinrich Drager discovered how hyperbaric oxygen therapy could be used to treat Caisson Disease. But it was only in 1937 when Albert Behnke and Louis Shaw started adding oxygen to the hyperbaric chambers, that they could be used on a larger scale to treat Caisson Disease (Butler et al., 2004).

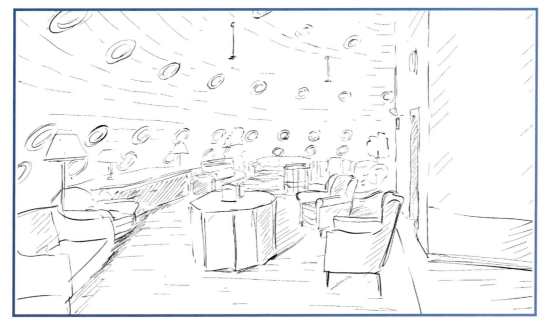

Figure 2: The Cunningham Sanatorium interior view

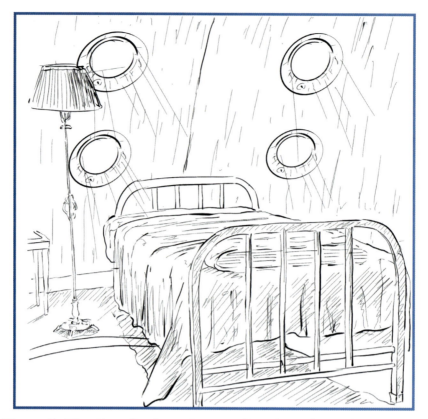

Figure 3: The Cunningham Sanatorium interior private room

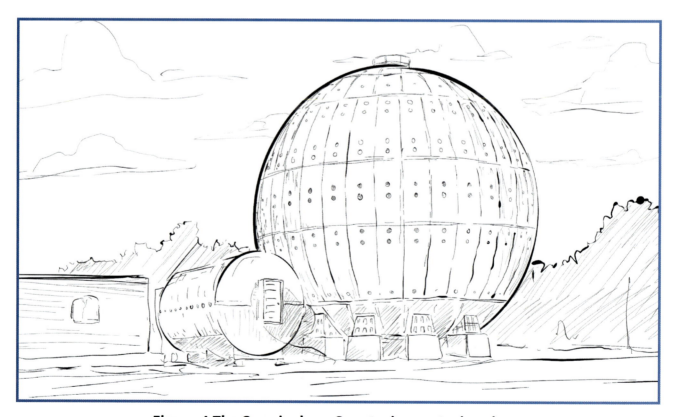

Figure 4: The Cunningham Sanatorium exterior view.

CHAPTER 16 - HYPERBARIC OXYGEN

How does hyperbaric oxygen treat Caisson Disease? Remember Boyle's Law from high school chemistry:

$$P_1V_1 = P_2V_2$$

If all else is constant, when the pressure on a gas increases, its volume will decrease. For example, if we were to place a balloon inside a hyperbaric chamber and increase the pressure from 1 to 2 atmospheres, the balloon's relative volume would decrease by 50%. If a person with Caisson's Disease with gas bubbles in his or her circulation were subjected to increased atmospheric pressure, the size of those bubbles would decrease proportionally.

Around the same time that the Dragers were studying Caisson Disease, Orval Cunningham, a physician at the University of Kansas, noticed that soldiers returning from World War I with "Spanish" Influenza were more likely to die if they lived at high altitudes. Cunningham postulated that this had to do with the lower oxygen saturation at higher elevations. He built a hyperbaric chamber and began using it to treat a variety of illnesses including diabetes and syphilis. He surmised that it was the presence of anaerobic bacteria that led to the complications from these illnesses. Cunningham's practice continued to grow, eventually culminating in the construction of the Cunningham Sanitorium in Cleveland, Ohio. Cunningham built a hyperbaric facility where patients could live and simultaneously receive hyperbaric oxygen therapy.

Unfortunately, he ignored multiple requests from the American Medical Association (AMA) asking him to publish his results. As a result, he received multiple criticisms and sanctions from the AMA, and his sanitorium was ultimately dismantled for steel and spare parts for World War II.

More mainstream applications of hyperbaric oxygen therapy came into play in 1956 when the Dutch surgeon, Ite Boerema, used it to facilitate cardiopulmonary surgery. His article, "Life Without Blood," described how patients could survive inside a hyperbaric chamber. His patients could tolerate a cardiopulmonary arrest if they had been pretreated with hyperbaric oxygen. At 1 atmosphere (sea level), we can only dissolve 2.1 vol% oxygen in plasma. Yet at 3 atmospheres, we can dissolve 6.6 vol% oxygen.

In 1961, Boerema's colleague, Willem Brummelkamp, found that hyperbaric oxygen therapy could treat anaerobic infections (Duff et al., 1970). How does hyperbaric oxygen therapy work for wounds? At increased atmospheric pressures, levels of interleukin 1 (IL-1), interleukin 6 (IL-6), and tumor necrosis factor alpha (TNF-alpha) decrease. There is evidence that hyperbaric oxygen may have as potent an anti-inflammatory effect as dexamethasone (Thom et al., 2009). Hyperbaric therapy can also promote collagen deposition and fibroblast and osteoblast proliferation (Thom et al., 2009). This could be because, during wound healing, there is greater demand for oxygen for cellular metabolism. However, oxygen has a harder time actually traveling to the area where it is most needed—either because of the direct injury to the blood vessels or because of inflammatory fluid in the extracellular space.Injuries and medical disease interfere with the body's ability to transport oxygen. At the same time, the body's demand for oxygen increases during times of wound healing and infection. Most of the oxygen in the blood is carried by hemoglobin. However, there is some oxygen carried in the plasma itself. It is theorized that at 2.5 atmospheres and 100% oxygen saturation, the amount of oxygen carried by the plasma increases 17 times—enough to oxygenate the tissues without hemoglobin (Singh et al., 2014).

One of the concerns about increased oxygenation is the formation of reactive oxygen and nitrogen species (a.k.a. free radicals). These are the byproducts of natural cellular metabolism and they can cause damage to tissues. However, they also have bactericidal effects. Moreover, Hypoxia Inducible Factor (HIF), these oxygen species can stimulate the bone marrow to release more stem cells. There is evidence that suggests that a single exposure to 100% oxygen at 2 atmospheres can cause the population of stem cells in the blood to double. After 20 treatments, the population of circulating stem cells may be 8 times higher. If the atmospheric pressure is increased from 2.0 to 2.5, the stem cell count might be between 1.9 and 3.0 times higher (Thom et al., 2006).

In addition, alterations in atmospheric pressure and oxygen saturation may affect up to 8000 genes (Godman et al., 2010). Both atmospheric pressure as well as the inhaled oxygen level, can independently cause these changes (Malek et al., 2013).

In current clinical practice, there are two different types of hyperbaric chambers: monoplace (for a single patient) and multiplace (for multiple patients). Monoplace chambers are clinical devices the size of a stretcher. They are typically pressurized with 100% oxygen and are the most common form of hyperbaric chamber.

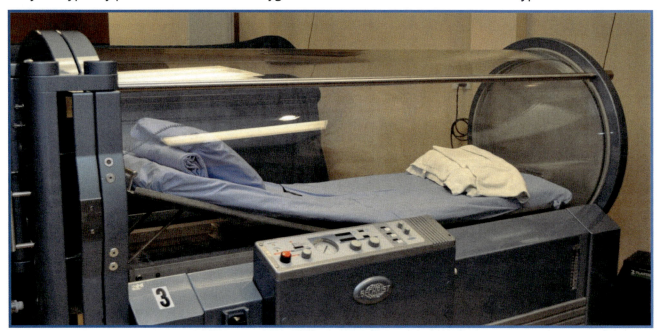

Figure 5: Example of monoplace chamber

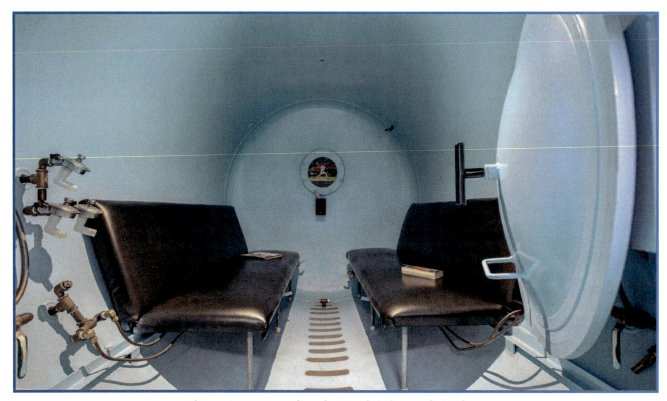

Figure 6: Example of a multiplace chamber

The multiplace chambers are room-sized, require both internal and external staff, and are much more costly. The patients have to wear oxygen hoods or masks. In a monoplace chamber, when the pressure changes, a patient might experience fullness in the ears—similar to what happens on an airplane during take-off and landing. The patient can swallow, yawn or use other techniques to mitigate this.

CHAPTER 16 - HYPERBARIC OXYGEN

Depending on the medical condition being treated, a patient may have anywhere from one to sixty of these 60 to 90 minute sessions. Additionally, the patient will receive scheduled air breaks to induce the effects of cellular mediators such as HIF (hypoxia inducible factor). This is referred to as the hyperoxic-hypoxic paradox. (Hadanny et al., 2020)

The risks of hyperbaric oxygen therapy are minimal. Patients may feel claustrophobic because of the enclosed space. They may experience temporary near-sightedness, where they have a hard time seeing objects in the distance. This is called myopia. They could also experience a sensation of ear fullness or mild ear barotrauma. Patients can experience insulin sensitivity, which can lead to acute hypoglycemic events. In rare cases, patients can experience oxygen toxicity with resultant seizures. An untreated pneumothorax could develop into a tension pneumothorax. Given the elevated oxygen levels, abundant precautions are required to mitigate any potential for fire.

In the U.S., FDA-approved indications for hyperbaric oxygen therapy include non-healing wounds, compromised skin grafts and flaps, necrotizing soft tissue infections, diabetic foot ulcers, refractory osteomyelitis, gas gangrene, acute traumatic ischemia, crush injury, radiation tissue damage, severe anemia and decompression sickness (Mitton et al., 1999). Hyperbaric oxygen therapy is used off-label for both anoxic and traumatic brain injuries, cancer, Crohn's disease, ulcerative colitis, Lyme Disease, multiple sclerosis, stroke, and spinal cord injury (Mitton et al., 1999). It is also used off-label to treat chronic pain from osteoarthritis, fibromyalgia, complex regional pain syndrome and migraine.

In rehabilitation medicine, sports medicine, and pain medicine, multidisciplinary care is often more effective than a single-therapy approach. In animal studies, hyperbaric oxygen therapy has been combined with regenerative medicine treatments to manage several conditions. Hyperbaric oxygen, in combination with platelet rich plasma, has improved bone healing (Neves et al., 2013). Hyperbaric oxygen, in combination with umbilical mesenchymal stem cells, has augmented recovery from traumatic brain injury (Zhou et al., 2016). Adult stem cells, as compared to fetal stem cells, are less resilient. Hyperbaric oxygen therapy may be a useful tool to improve their efficiency.

In some animal studies, acetic acid is injected intraperitoneally into mice. The number of times they wince in pain, called abdominal constrictions, is measured (Emmanouil et al., 2008). In one study, a group of mice were pre-treated with 60 minutes of 100% oxygen at 3.5 atmospheres. The others received sham treatment with air. The number of abdominal constrictions decreased by 80-95% for 90 minutes suggesting that hyperbaric oxygen therapy has analgesic effects (Zelinski et al., 2009).

Hyperbaric oxygen therapy decreases pain and inflammation. This has been studied in mice injected with carrageenan, a chemical that induces arthritis-like pain and swelling. In at least two studies, the amount of swelling in the hind paws of these mice decreased with hyperbaric oxygen (Sumen et al., 2001; Wilson et al., 2006). In one study, the number of mechanical paw withdrawals, a surrogate measure for pain, was decreased by hyperbaric oxygen (Wilson et al., 2006). In another study of knee pain in mice, hyperbaric therapy was as effective as aspirin in relieving the arthritis-like symptoms (Wilson et al., 2007).

There is some evidence from animal studies that hyperbaric oxygen therapy can decrease both mechanical and thermal sensitivity and pain (Sutherland et al., 2016). One randomized controlled trial of patients with fibromyalgia suggested that hyperbaric oxygen could decrease the pain threshold and number of tender points in as little as one session (Yildiz et al., 2004). One randomized controlled trial of patients with complex regional pain syndrome showed that hyperbaric oxygen therapy could provide analgesia—but it might require up to 15 sessions (Kiralp et al., 2004). There have been at least five randomized controlled studies assessing hyperbaric oxygen therapy for migraine (Eftedal et al., 2004; Fife et al., 1992; Hill et al., 1992; Myers et al., 1995; Wilson et al., 1998; Bennett et al., 2008). Generally, the evidence suggests that it is effective at treating a migraine in progress. However, it does not appear to prevent future migraines (Bennett et al., 2008).

There is some evidence from animal studies that hyperbaric oxygen therapy can decrease both mechanical and thermal sensitivity and pain (Sutherland et al., 2016). One randomized controlled trial of patients with fibromyalgia suggested that hyperbaric oxygen could decrease the pain threshold and number of tender points in as little as one session (Yildiz et al., 2004). One randomized controlled trial of patients with complex regional pain syndrome showed that hyperbaric oxygen therapy could provide analgesia—but it might require up to 15 sessions (Kiralp et al., 2004). There have been at least five randomized controlled studies assessing hyperbaric oxygen therapy for migraine (Eftedal et al., 2004; Fife et al., 1992; Hill et al., 1992; Myers et al., 1995; Wilson et al., 1998; Bennett et al., 2008). Generally, the evidence suggests that it is effective at treating a migraine in progress. However, it does not appear to prevent future migraines (Bennett et al., 2008).

CHAPTER 16 - HYPERBARIC OXYGEN

References:

Sutherland AM, Clarke HA, Katz J, Katznelson R, Hyperbaric Oxygen Therapy: A New Treatment for Chronic Pain?, Pain Practice 2016; 16(5): 620-8

Jain KK. Textbook of Hyperbaric Medicine, 3rd Ed. Seattle, WA. Hogrefe and Huber Publishers; 1999

Thom SR. Hyperbaric oxygen: Its mechanisms and efficacy. Plast Reconstr Surg 2011; 127 (Suppl 1): 131S-141S

Henshaw N. Aero-chalinos, or, A register for the air for the better preservation of health and cure of diseases, after a new method. Dublin: Printed for Samuel Dancer, 1664

Gill AL, Bell CAN. Hyperbaric oxygen: its uses, mechanisms of action and outcomes. QJM: An International Journal of Medicine 2004; 97(7): 385-95

American Chemical Society International Historic Chemical Landmarks. Discovery of oxygen by Joseph Priestley. http://www.acs.org/content/acs/en/education/whatischemistry/landmarks/josephpriestleyoxygen.html [Accessed April 29, 2019]

Fontaine R, Kim M, Kieny R, et al., Die chirugische behandlung der peripheren durchblutungsstorungen (Surgical treatment of peripheral circulation disorders). Helvetica Chirurgica Acta (1954)

Williams CT. Lectures on the compressed air bath and its uses in the treatment of disease. The British Medical Journal 1885; 1(1268): 769-72

Gorelick PB and Zych D. James Leonard Corning and the early history of spinal puncture. Neurology 1987; 37(4): 672-4

Knight, Edward Henry. "Caisson" def. Knight's American mechanical dictionary: A description of tools, instruments, machines, processes and engineering: History of inventions; General technological vocabulary; and digest of mechanical appliances in science and the arts. Vol 1. Boston: Houghton, Mifflin and Co., 1977, 420

Butler WP. Caisson disease during the construction of the Eads and Brooklyn Bridges: A review. Undersea Hyperb Med 2004; 31(4): 445-59

Photos courtesy of Cunningham Sanitorium: https://clevelandhistorical.org/index.php/items/show/378

Duff JH, McLean APH, MacLean LD. Treatment of Severe Anaerobic Infections. Arch Surg 1970;101(2):314–318.

Thom SR. Oxidative stress is fundamental to hyperbaric oxygen therapy. J Appl Physiol 2009; 106(3): 988-95

Singh S and Gambert SR. Hyperbaric oxygen therapy: A brief history and review of its benefits and indications for the older adult patient. Annals of Long-Term Care 2014; 22(7-8): 37-42

Thom SR, Bhopale VM, Velazquez OC, et al., Stem cell mobilization by hyperbaric oxygen. Am J Physiol Heart Circ Physiol 2006; 290(4): H1378-86

Godman CA, Chheda KP, Hightower LE, et al., Hyperbaric oxygen induces a cytoprotective and angiogenic response in human microvascular endothelial cells. Cell Stress Chaperones 2010; 15(4): 431-42

Malek M, Duszczyk M, Zyszkowski M, et al., Hyperbaric oxygen and hyperbaric air treatment result in comparable neuronal death reduction and improved behavioral outcome after transient forebrain ischemia in the gerbil. Exp Brain Res 2013; 224(1): 1-14

Mitton C and Hailey D. Health technology assessment and policy decisions on hyperbaric oxygen treatment. Int J Technol Assess Health Care 1999; 15(4): 661-70

Neves PC, Abib SC, Neves RF, et al., Effects of hyperbaric oxygen therapy combined with autologous platelet concentrate applied in rabbit fibula fraction healing. Clinics (Sao Paolo) 2013; 68(9): 1239-46

Zhou HX, Liu ZG, Liu XJ, et al., Umbilical cord-derived mesenchymal stem cell transplantation combined with hyperbaric oxygen treatment for repair of traumatic brain injury. Neural Regen Res 2016; 11(1): 107-13

Emmanouil DE, Dickens AS, Heckert R et al., Nitrous oxide- Antinociception is mediated by opioid receptors and nitric oxide in the periaqueductal gray region of the midbrain. Eur Neuropsychopharmacol 2008; 18: 194-9

Zelinski LM, Ohgami Y, Chung E, et al., A prolonged nitric oxyide- dependent, opioid-mediated antinociceptive, effect of hyperbaric oxygen in mice. J Pain 2009; 10: 167-72

Sumen G, Cimsit M, Eroglu L. Hyperbaric oxygen treatment reduces carrageenan-induced acute inflammation in rats. Eur J Pharmacol 2001; 431: 265-8

Wilson HD, Wilson JR, Fuchs PN. Hyperbaric oxygen treatment decreases inflammation and mechanical hypersensitivity in an animal model of inflammatory pain. Brain Res 2006; 1098: 126-8

Wilson HD, Toepfer VE, Senapati AK, et al., Hyperbaric oxygen treatment is comparable to acetylsalicylic acid in treatment of an animal model of arthritis. J Pain 2007; 8: 924-30

Yildiz S, Kiralp MA, Akin A et al., A new treatment modality for fibromyalgia syndrome: Hyperbaric oxygen therapy. J Int Med Res 2004; 32: 263-7

Kiralp MZ, Yildiz S, Vural D, et al., Effectiveness of hyperbaric oxygen therapy in the treatment of complex regional pain syndrome. J Int Med Res 2004; 32: 258-62

Effedal OS, Lydersen S, Helde G, et al., A randomized double-blind study of the prophylactic effect of hyperbaric oxygen therapy on migraine. Cephalalgia 2004; 24: 639-44

Fife CEM, Meyer JS, Berry JM, et al., Hyperbaric oxygen and acute migraine pain: Preliminary results of a randomised blinded trial. Undersea Biomed Res 1992; 19: 106-7

Hill RK. A blinded, crossover controlled study of the use of hyperbaric oxygen in the treatment of migraine headache. Undersea Biomed Res 1992; 19:106

Myers DE and Myers RA. A preliminary report on hyperbaric oxygen in the relief of migraine headache. Headache 1995; 35: 197-99

Wilson JR, Foresman BH, Gamber RG, et al., Hyperbaric oxygen in the treatment of migraine with aura. Headache 1998; 38: 112-5

Bennett MH, French C, Schnabel A, et al., Normobaric and hyperbaric oxygen therapy for migraine and cluster headache. Cochrane Database Syst Rev 2008; 3: CD005219

A Hadanny, S Efrati, The Hyperbaric-Hypoxic Paradox. Biomolecules. 2020; 10(6): 958.

CHAPTER 17 Basics of Needle Technique

Devi Nampiaparampil, Pradeep Albert & Sairam Atluri

CHAPTER PREVIEW

Proper needle technique is an important part of getting to the right "spot" anatomically. This chapter will review the basics of injection technique.

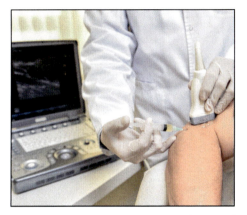

In superficial tissues like the skin and subcutaneous fat, a needle will move in the direction it is aimed. In deeper tissues, the needle can start to bend. This is because of the density of the tissue and the resistance the needle encounters. If a patient is tense and contracts the muscle, you may also feel the needle pulling in a certain direction.

For deeper injections, you can use beveled tip needles to overcome this resistance.

The notch on a beveled tip needle corresponds to the bevel opening. Because of its increased surface area, more tissue will push on the beveled side as you advance the needle. That means that if you push the needle forward—seemingly in a straight line—the needle will move away from the direction of the bevel. It will start to move in a direction opposite to the notch. If your entry point is close to the desired target, you can use this property of beveled needles to steer them into place. The notch on

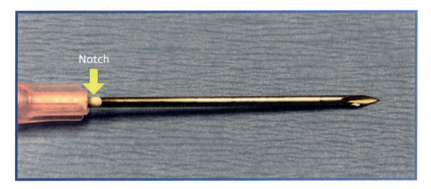

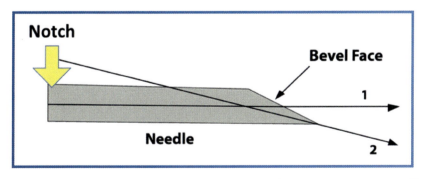

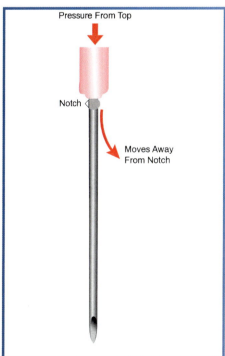

Bevel Up 18 Gauge Needle

A COMPLETE GUIDE TO REGENERATIVE MEDICINE ©

a beveled tip needle corresponds to the bevel opening. Because of its increased surface area, more tissue will push on the beveled side as you advance the needle. That means that if you push the needle forward—seemingly in a straight line—the needle will move away from the direction of the bevel. It will start to move in a direction opposite to the notch. If your entry point is close to the desired target, you can use this property of beveled needles to steer them into place.

Some needles are stylletted. That means that the needle has two parts. The outer portion is a hollow tube or cannula that can deliver medication to a site. The inner portion is a plug or stylet that prevents tissue from entering the cannula as the needle moves through deeper tissues. Having the stylet in place can also make it easier to maneuver the needle.

There are multiple ways to inject joints. In this text, we provide some possible injection techniques. We recommend reading this textbook, attending some courses, and watching some live demonstrations. Everyone has to start somewhere.

We strongly recommend image guidance for all injections. It is also important to look at the physical anatomy and the patient first as opposed to looking at the screen at all times, especially for the novice injector. For those of you that are already using image guidance for injections, the technique is very similar. The injectate is different. Instead of using local anesthetic and steroid products, you are injecting PRP or another substance.

For large joints, we typically inject at least 10 milliliters of platelet-rich plasma, stem cell products or amniotic fluid. For smaller joints approximately 2-3 milliliters may be enough.

Basic techniques:

Direct (in-plane) Injection- we visualize the needle along the entire screen as we inject.

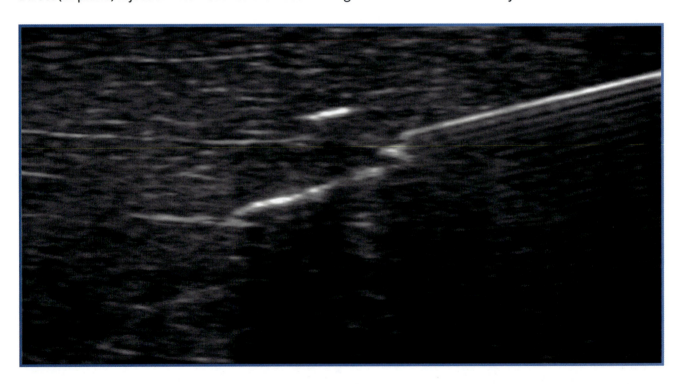

This is an example of an in-plane injection technique under ultrasound guidance where the length of the needle is visualized

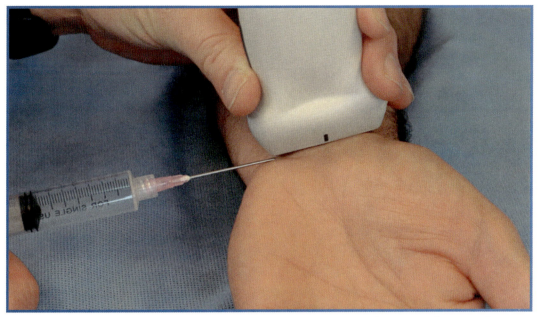

Needle position of an in-plane injection into the carpal tunnel

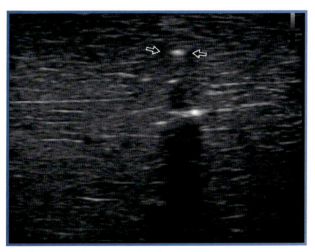

Out of plane technique advancement

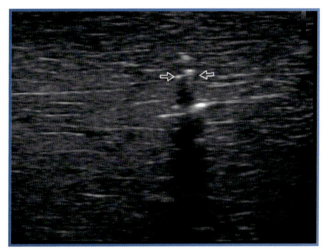

Out of plane "step down" technique advancing

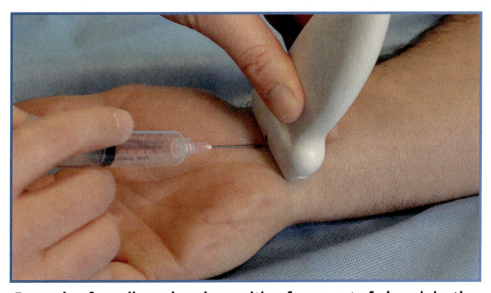

Example of needle and probe position for an out of plane injection

CHAPTER 18 The Shoulder

Colin Rigney, Pradeep Albert & Devi Nampiaparampil

> **CHAPTER PREVIEW**
>
> In this chapter we will cover sonoanatomy of the shoulder as well as patient and probe positions for proper evaluation. Additionally, the chapter will include common pictorial examples and explanations of pathology found with ultrasound as well as basic ultrasound-guided injection techniques.

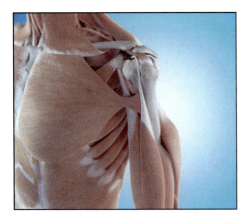

The common pain generators in the shoulder are the rotator cuff, the biceps tendon, the labrum, the acromioclavicular (AC) joint and the glenohumeral joint.

The type of procedure performed depends on the patient's clinical signs and symptoms.

For intra-articular injections:
Pain with all movements of the shoulder
Limited range of motion
Labral tear or glenohumeral arthritis on x-ray, CT scan, MRI, or ultrasound

For supraspinatus injection:
Pain with overhead activities
Pain with forward flexion and/ or abduction above 90 degrees
Subscapularis partial tear or tendinosis on MRI or ultrasound

For subscapularis injection:
Pain at the anterior aspect of the shoulder
Pain with internal rotation of the shoulder ex. putting arm in jacket or closing bra
Subscapularis partial tear or tendinosis on MRI or ultrasound

For biceps tendon injection:
Pain at the anterior aspect of the shoulder
Pain with lifting objects
Pain exacerbated with resisted flexion and/ or supination of the elbow
Bicipital partial tear or tendinosis on MRI or ultrasound

Contraindications to Injection:
Systemic infection
Infection or rash over the puncture site
Coagulopathy (International Normalized Ratio [INR] > 1.3 or platelets < 50,000/ mm3)
Inability to reach target site because of prior surgery or scar tissue

Equipment and Supplies:
Alcohol swabs
Tourniquet
18G or 20G needle for blood draw
Tubing
PRP Kit
Gauze

Betadine or Chlorhexidine
Sterile drapes
Sterile gloves
Sterile ultrasound gel
Tuberculin syringe with needle (optional for local anesthetic in the skin)
Syringes
Bandaid
Positioning aids
Imaging Requirements for Procedure:
Ultrasound with linear high frequency probe

Precautions:
1% lidocaine can be used for a skin wheal; avoid injecting lidocaine into the deep tissues or mixing it with the PRP

Potential Complications:
Bleeding
Infection
Post-procedural pain
Nerve injury
Risk of pneumothorax for scapulo-thoracic procedures
Vasovagal reactions and ataxia

Post-Procedure Care/ Follow-Up
After the procedure, the patient is observed and questioned about nausea and lightheadedness. If there are no signs of a vasovagal reaction, the patient can sit and then stand. The affected area can be actively mobilized in a gentle fashion to spread the PRP.

If a procedural complication occurs, the physician and/ or staff should observe the patient until the symptom resolves. If the patient is vasovagal, consider giving them a snack and some fluids.

The most commonly treated structures in the shoulder are the acromioclavicular joint, the biceps tendon sheath, the supraspinatus tendon, the subscapularis tendon, and the glenohumeral joint.

We must first cover the anatomy of the shoulder complex before considering intervention. The osseous anatomy is relatively straightforward (Figure 1.1). The clavicle, scapula, and humerus intersect to form the bony shoulder. The junction between the clavicle and the acromion of the scapula is known as the acromio-clavicular (AC) joint. The area where the glenoid of the scapula and the humerus meet is the glenohumeral joint.

CHAPTER 18 - THE SHOULDER

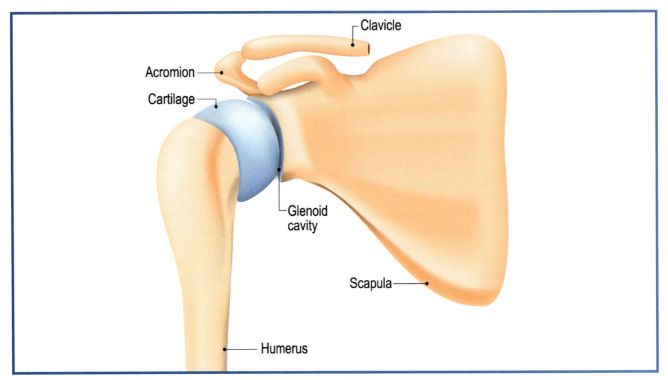

Figure 1.1: Osseous shoulder anatomy

Four tendons make up the rotator cuff: supraspinatus, infraspinatus, teres minor and subscapularis (SITS). These are the muscles that stabilize the shoulder during movement.

These are easy to remember as they are named by their position on the scapula and looking at the POSTERIOR and ANTERIOR aspects of the shoulder we can see why these muscles and tendons are named in this manner (figure 1.2)

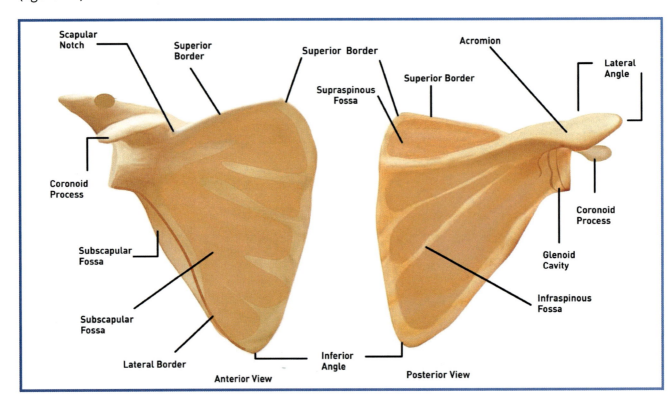

Figure 1.2: Anterior and posterior view of scapular osseous anatomy

The supraspinatus tendon originates in the supraspinous fossa and attaches to the superior facet of the greater tuberosity of the humerus. The infraspinatus originates in the infraspinous fossa of the scapula and attaches onto the middle facet of the greater tuberosity of the humerus as well as the teres minor which originates at the infraspinous fossa of the scapula more inferiorly than infraspinatus and inserts to the inferior facet of the humeral greater tuberosity. The teres minor inserts more posterior than the supraspinatus and infraspinatus. The teres minor carries very little clinical significance because it is not often involved in rotator cuff pathology so we will not discuss it beyond the relevant anatomy. Functionally, the supraspinatus, infraspinatus, and teres minor make up the posterior rotator cuff acting as force coupling stabilizers to initiate shoulder abduction, flexion and external rotation providing the essential "fine tuning" movements of the humeral head on the glenoid (figure 1.3). The subscapularis originates from the anterior fossa of the scapula and inserts to the lesser tuberosity of the humerus (figure 1.4). The subscapularis has the largest footprint of all the rotator cuff tendon insertions measuring roughly 22-32mm cephalocaudal with an average width of 18.1mm (L D'Adessi et al., 2006).

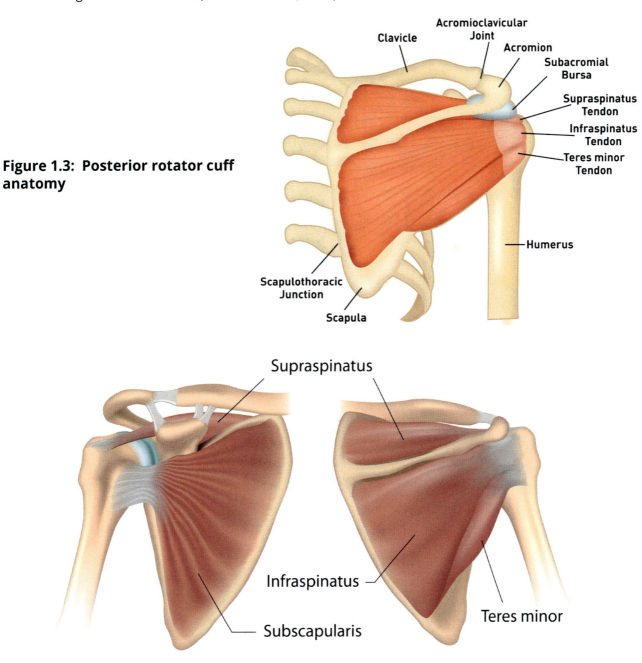

Figure 1.3: Posterior rotator cuff anatomy

Figure 1.4: Anterior and posterior view of rotator cuff anatomy

CHAPTER 18 - THE SHOULDER

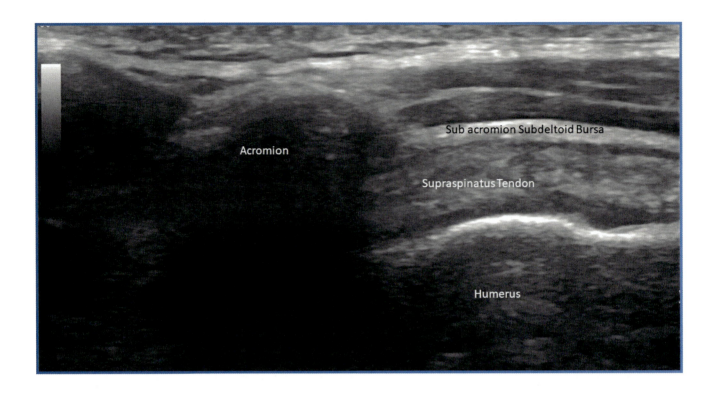

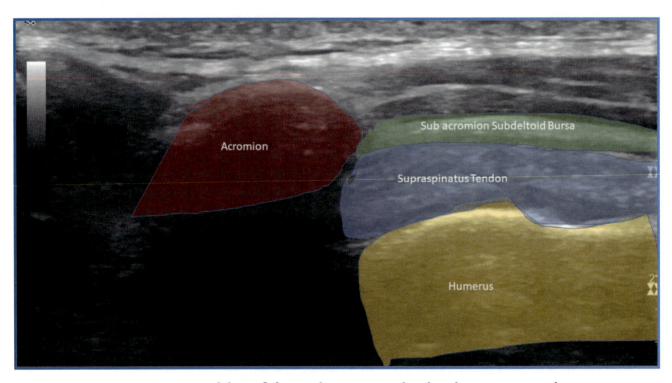

Image: Start position of dynamic compressive impingement testing.

To inject and/or diagnostically assess the supraspinatus tendon or the subscapularis tendon one needs to unfurl them and bring into view.

Unfurling the supraspinatus tendon is done by placing the patient's hand on their affected hip. This position effectively places the patient's extremity into shoulder extension, internal rotation and slight abduction; this is known as the Crass position. This position exposes the supraspinatus and subacromial-subdeltoid bursa from underneath the acromion (figure 1.5, 1.6, 1.7). When performing percutaneous procedures here, some people find that having the patient facing away from the provider is easier because there is less chance of the patient becoming anxious. To unfurl the subscapularis tendon and bring it into view, the patient needs the shoulder to be externally rotated to expose the footprint from underneath the coracoid.

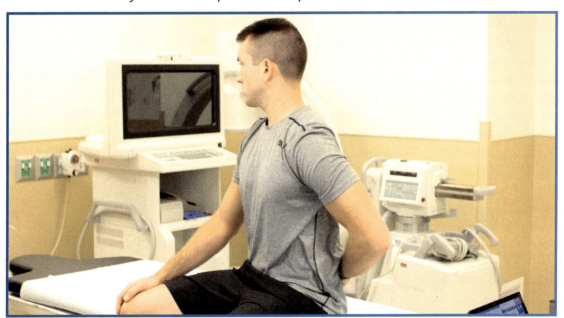

Figure 1.5: Example of full crass position of patient with hand behind the back. This places maximal stress on the supraspinatus insertion.

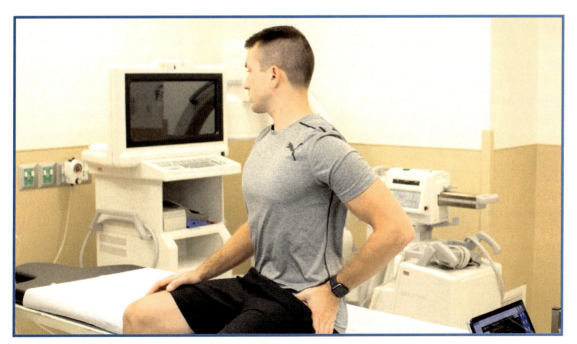

Figure 1.6: Modified crass position. Patient is instructed to "place your hand on your hip." This position is usually better tolerated in patients with shoulder pain.

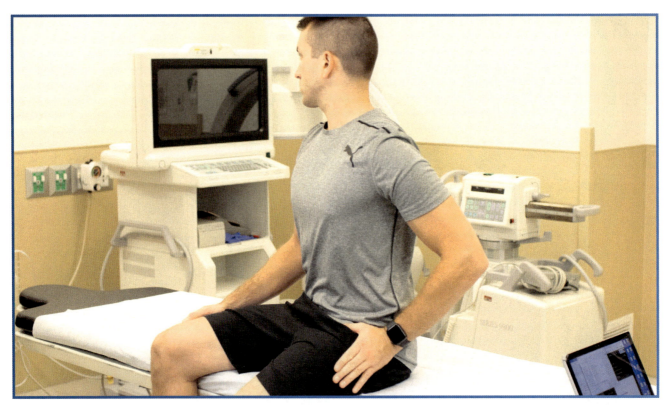

Figure 1.7: The "gunslinger position" can be an option in cases of severe shoulder pain from rotator cuff pathology. It is not the ideal position to evaluate the supraspinatus because it doesn't expose the tendon far enough from under the acromion.

Supraspinatus

The supraspinatus is the most commonly involved rotator cuff tendon in musculoskeletal disorders. It inserts anterior to the infraspinatus and teres minor on the greater tuberosity and posterior to the biceps long head tendon. The supraspinatus muscle functions as a fastener attaching muscle to bone, crossing the glenohumeral joint. It is a dynamic stabilizer and its primary action is to perform abduction of the arm, pulling the head of the humerus medially towards the glenoid cavity creating a suction effect. The supraspinatus also works to prevent the head of the humerus from slipping inferiorly and works in cooperation with the deltoid muscle to perform the first 15 degrees of abduction beginning from an adducted position (Ruotolo, et al., 2004). Beyond the first 15 degrees, the deltoid muscle becomes increasingly more effective at abducting the arm and becomes the main propagator of this action while the supraspinatus maintains secondary activity throughout (Ruotolo, et al., 2004). The supraspinatus is a relatively small muscle with a footprint attachment of roughly 25mm anterior to posterior to the superior facet of the greater tuberosity with an average superior to inferior attachment being 11.5-12mm (Ruotolo, et al., 2004). It is susceptible to injury because of the delicate nature of its makeup and its relatively small bulk. Due to the large amount of motion the shoulder is capable of, it has higher odds to be mechanically exposed in bad positions. Repetitive overhead motions such as manual labor and weightlifting (pressing) are two very common mechanisms of which the supraspinatus can become injured.

Ultrasound is very dynamic in nature and it carries advantages that other soft tissue imaging modalities do not possess. The operator can dynamically assess whether or not the supraspinatus is intact or whether or not there is subacromial impingement. To dynamically assess the supraspinatus and evaluate compressive impingement disorders, place the probe over the acromial shelf directly where it lies over the rotator cuff with the patient starting shoulder neutral in a seated, rested position (Figure 1.8). From here, the operator needs to coach the patient to actively, or actively-assisted with help from the provider, abduct the shoulder while keeping the probe focused on the acromial relationship with the tendon and bursa and assess quality of gliding and/or integrity of the tendon-bone relationship of the rotator cuff during the motion. Bursal bunching or "catching" that matches the patient's signs and symptoms is considered a positive test as well as the observation of paradoxical motion at the tendon-bone interface where at any point during abduction the tendon moves one way and the bone moves another, is a sign of a large rotator cuff tear. Cases where the tendon and bone move at the same rate indicate an intact rotator cuff. The most common sono pathologic findings of a supraspinatus tear are cortical irregularity and hypoechoic clefting adjacent to the cortical irregularity (Flgure 1.9 and 1.10).

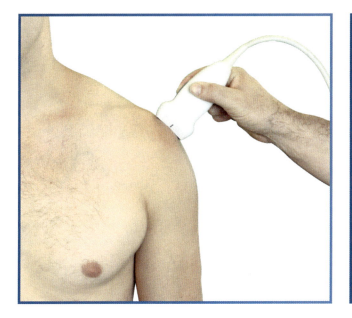
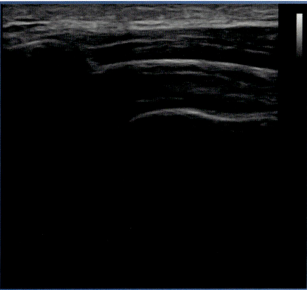
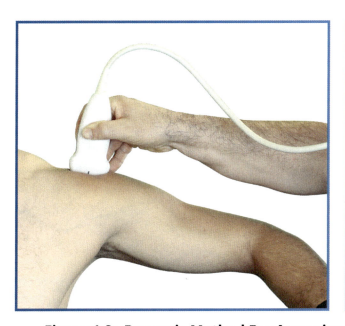
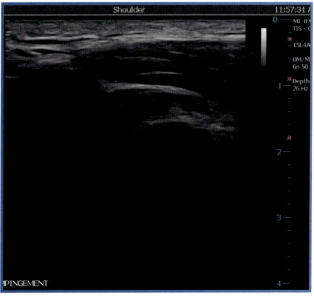

Figure 1.8: Dynamic Method For Assessing Compressive Subacromial Impingement

The patient's arm is flexed 90° with a prone wrist. The probe is placed in the coronal plane so that the rotator cuff tendon can be visualized traveling underneath the acromion. The supraspinatus tendon should be visualized below the acromion. Ask the patient to slowly raise his arm and evaluate the supraspinatus and subacromial and subdeltoid bursa as it glides under the coracoacromial arch. Top left: start position. Bottom left: finish position. Top right: Ultrasound image of start position. Bottom right: Ultrasound image of finish position.

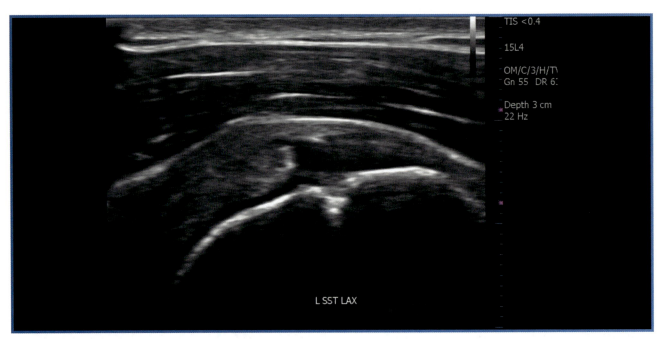

Figure 1.9: Long axis ultrasound image of a partial thickness, articular surface supraspinatus tear as evidenced by the cortical defect at the anatomic footprint and adjacent hypoechoic defect of the tendon.

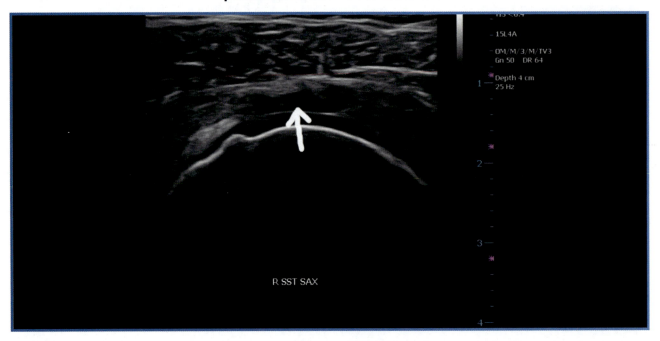

Figure 1.10: Short axis ultrasound image of a full thickness supraspinatus tendon tear. Arrow is pointing to the defect.

There are multiple ways to access the supraspinatus tendon when performing diagnostics or ultrasound guided procedures. Figure 1.11 and 1.12 detail scanning positions for diagnostic evaluation of the supraspinatus. When performing an ultrasound guided procedure, we recommend visualizing the supraspinatus in the short axis with the patient seated in the crass position. We recommend this technique because the full bulk of anterior to posterior bundle of the supraspinatus can be appreciated, giving the operator full visualization of its dimension that we cannot see in the long axis position. Once the bulk of the tendon is visualized and the operator has a clear grasp of the pathologic region, the needle is then moved from lateral to medial in plane with the probe (1.11 and 1.12).

Figure 1.11: Supraspinatus Tendon: Long Axis and Short Axis

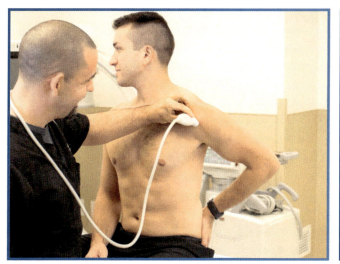
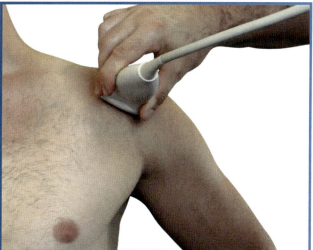
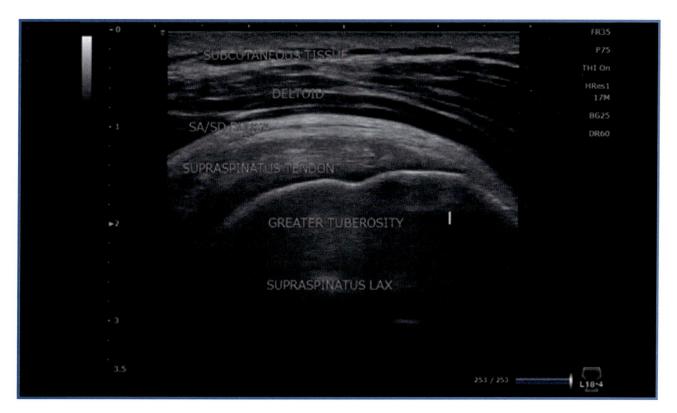

Long axis: The patient is seated. The clinician will instruct the patient to "place your hand on your hip", this is known as the modified crass position. Place the probe in the sagittal or long axis on the greater tuberosity in line with the shaft of the humerus.

Clinical Pearl: The crass position is a good position to see the supraspinatus on full tension and see defects in the fibers. The full crass position has the patient place the arm fully behind the back. The modified crass position has the patient place the hand on the ipsilateral hip.

Short axis: Place the patient's arm posteriorly with the elbow flexed in the full or modified crass position. The probe is positioned across the anterior and middle deltoid. Imagine drawing a line across the patient's chest from the humeral greater tuberosity to the contralateral hip and placing the probe in that line. The ultrasound image should have the metaphoric "tire and wheel" appearance.

CHAPTER 18 - THE SHOULDER

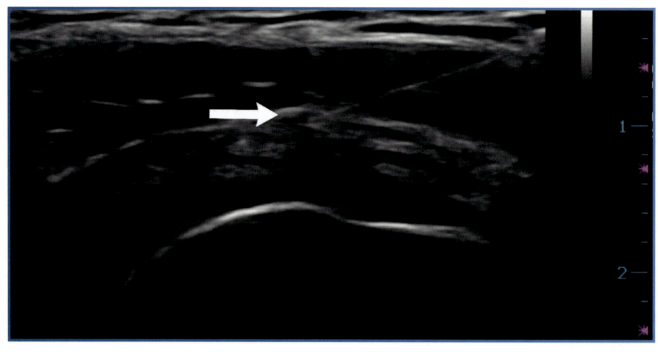

Figure 1.12: Ultrasound image of the supraspinatus in short axis with the needle moving from lateral to medial in plane with the probe

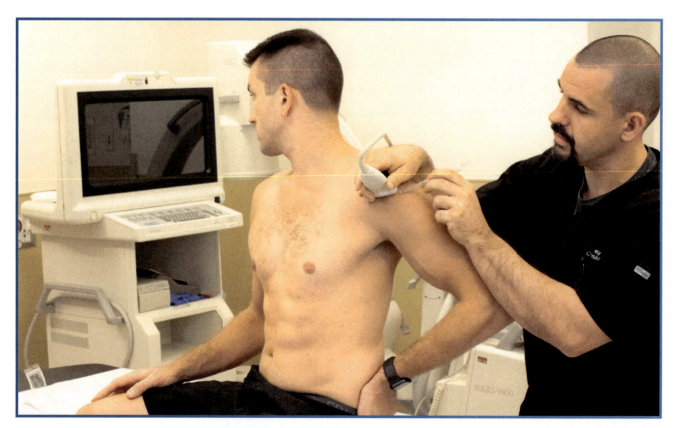

Figure 1.13: Ultrasound guided injection technique to the subacromial-subdeltoid bursa. Probe is placed for a short axis image of the supraspinatus, the needle is moved lateral to medial, in-plane with the probe.

CHAPTER 18 - THE SHOULDER

Figure 1.14: Infraspinatus Tendon: Long axis

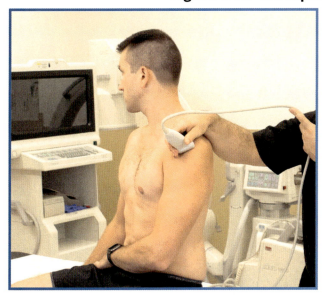
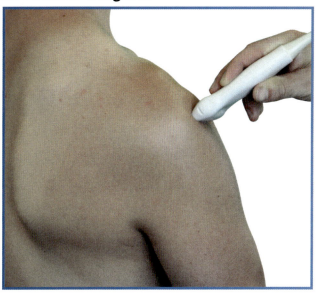
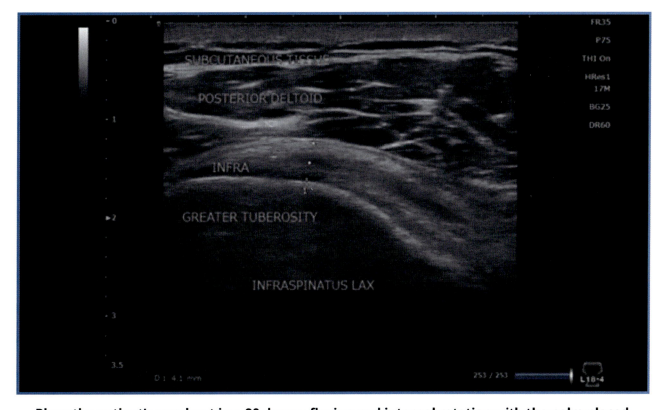

Place the patient's arm bent in a 90 degree flexion and internal rotation with the palm placed on the abdomen or on the contralateral thigh to place the infraspinatus on a stretch. The probe is positioned in line with the posterior deltoid and perpendicular to the triceps muscle. The infraspinatus will have the appearance of a fibrillar "bird beak" in this view.

A COMPLETE GUIDE TO REGENERATIVE MEDICINE ©

Figure 1.15: Infraspinatus Tendon: Short Axis

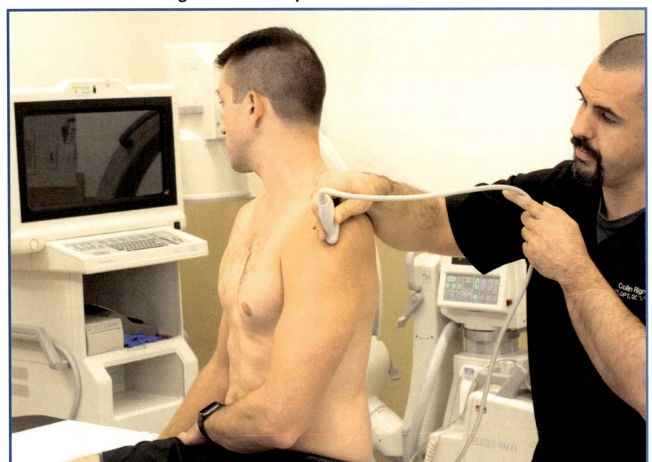

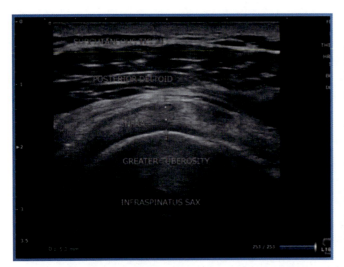

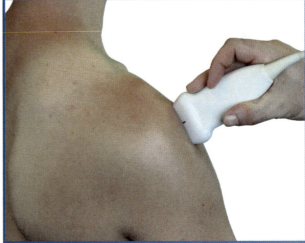

The patient is positioned in the seated position with the affected arm in neutral or reaching to the contralateral thigh, this places the tendon on a stretch. The probe is positioned along the middle deltoid parallel to the triceps muscle. The ultrasound image should show a bone-tendon relationship with a "tire and the wheel" appearance.

CHAPTER 18 - THE SHOULDER

The subscapularis tendon

The subscapularis tendon is not as commonly involved in shoulder pathology as the supraspinatus; however, it has been found to be more prevalent in cases of rotator cuff pathology than what was previously thought. With the advancement of radiologic detection and arthroscopic techniques, there is a renewed focus on recognition and repair of the affected tendon (Lenart et al., 2017). The subscapularis originates from a wide area on the anterior facing portion of the scapula and inserts to the lesser tuberosity. The subscapularis footprint at the lesser tuberosity measures 18mm in width has been found, on average, to be larger than that of the infraspinatus and the supraspinatus (Dugas et al, 2002 and Defranco et al., 2009) and has been identified to have a distinct interdigitation of fibres (along with the supraspinatus on the opposite side of the bicipital groove) to form the floor of the bicipital groove (Clark et al., 1992). The more experienced and advanced the user, the more sensitive ultrasound is in detecting small subscapularis tendon tears. To best evaluate the subscapularis tendon, it needs to be unfolded from underneath the coracoid. The best way to do this is to externally rotate the shoulder and place the tendon on a stretch (Figure 1.17 and 1.18). Because of its relationship with the bicipital groove and because it is a subsequent secondary stabilizer of the biceps long head, the subscapularis is often torn in cases with biceps long head dislocations or biceps long head split tears, where a portion of the biceps slips over the lesser tuberosity (Clark et al., 1992). This type of pathology with the biceps long head is, in many cases, pathognomonic with a subscapularis tendon tear and it is up to the provider to correlate the extent of its involvement (Pfirrmann et al., 1999) (Figure 1.21). These tears have classically been discovered using magnetic resonance with arthrogram; however, with recent technological advancements in resolution and training, musculoskeletal ultrasound has become a reliable diagnostic tool to detect larger, high grade subscapularis tendon tears although it must be said that smaller tears are often missed (Narasimhan et al., 2015). This is because the interrater reliability is not as consistent as that of static soft tissue imaging modalities such as an MRI; and like many other things with ultrasound, is a user and experience-dependent skill.

When injecting the subscapularis tendon, the patient is positioned supine on the table with the head turned away from the provider so they do not breathe directly onto the field which can help prevent infection (Figure 1.19). To best access and visualize the subscapularis insertion at the lesser tuberosity of the humerus for injection, place the affected shoulder into external rotation to unfold the tendon from underneath the coracoid, the needle is moved from distal to proximal, in-plane with the probe (Figure 1.20).

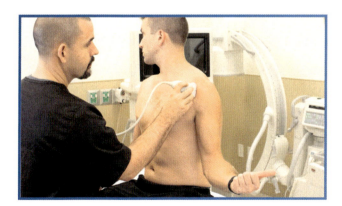

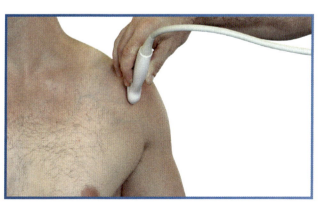

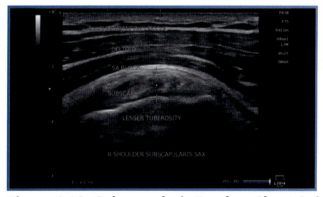

Figure 1.16: Subscapularis Tendon: Short Axis

With the patient sitting and arm placed in 90° flexion and rotating externally. The probe is positioned across the anterior deltoid and perpendicular the clavicle.

Locate the coracoid process and sweep the probe laterally until the lesser tuberosity is located. The short axis ultrasound image of the short axis should be mixed hyperechoic/hypoechoic secondary to the multipennate muscle structure of the subscapularis

Figure 1.17: Subscapularis Tendon: Long axis

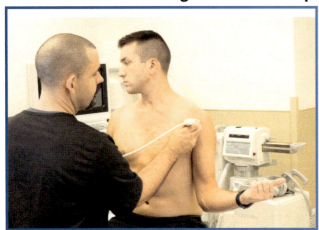
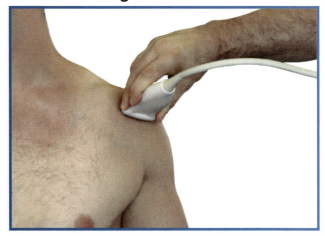
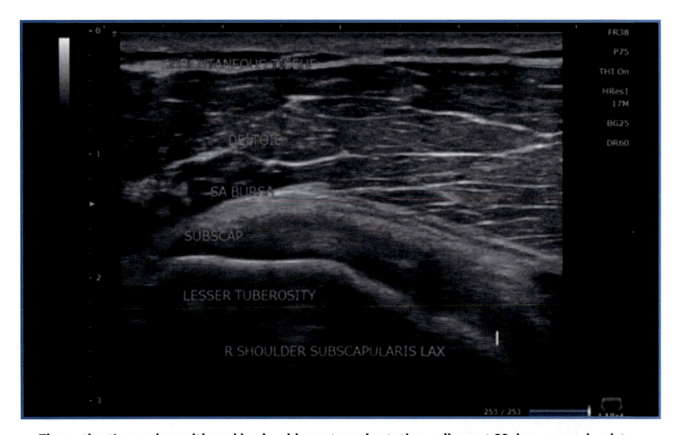

The patient's arm is positioned in shoulder external rotation, elbow at 90 degrees and wrist in full supination. The probe is positioned across the anterior deltoid perpendicular to the clavicle. Locate the coracoid process and sweep the probe laterally until the lesser tuberosity is located. The short axis ultrasound image of the short axis should be mixed hyperechoic/hypoechoic secondary to the multipennate muscle structure of the subscapularis

CHAPTER 18 - THE SHOULDER

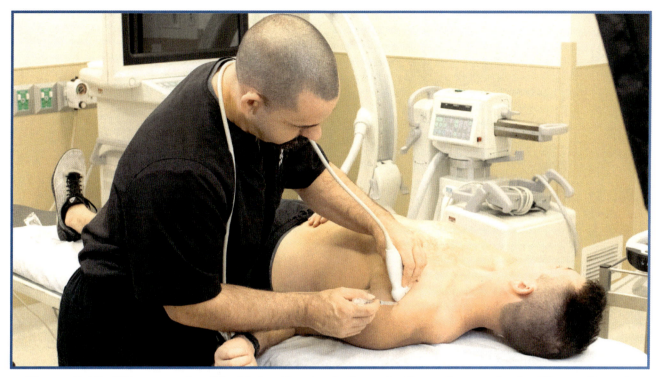

Figure 1.18: Ultrasound guided injection technique to the subscapularis. The patient is positioned supine with the head turned away. The probe is placed in the long axis to the subscapularis tendon and the needle is moved distal to proximal, in-plane with the probe.

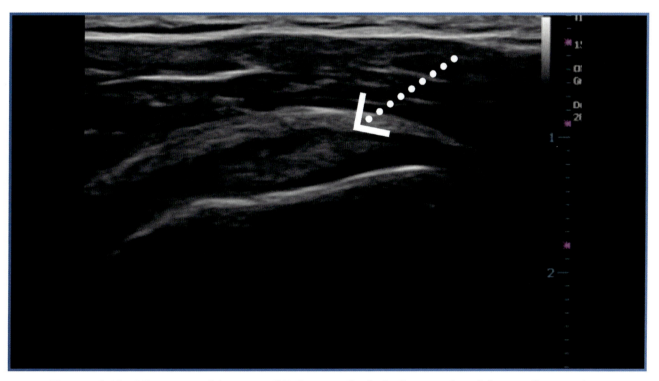

Figure 1.19: Ultrasound Image of Subscapularis in long axis with needle moving lateral to medial in-plane with the probe

A COMPLETE GUIDE TO REGENERATIVE MEDICINE ©

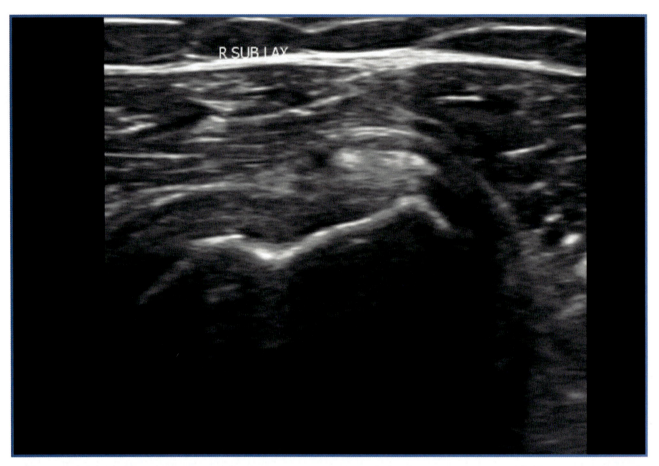

Figure 1.20: Long axis ultrasound image of a partial thickness subscapularis tendon tear. Note the dislocated biceps long head in the short axis over the distal portion of the tendon insertion, as described in the text, this is pathognomonic for a subscapularis disruption.

Biceps long head

Another pain generator in the anterior shoulder is the long head of the biceps tendon. The biceps long head can be analogized as "the window into the shoulder" because of its synovial sheath and communication with the glenohumeral joint where it attaches to the superior rim of the glenoid. The intra articular portion of the biceps is stabilized by the superior glenohumeral ligament and coracohumeral ligament at the rotator cuff interval and functions as a dynamic stabilizer of the glenohumeral joint as well as a depressor of the humeral head (Warner JJ et al., 1995). The short head of the biceps is usually not considered a pain generator in the shoulder region, does not have significant biomechanical influence on shoulder motion and is clinically not involved in many cases where musculoskeletal medicine is applied. The biceps short head originates at the coracoid process and conjoins with the long head distally toward its radial attachment. Clinically, the most common region where the biceps long head tendon becomes thickened and hypoechoic is the proximal aspect of the bicipital groove or the "magic angle" where the tendon turns and angles toward its attachment to the superior glenoid. Biceps tendon pathology can range from tenosynovitis, intrasheath tendon thickening, fraying or split tear such as Figure 1.26. Fluid found within the biceps long head tendon sheath can be an indirect sign of a rotator cuff tear and not just tenosynovitis (10). Because the long head of the biceps brachii tendon and it's sheath both communicate with the glenohumeral joint, increased joint fluid will collect in this extension of the joint. A small amount of fluid at one side of the biceps tendon is often seen normally, but fluid greater in diameter of the tendon is considered abnormal, especially if it is seen circumferential to the biceps tendon (the bullseye sign) (Jacobsen j. 2017). This is why it is important to examine the entire shoulder and not stop at the biceps as the fluid can be coming from somewhere else. Figure 1.22 and 1.23 detail the scanning positions to evaluate the biceps long head using diagnostic ultrasound.

CHAPTER 18 - THE SHOULDER

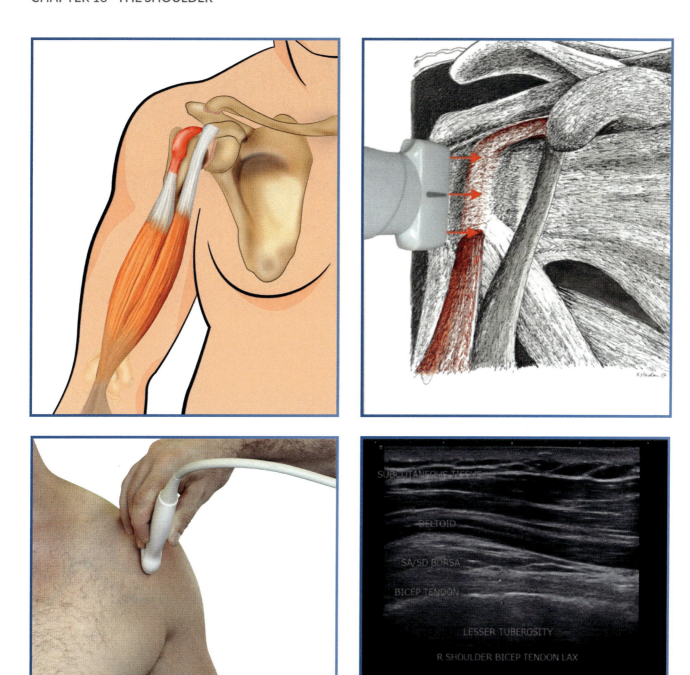

Figure 1.21: Biceps Tendon: Longitudinal/LAX

The patient is seated with elbow in 90 degrees flexion, wrist in full supination and shoulder hanging by their side in neutral. The probe is positioned across the line with the anterior deltoid and parallel to the humeral shaft.

A COMPLETE GUIDE TO REGENERATIVE MEDICINE ©

Figure 1.22: Biceps Tendon: Transverse/SAX

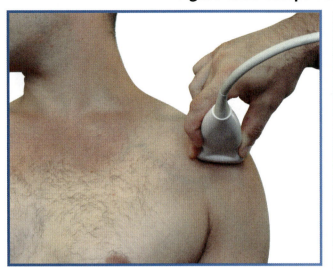
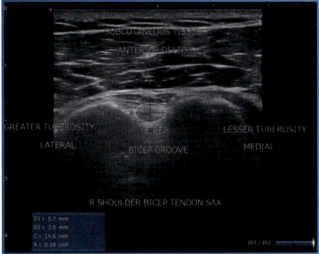

The patient is seated with the affected arm in neutral, elbow flexed to 90 degrees and wrist in full supination. The probe is positioned across the anterior deltoid, perpendicular to the biceps tendon.

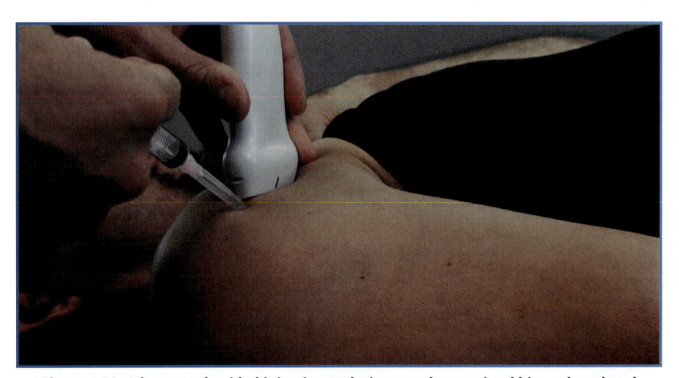

Figure 1.23: Ultrasound guided injection technique to the proximal biceps long head tendon. Patient is positioned supine with the shoulder in neutral. Probe is positioned in the short axis to the biceps tendon and bicipital groove, needle is moved lateral to medial, in-plane with the probe.

The biceps long head tendon sheath is best accessed for percutaneous intervention by using a direct, in-plane approach. The patient is positioned lying flat, palm up, with the shoulder externally rotated (Figure 1.23). With this approach, the transducer is placed in the short axis to the bicipital groove and the needle is moved from lateral to medial in plane with the probe to the bicipital sheath (Figure 1.24).

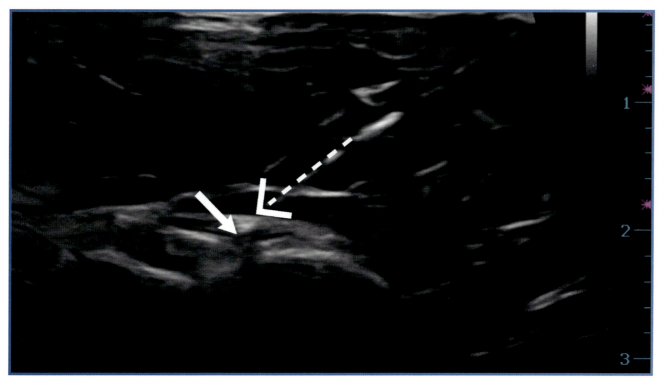

Figure 1.24: Short axis image of the proximal biceps tendon in its sheath with the needle moving lateral to medial in-plane with the probe

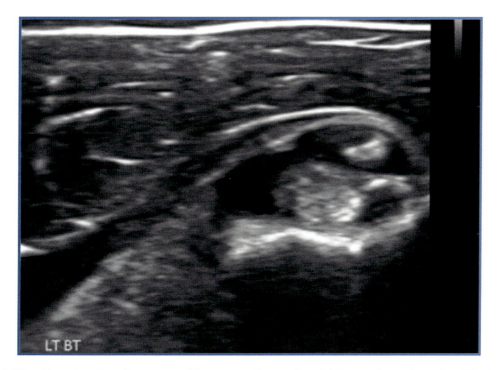

Figure 1.25: Short axis ultrasound image of proximal biceps long head split tear with tenosynovitis as evidenced with hypoechoic effusion within the bicipital groove and atypical bi-lobed appearance of the tendon proper.

ACROMIOCLAVICULAR JOINT

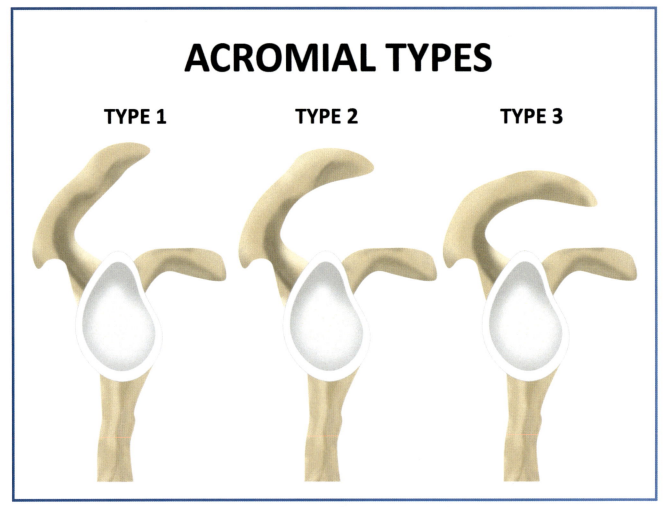

Figure 1.26: Acromial Types I, II, and III.

There are three different types of acromion that are clinically important : The flat acromion, which is a type I acromion, there is a type II acromion which is curved, there is a type III hooked acromion (Figure 1.26).

The reason these types of acromion are clinically important is that when they progress to types II and III, it encroaches the roof of the subjacent rotator cuff and the subacromial-subdeltoid bursa via bony outgrowth and osteophytic change.

The acromion is part of the scapula and the scapula has multiple bony landmarks we must remember. The acromion interfaces with the lateral edge of the clavicle forming the acromioclavicular joint. The acromioclavicular joint is a plane-style synovial joint that is held together by a ligamentous complex (Dutton, et al., 2008). The AC Joint has a thin capsule lined with synovium. The capsule is weak and is strengthened by capsular ligaments both inferiorly and superiorly, which in turn are reinforced through attachments from the deltoid and trapezius (Neumann et al., 2009). Without the superior and inferior capsular ligaments, the AC Joint capsule would not be strong enough to maintain the integrity of the joint (Neumann et al., 2009). The articular surfaces of the interfacing joint are lined with fibrocartilage and the joint cavity is partially divided by an articular disc (also fibrocartilage) wedged and suspended from the upper part of the capsule (Levangie et al., 2005). The acromioclavicular joint is a common pain generator in the shoulder complex. Potential causes of acromioclavicular joint pain could be an acute sprain and subsequent instability or from chronic arthropathy secondary to repetitive overuse over the course of time.

CHAPTER 18 - THE SHOULDER

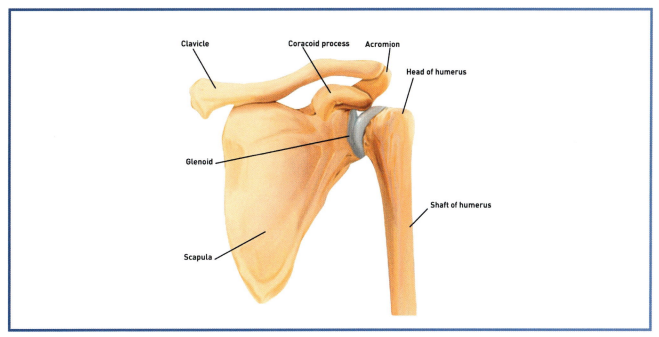

Figure 1.27: Osseous Anatomy of the shoulder complex

Another scapular landmark to be mindful of is the coracoid process located anteriorly on the scapula. The Coracoid is a Greek word and it means "raven." It looks like the outpouching or raven-like beak that sits anteriorly on the scapula. The coracoid serves as a ligamentous attachment site that connects it to the acromion (Figure 1.27). This ligament is called the coracoacromial ligament and it functions as a bone-to-bone stabilizer as well as serves as the "roof of the rotator cuff" housing the subacromial bursa. The coracoacromial ligament forms an osteoligamentous static restraint to superior humeral head displacement (Rothenberg et al., 2017) that also provides coverage for the rotator cuff tendons from bony prominences of the undersurface acromion during dynamic movements of the shoulder. There is much variance across literature in the morphologic mechanism of the coracoacromial ligament in musculoskeletal disorders (Rothenberg et al., 2017). Adjacently located between the coracoacromial ligament and the rotator cuff is the subacromial bursa which provides cushion and protection for the rotator cuff from the bony prominences (Figure 1.28). The subacromial bursa, which is a friction transducer, can be a pain generator in

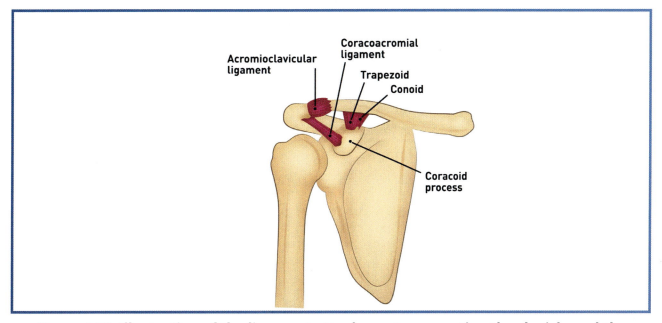

Figure 1.28 Illustration of the ligament attachments connecting the clavicle and the scapula

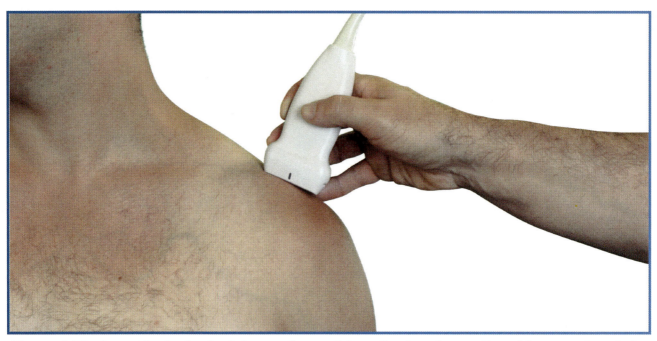

Figure 1.29: Acromioclavicular joint probe position: Patient is comfortably seated and the probe is placed in the coronal plane in long axis with the acromioclavicular joint

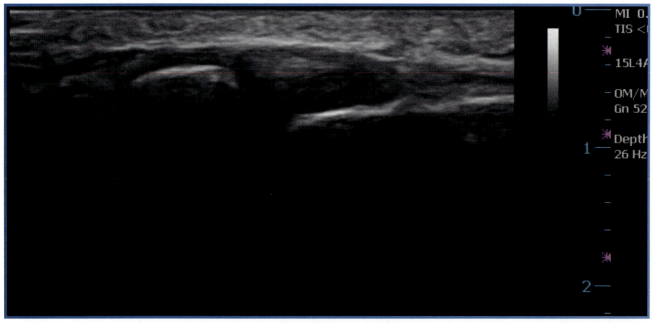

Figure 1.30: Long axis ultrasound image of the acromioclavicular joint. Clavicle is on the left and acromion is on the right

rotator cuff pathology and acromial morphology because of its location and is often involved concurrently with acromioclavicular joint pathology, rotator cuff pathology and; although more rare, sometimes in isolation. Over time, the acromioclavicular joint is susceptible to chronic friction from repetitive activity or repeated overloading that cause irregular bony formation and/or instability. Probe positioning and normal sonoanatomy of the acromioclavicular joint is referenced in Figure 1.29 and 1.30.

When performing an injection to the acromioclavicular joint the patient is positioned supine with the acromioclavicular joint visualized in the long axis with the needle moving from superior to inferior using an indirect or out-of-plane approach (Figure 1.31-1.33).

CHAPTER 18 - THE SHOULDER

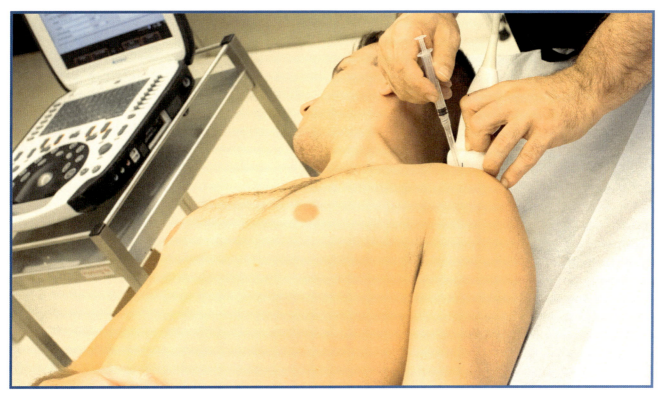

Figure 1.31: Ultrasound guided injection technique to the acromioclavicular joint. Patient is positioned supine with the joint visualized in long axis, the needle is moved superior to inferior, out-of-plane with the probe

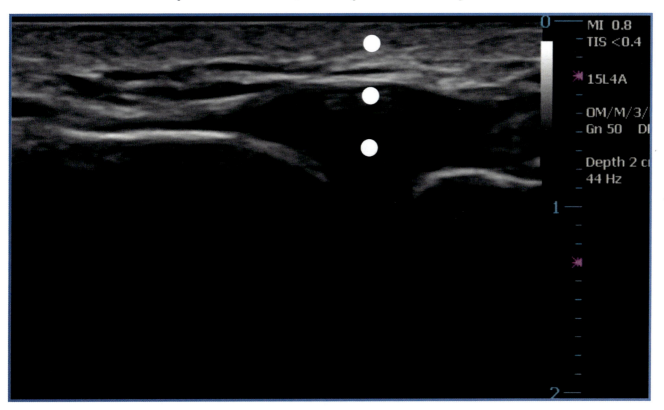

Figure 1.32: Long axis image of the acromioclavicular joint with the needle moving superior to inferior out-of-plane with the probe

A COMPLETE GUIDE TO REGENERATIVE MEDICINE ©

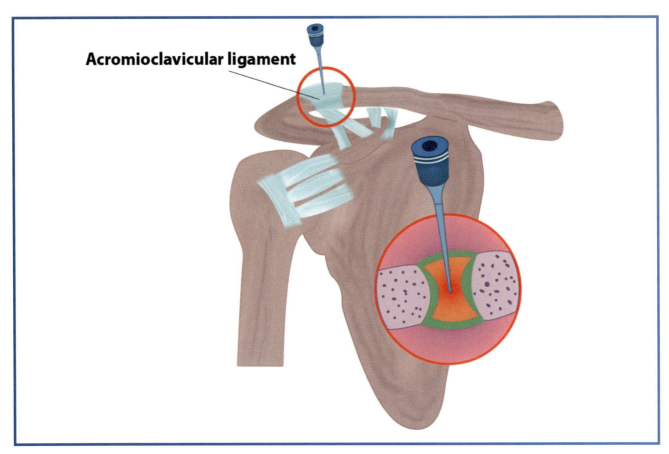

Figure 1.33: Out of plane needle approach to the acromioclavicular joint

Sono pathologic features of acromioclavicular joint arthropathy include capsular bowing, bony outgrowth, and joint space narrowing (Figure 1.34). These features can vary widely across the patient population, take care when evaluating with ultrasound and be sure to perform a thorough physical exam and history to best correlate the sonographic features.

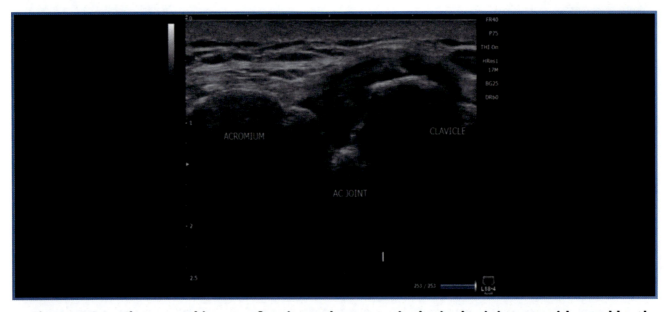

Figure 1.34: Ultrasound image of an irregular acromioclavicular joint as evidenced by the capsular effusion as well as offset joint angle where the clavicle is slightly elevated compared to the acromion secondary to ligament sprain

GLENOHUMERAL JOINT

The glenohumeral joint is the most inherently unstable joint in the body because it has the most range of motion. When looking at glenoid and the humerus alone, you might wonder how the humerus stays in place? Given that the shoulder complex is less "ball and socket" and more "golf ball and tee" why wouldn't it constantly dislocate? The combination of capsular ligaments, labrum and the rotator cuff/biceps long head force coupling system all have a suction cup effect on the glenoid, keeping the humerus in place. The glenoid is a part of the scapula where the humerus sits and it keeps itself positioned to the humerus almost like a "suction cup on glass."

The glenohumeral articulation is hard to inject blindly with a consistent level of accuracy. Ultrasound guidance is the new standard of practice when performing intervention in this region and the posterior injection technique offers an easier and a more effective approach to the glenohumeral joint with less extravasation rate compared with the anterior approach (Ogul et al., 2014). The posterior approach also avoids the potential risk of accidental puncture or injection into the axillary neurovascular structures (Ogul et al., 2014). One structure to be aware of in the posterior glenohumeral joint region is the spinoglenoid notch which houses the suprascapular nerve. The spinoglenoid notch probe position is optimally visualized slightly posterior to the glenohumeral joint (Figure 1.35 and 1.36).

To set up the posterior approach for an ultrasound guided procedure to the glenohumeral joint, the patient will lie in the lateral decubitus on the unaffected side and give themselves a hug with the affected extremity. This position gaps the glenohumeral joint for better visualization. Our preference is the performance of an in-plane injection keeping the probe focused over the posterior aspect of the glenohumeral joint so that the infraspinatus and posterior deltoid are in the long axis (Figure 1.37 and 1.38). The needle is moved from posterior to anterior toward the capsule.

Figure 1.35: Glenohumeral Joint

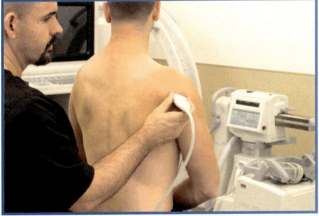

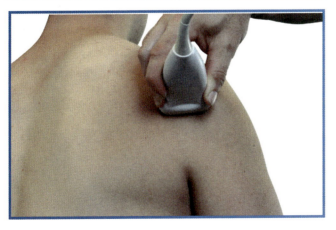

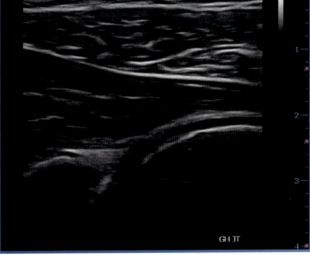

The patient is positioned seated with the affected shoulder in neutral or position the patient's arm across their body to place a stretch on the infraspinatus and gap the posterior glenohumeral joint. The clinician may alternatively have the patient reach the affected hand to the contralateral hip or opposite thigh to gap the joint and stretch the infraspinatus. The probe is positioned perpendicular to the posterior deltoid and perpendicular to the triceps muscle.

CHAPTER 18 - THE SHOULDER

Figure 1.36: Spinoglenoid notch

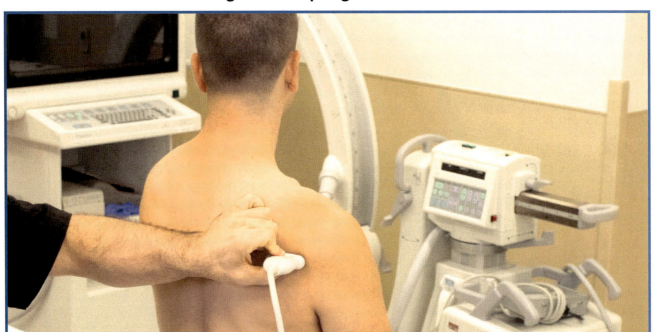
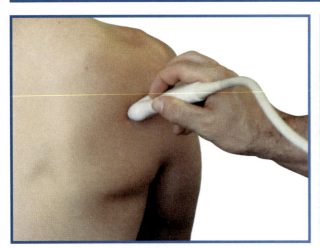
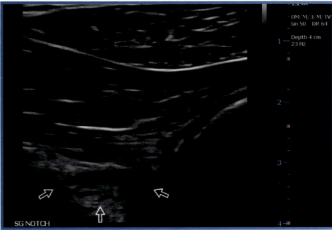

The patient is in the seated position with the affected arm in neutral or to better gap the posterior glenohumeral joint the clinician can tell the patient to reach for the opposite thigh to put the infraspinatus on a stretch. To best visualize the spinoglenoid notch and posterior glenohumeral joint, the probe is positioned parallel to the posterior deltoid and perpendicular to the triceps muscle.

CHAPTER 18 - THE SHOULDER

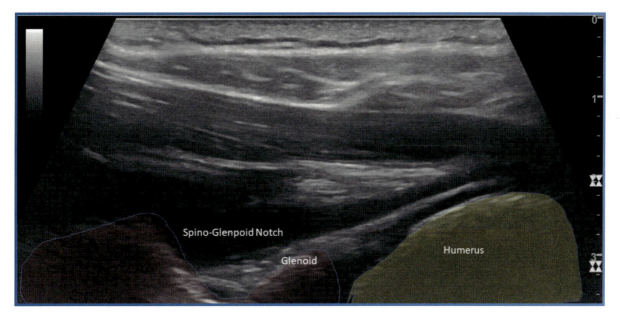

Figure 1.36: The spinoglenoid notch is located just posterior to the posterior aspect of the glenohumeral joint

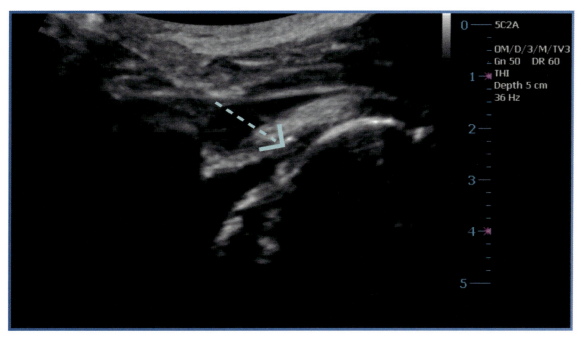

Figure 1.37: Short axis ultrasound image of the glenohumeral joint with the needle moving from posterior to anterior toward the posterior capsule

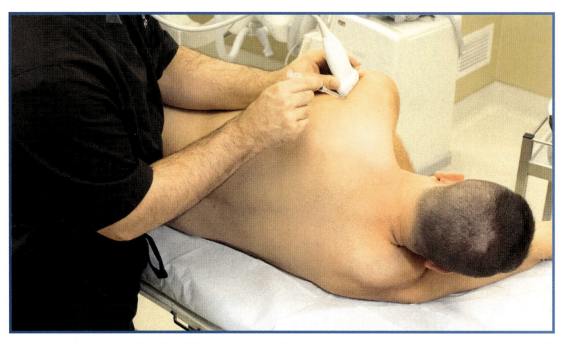

Figure 1.38: Ultrasound guided injection technique to the posterior glenohumeral joint. The patient is positioned in the lateral decubitus on the patient's contralateral side. The glenohumeral joint is visualized in the short axis.

Sample Dictation/Note:

Sample Dictation for PRP for Rotator Cuff Injection:
The procedure and potential complications were discussed with the patient. After written and verbal consent were obtained, the patient was placed in the seated position. A tourniquet was placed on the right arm and the area was surveyed for large palpable veins. The antecubital area was prepped and draped in the usual sterile fashion using alcohol. Using an 20G needle, approximately [ ] ccs of blood was drawn from the patient and transferred to a specially prepared PRP tube containing anticoagulants. After the needle was removed, and a sterile bandage was placed over the entry site, the tube was vertically rotated back and forth five times.

The tube was placed in a centrifuge with an opposing counter-weight. After five minutes, the tube was removed and inspected. There was a visible gel, a buffy coat, and a golden liquid layer of PRP. The tube was vertically rotated back and forth five times. Afterwards, the PRP and buffy coat were gently extracted and transferred to a 10 cc syringe. The syringe was attached to a 22G 1.5" needle.

[Patient positioning as described above depending on the type of injection and approach]

The shoulder was prepped and draped in the usual sterile manner using three coats of betadine. The area of interest was identified using sonography. With the probe held in place, a ½ a cc of 1% lidocaine was used to create a wheal at the entry site alongside the probe. The needle guidance software package was turned on. After a moment, with the probe held in place, the needle and syringe containing the PRP was advanced through the skin and the deeper tissues towards the target area. Under ultrasound guidance, the PRP was injected. The final image was recorded. The probe was moved, the needle was removed and a sterile gauze was held over the injection site with gentle pressure. A sterile bandage was applied. The patient was repositioned for comfort. The patient tolerated the procedure well with no apparent complications.

References:

D'Adessi, L., Calandra, J. J., Bannwarth, B., Planchamp, F., & Gonzalez, J. F. (2006). The subscapularis footprint: an anatomic study of the subscapularis tendon insertion. Arthroscopy: The Journal of Arthroscopic & Related Surgery, 22(7), 762–768. doi: 10.1016/j.arthro.2006.04.101

Ruotolo, C., Nottage, W. M., & McGarry, M. H. (2004). The supraspinatus footprint: an anatomic study of the supraspinatus insertion. Arthroscopy: The Journal of Arthroscopic & Related Surgery, 20(3), 246–249. doi: 10.1016/j.arthro.2004.01.002

Lenart, B. A., Martens, K. A., Kearns, K. A., & Gillespie, R. J. (2017). Subscapularis tendon tears management and arthroscopic repair. Journal of Orthopaedics, 14(3), 492–496. doi: 10.1016/j.jor.2017.06.017

Dugas, J., Campbell, D., Warren, R., Robie, B., & Millet, P. (2002). Anatomy and dimensions of the rotator cuff. Journal of Shoulder and Elbow Surgery, 11(5), 498–503. doi: 10.1067/mse.2002.126613

DeFranco, M. J., & Cole, B. J. (2009). Current perspectives on rotator cuff anatomy. Arthroscopy: The Journal of Arthroscopic & Related Surgery, 25(3), 305–320. doi: 10.1016/j.arthro.2008.11.017

Clark, J. M., & Harryman, D. T. (1992). Tendons, ligaments, and capsule of the rotator cuff. Gross and microscopic anatomy. The Journal of Bone & Joint Surgery, 74(5), 713–725. doi: 10.2106/00004623-199274050-00014

Pfirrmann, C. W., Zanetti, M., Weishaupt, D., Gerber, C., Hodler, J. (1999). Residual defects of the rotator cuff after repair: assessment with MR imaging. Acta Orthopaedica Scandinavica, 70(6), 571–576. doi: 10.

Narasimhan, R., Kukke, S. N., Fong, B., & Birdsell, D. C. (2016). Prevalence of subscapularis tears and accuracy of shoulder ultrasound in pre-operative diagnosis. International Orthopaedics (SICOT), 40(5), 975–979. doi: 10.1007/s00264-015-3038-5

Warner, J. J., Allen, A., Marks, P. H., & Wong, P. (1995). The role of the long head of the biceps brachii in superior stability of the glenohumeral joint. The Journal of Bone & Joint Surgery, 77(3), 366–372. doi: 10.2106/00004623-199503000-00006

Dutton, A. Q., Yeo, S. J., Yang, K. Y., & Lo, N. N. (2008). Computer-assisted minimally invasive total knee arthroplasty compared with standard total knee arthroplasty. A prospective, randomized study. The Journal of Bone & Joint Surgery, 90(1), 2–9. doi: 10.2106/JBJS.F.01148

Levangie, P. K., & Norkin, C. C. (2005). Joint Structure and Function: A Comprehensive Analysis. 4th ed. Philadelphia, PA: F.A. Davis Co.

Rothenberg, J. B., Gerber, C., & McFarland, E. G. (2017). The coracoacromial ligament: anatomy, function, and clinical significance. Orthopaedic Journal of Sports Medicine, 5(4), 2325967117703398. doi: 10.1177/2325967117703398

Ogul, H., Uysal, M. A., Genc, H., Kaya, E., Yilmaz, G., & Akgun, K. (2014). Ultrasound-guided shoulder MR arthrography: comparison of rotator interval and posterior approach. Clinical Imaging, 38(1), 11–17. doi: 10.1016/j.clinimag.2013.07.006

CHAPTER 19 The Elbow

Colin Rigney & Pradeep Albert

CHAPTER PREVIEW

This chapter will cover sonoanatomy of the elbow as well as patient and probe positions for proper evaluation. The chapter will also include common pictorial examples and explanations of sono-pathology found as well as basic ultrasound-guided injection techniques.

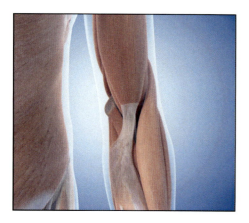

The type of procedure performed depends on the patient's clinical signs and symptoms.

For intra-articular injections:
Pain with all movements of the elbow
Limited range of motion
Radiocapitallar osteoarthritis on x-ray, CT scan, MRI, or ultrasound

For bicipital tendon injection:
Pain with flexion and supination
Pain with resisted flexion
Biceps partial tear or tendinosis on MRI or ultrasound

For lateral epicondylitis injection:
Pain at the lateral aspect of the elbow over the lateral epicondyle
Pain with resisted extension of the wrist

For medial epicondylitis injection:
Pain at the medial aspect of the elbow over the medial epicondyle
Pan with resisted flexion of the wrist

Contraindications to Injection:
Systemic infection
Infection or rash over the puncture site
Coagulopathy (International Normalized Ratio [INR] > 1.3 or platelets < 50,000/ mm3)
Inability to reach target site because of prior surgery or scar tissue

Equipment and Supplies:
Alcohol swabs
Tourniquet
18G or 20G needle for blood draw
Tubing
PRP Kit
Gauze
Betadine or Chlorhexidine
Sterile drapes
Sterile gloves
Sterile ultrasound gel
Tuberculin syringe with needle (optional for local anesthetic in the skin)
Syringes
Bandaid
Positioning aids

Imaging Requirements for Procedure:
Ultrasound with linear high frequency probe

Precautions:
1% lidocaine can be used for a skin wheal; avoid injecting lidocaine into the deep tissues or mixing it with the PRP

Potential Complications:
Bleeding
Infection
Post-procedural pain
Nerve injury
Risk of pneumothorax for scapulo-thoracic procedures
Vasovagal reactions and ataxia

Post-Procedure Care/ Follow-Up
After the procedure, the patient is observed and questioned nausea and lightheadedness. If there are no signs of a vasovagal reaction, the patient can sit and then stand. The affected area can be actively mobilized in a gentle fashion to spread the PRP.

If a procedural complication occurs, the physician and/ or staff should observe the patient until the symptom resolves. If the patient is vasovagal, consider giving them a snack and some fluids.

Anatomic Considerations:

How do we identify pathology in the elbow? Tendons go through a degradation process usually from chronic overuse or can often be precipitated from an old injury. The typical sonographic appearance of an inflamed tendon is the loss of fibrillar pattern, where tendon shapes become heterogeneous, thickened and hypoechoic. In the case of long-term tendinopathy, tendons can become calcified with mixed hyperechoic foci interspersed throughout (lighter compared to the background) and in the case of frank tearing or rupture the space where the tendon should be hyperechoic can become anechoic (dark) due to effusion. If a tendon is completely torn and does not have viable attachment fibers left, the provider isn't doing the patient any favors by injecting the structure with PRP or stem cells because the patient may need surgery in those cases so please keep that in mind.

If a patient has chronic bursitis, treat the root cause first which is usually the adjacent tendon. Consider consulting a rheumatologist to ensure that the patient does not have gout or other treatable conditions. If autoimmune disease is the underlying cause, the patient will likely not get relief with PRP injections.

Regenerative medicine has potential for application in the treatment of osteoarthritis but it is important to correctly identify typical osteoarthritis versus atypical osteoarthritis. Usually, degenerative arthritis in young people is due to trauma or crystal deposition. There could also be systemic underlying neuropathy or metabolic abnormality or hemophilia. In the case of inflammatory arthritis, usually it is in one joint, and infection should be a concern. If the patient is affected in multiple joints, the provider should consider either rheumatoid arthritis or a class of inflammatory arthropathy.

Synovitis, inflammation of the synovium, can also be treated with PRP to potentially bring down inflammation and it is something to consider in patients who are recalcitrant to typical treatment. There are five grades for synovitis on ultrasound. 0 is normal, grade 1 is a joint effusion with capsular distention, grade 2 is small erosions in the radial head with irregular cartilage, grade 3 is cortical defect and bony erosion of the humeral capitellum. Bony erosions typically occur on the radius first and capitellum second. If there is a cortical defect of the radial head and humeral capitellum combined with synovial hypertrophy and capsular thickening, this could be defined as grade 4, and complete destruction of the joint would be grade 5. The grading scale for synovitis of the elbow can be technically challenging and is user and experience-dependent, if the provider is novice or uncomfortable utilizing a grading scale with ultrasound then the MRI can always be used as a fallback option.

What type of needles are you going to use? You can use anything from an 18-gauge to a 22-gauge. We don't advise using anything smaller than a 25-gauge. We want to encourage a healthy inflammatory process with the elbow joint with use of PRP. It is not advisable to inject more than 5 cc of PRP; and when using a significant amount of volume, the provider should use a face mask and eye goggles. Adherence to universal precautions, which includes the use of sterile procedure with gloves, facemask, goggles and gown is encouraged when incorporating PRP and stem cell use into your practice.

Medial epicondyle – 2-4 cc of PRP or stem cells. Low volume, 18-22 gauge needle. Lateral epicondyle is the same – typically 2-4cc of PRP or stem cell with 18-22 gauge needle. Biceps brachii -- 2-4cc of PRP or stem cells in a 18-22g needle. In the radiocapitellar joint we advise 3-5cc of PRP or stem cell. Since the radiocapitellar is a small joint, it is not advisable to inject more than 5 cc as this can cause significant distention which can cause significant irritation. There are some manufacturers who use large amounts of platelet rich plasma who produce it and ideally, we occasionally use systems that have lower volumes and higher concentrations of platelet rich plasma as well as stem cell concentrations so as not to put too much in because may not be able to tolerate the procedure which is obviously counterproductive. The triceps tendon insertion is also approximately 4-5 cc of PRP or stem cell using 18-22g needle.

The most common injections in the elbow region are the medial epicondyle, (golfers elbow), lateral epicondyle (tennis elbow) and the biceps tendon insertion for tendinopathy. You can also inject the radiocapitellar joint space via sonography.

Now we dive into the anatomy.

The elbow functions both as a hinged and a rotational joint. The radius and the capitellum provide the major rotational component into pronation-supination and the humeroulnar joint primarily functions as a hinged joint where it performs flexion-extension. Grossly, the functional movements of the elbow are pronation, supination, flexion and extension.

Orientation to the elbow; as the patient is lying down with the thumbs pointing away from the body, the thumb is radial and the pinky is ulnar with the palm up. Directionally, ulnar is medial and radial is lateral.

To avoid mistakes, remember anatomic positioning. Please see the ultrasound images and diagrams below (figure 2.1 and 2.2).

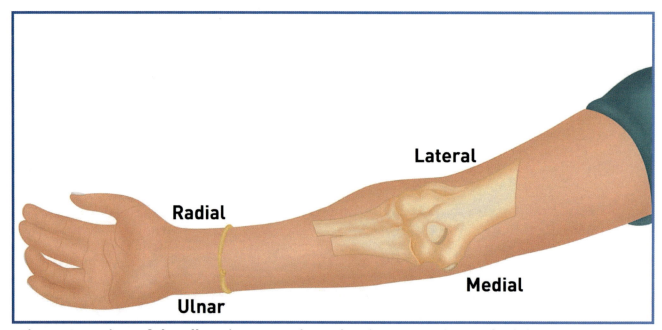

Figure 2.1: View of the elbow in anatomic supination. Superior to the joint it is universal to label direction either lateral or medial. Below the joint is is more universal to directionally label radial or ulnar.

CHAPTER 19 - THE ELBOW

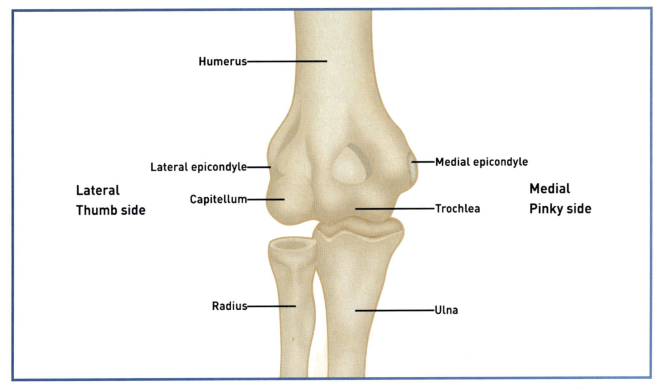

Figure 2.2: Osseous anatomy of the elbow joint from an anterior to posterior direction

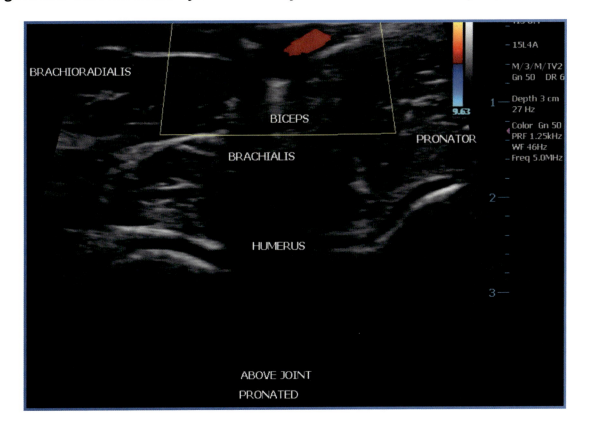

A COMPLETE GUIDE TO REGENERATIVE MEDICINE ©

Distal Biceps Brachii

The biceps brachii lies anteriorly and crosses the elbow joint itself. The brachioradialis sits laterally (radially) while the pronator teres and forearm flexors lie medially (ulnarly). With the patient in anatomic neutral, the cross sectional diagram of the elbow is analogous to a pyramid. The base of the pyramid is formed by the ulna, radius and humerus. In the middle section of the pyramid from ulnar to radial, the muscle cross sections are brachioradialis, brachialis and pronator teres. The biceps brachii tendon, vessels and median nerve all sit at the apex of the pyramid.

The biceps brachii has two heads. The short head originates at the coracoid process and the long head originates at the superior rim of the glenoid. The long head and short head biceps brachii conjoint at the humerus and travel distally to the radial tuberosity and the fascia in the form of bicipital aponeurosis. At the level of the elbow, the biceps tendon is primarily an elbow flexor and supinator. It is innervated by C5 and C6 and vascularly supplied by the brachial artery.

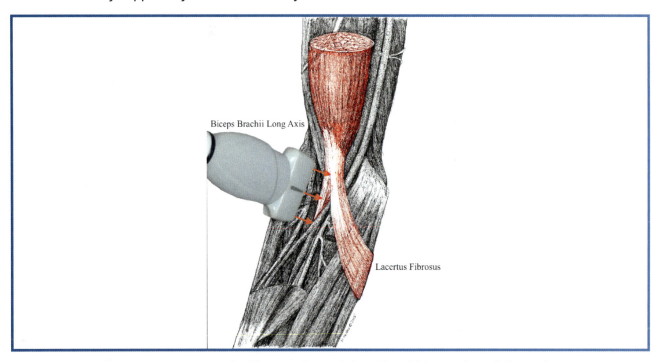

Figure 2.3: Anatomic illustration of the distal biceps brachii tendon

A significant structure located near the biceps brachii insertion is called the lacertus fibrosus; it wraps around the radial tuberosity and serves as an additional stabilizing structure of the biceps insertion at the insertion site. There are 4 acoustic windows to visualize the biceps brachii insertion: anterior, medial, lateral, and posterior(Jacobsen J. 2017). For the purposes of this book we are going to detail the anterior, lateral and posterior window approach to sonographically evaluate the distal biceps brachii (Figures 2.3-2.5). Scanning the insertion of the distal biceps brachii in the anterior window is one of the most difficult exams to perform in the field of musculoskeletal ultrasound because of the way the tendon dives deeply as it crosses the joint to its insertion to the radial tuberosity. To become a good interventionist for distal biceps brachii pathology, the provider must learn how to identify the region accurately and reliably.

Figure 2.4: Distal Biceps Tendon: Anterior Window

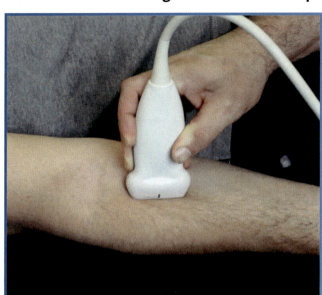 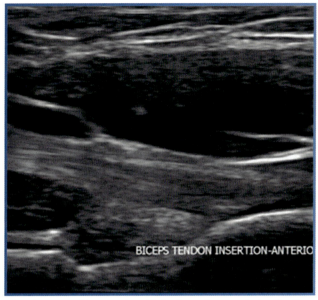

The patient is positioned in supine with elbow in full extension and full supination. The probe is in line or long axis to the fibers of the biceps brachii.

The ultrasound image should display a hyperechoic, fibrillar tendon at its insertion to the radial tuberosity. Bicipital-radial bursa is located between the deep aspect of the radius and the biceps tendon

If there is suspicion for a complete rupture of the biceps tendon, it can be confirmed by ultrasound and/or MRI. Regenerative medicine techniques are not going to regenerate complete tears and thus most often require surgical intervention. If unsure whether you are dealing with a complete tear on ultrasound imaging, you can always get an MRI and then review the images to confirm.

The flexor surfaces of the body are more difficult to inject because the anterior forearm is sensitive to needle puncture and patients are often anticipating pain. So how do we manage this? With the biceps tendon injection, there are multiple approaches to consider, we prefer to use the posterior approach. The reason for this is twofold: 1) the posterior aspect of the forearm is not as sensitive as the volar surface and does not elicit the same sensory effect as the volar surface would and 2) The posterior approach mitigates risk for penetrating neurovascular structures found anteriorly. For the posterior approach, the patient is positioned supine with the elbow flexed and wrist in pronation (Figure 2.5). The needle is moved from radial to ulnar in-plane with the probe (Figure 2.6).

CHAPTER 19 - THE ELBOW

Figure 2.5: Distal Biceps Tendon: Posterior approach

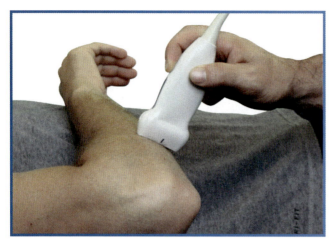
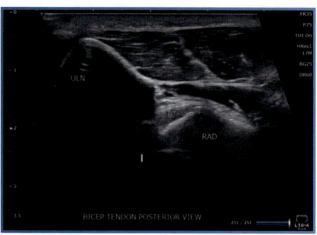

The patient is positioned Supine with shoulder slight abduction, and elbow flexed to 90 degrees, with full pronation.

Place the probe perpendicular to the radius and ulna in the mid forearm in the short axis. From here, sweep proximally until the "bird's beak" appearance of the distal biceps is visualized. (ULN=Ulna, RAD=Radius, BT=Biceps Tendon)

Figure 2.6: Distal Biceps Tendon: Lateral Window

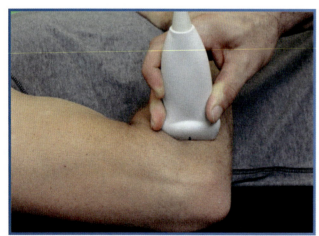
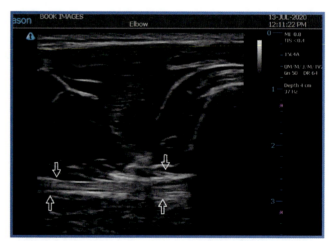

The patient is positioned in supine or seated with the elbow flexed to 90 degrees with the forearm in neutral. The probe is placed perpendicular to the radius and supinator muscle and in plane/longitudinal with the humeral shaft.

The ultrasound image of the biceps brachii lateral window should produce a hyperechoic/fibrillar and linear structure. The radius is visualized in the short axis with the supinator muscle cross section adjacently located to it. To best visualize the tendon have the patient actively or passively pronate-supinate the forearm to confirm tendon visualization.

EXOSOMES, PRP, AND STEM CELLS IN MUSCULOSKELETAL MEDICINE ©

CHAPTER 19 - THE ELBOW

Figure 2.7: Posterior approach to the biceps brachii

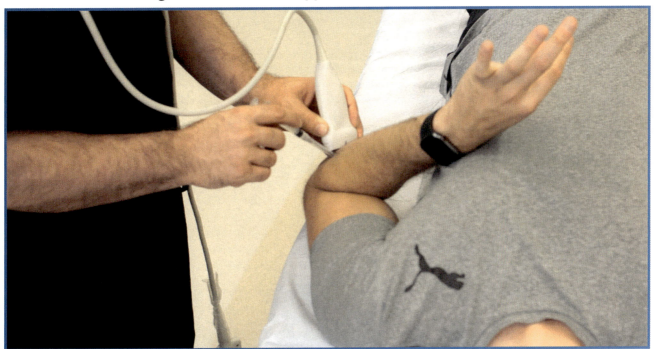

The patient is positioned supine with the elbow flexed and forearm pronated to expose the tendon insertion. The ultrasound is in the long axis to the insertion and the needle is moved radial to ulnar, in-plane with the probe.

Figure 2.8: Ultrasound image of the distal biceps in the posterior window

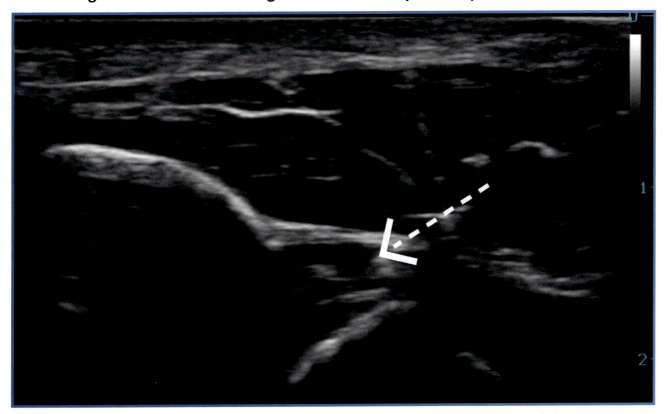

The ulna is on the left and the radius is on the right. The needle is visualized moving from radial to ulnar in-plane with the probe.

The lateral approach can also be used to insert the needle to the biceps insertion. The lateral window to the biceps brachii is not the preferred approach because the distal tendon-bone insertion cannot be visualized. It can still be a very effective means of treating the distal biceps brachii 1-2cm proximal to the insertion but also through the "downstream" effect it can have to the distal tendon-bone relationship. This approach also mitigates risk for penetration of neurovascular structures as well as being very patient-friendly. To perform an injection using this approach, the patient is positioned supine with the elbow flexed and palm to their belly button (Figure 2.7). The provider can confirm this is the biceps tendon by pronating and supinating the wrist either passively or actively. Once the biceps tendon has been located, the needle will move proximal to distal in relation to the tendon in-plane with the probe (Figure 2.9).

Figure 2.9: The lateral approach to the distal biceps brachii

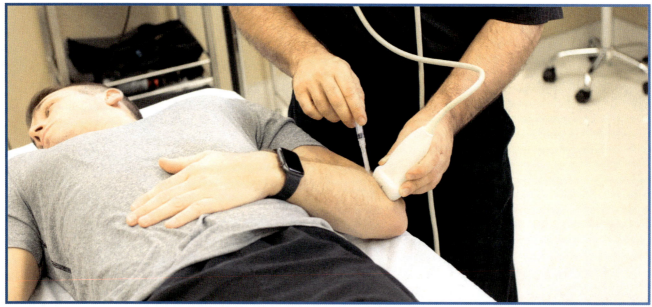

The patient is positioned supine with the elbow flexed and resting on the abdomen. The biceps tendon is visualized in the long axis in the lateral window and the needle is moved proximal to distal, in-plane with the probe.

Figure 2.10: Distal biceps tendon in the long axis lateral window

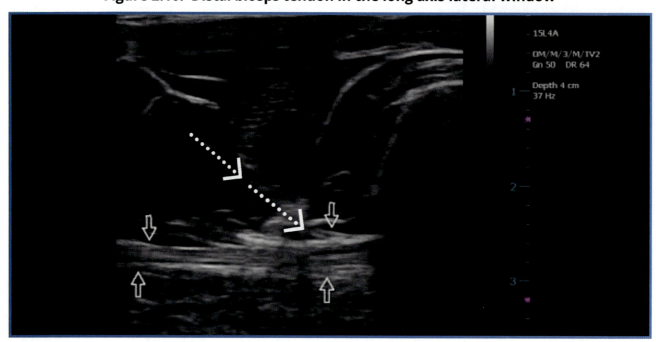

The needle is moving proximal to distal in-plane with the probe

CHAPTER 19 - THE ELBOW

Bicipital Radial Bursa

In the region of the biceps brachii insertion, the provider needs to be familiar with a piece of anatomy called the bicipital radial bursa. The bicipital radial bursa changes with flexion and extension and provides some cushion between the biceps brachii tendon and the radius (Sofka et al., 2004). If the patient pronates the arm, the bicipital radial bursa gets bigger and when the patient supinates, it gets smaller. Look at the graphic below, with an injury to the distal biceps the bursa can fill with fluid (Figure 2.9). Care needs to be taken to first assess the health of the biceps brachii insertion. Often when there is a lot of fluid extravasation it is secondary to a large biceps rupture. In these cases, PRP and stem cells would not help the patient because there aren't enough intact fibers to generate new tissue. When imaging the bicipital radial bursa anteriorly in preparation for an ultrasound guided procedure a direct approach can be taken from distal to proximal from radial to ulnar making sure to visualize the lateral aspect of the biceps brachii insertion as this is where the bursa lies (Figure 2.10 and 2.11). Take extra care to avoid the neurovascular structures that lie in this region by using the Doppler feature on the ultrasound as a guide.

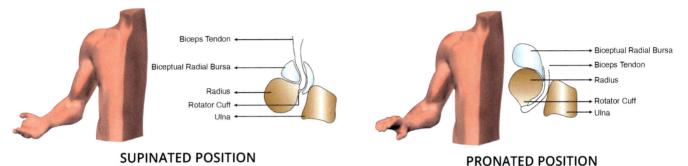

Figure 2.11: The bicipital radial bursa becomes impinged and can get larger in wrist/forearm pronation which becomes more pronounced with a large injury to the distal biceps brachii.

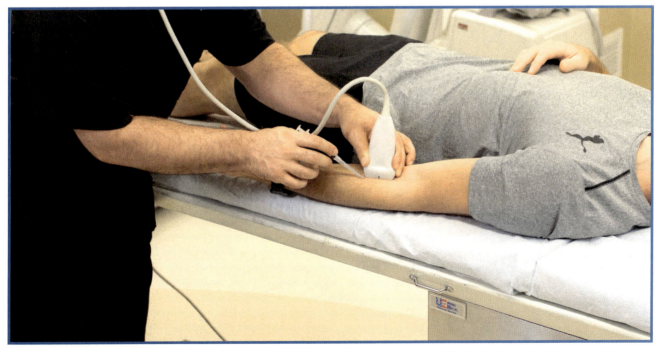

Figure 2.12: Ultrasound guided injection technique to the bicipital radial bursa. The patient is positioned supine with the elbow in full extension and supination. The bursa and biceps tendon is visualized in the long axis and the needle is moved distal to proximal, in-plane with the probe taking careful attention to locate the neurovascular bundle prior to the procedure.

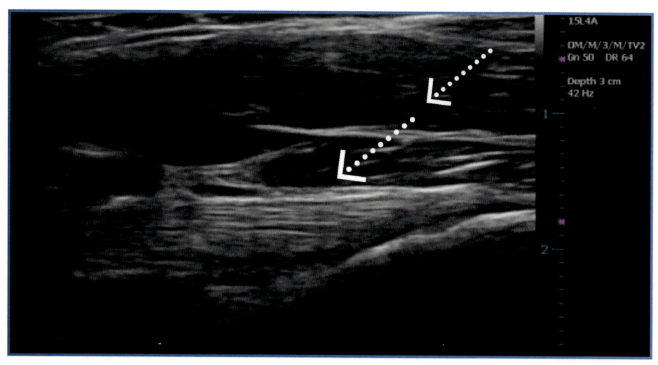

Figure 2.13: Ultrasound image of distal biceps tendon anterior window. Needle is moving towards the bicipital radial bursa from distal to proximal in-plane with the probe.

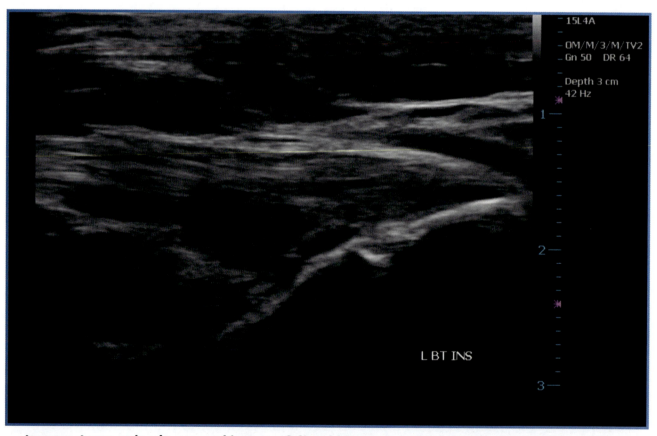

Image: Long axis ultrasound image of distal biceps brachii insertional tendinopathy in the anterior window as evidenced with atypical tendon-bone relationship at the radial tuberosity

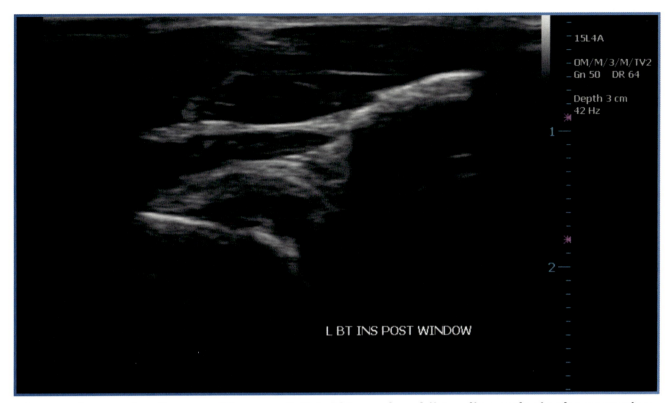

Image: Long axis ultrasound image of distal biceps brachii tendinopathy in the posterior window as evidenced by hypoechoic clefting and cortical irregularity of the bony attachment site.

Anterior Elbow Musculature

As mentioned earlier, cross sectional anatomy of the soft tissue anatomy in the anterior elbow is analogous to a pyramid (Figure 2.12). The base of the pyramid is formed by the ulna, radius and humerus. In the middle section of the pyramid from ulnar to radial the muscle cross sections are brachioradialis, brachialis and pronator teres. The biceps brachii tendon, vessels and median nerve all sit at the apex of the pyramid (Figure 2.13). The brachialis muscle originates at the mid portion of the humerus and inserts to the coronoid process of the ulna and is innervated by C5 and C6 and, also like the biceps brachii, is supplied by the brachial artery. Sonographically, the brachialis and biceps brachii insertion look very similar (Figure 2.14). When performing percutaneous procedures to the biceps brachii, extra care should be taken to confirm that you aren't in the brachialis and store the images accordingly.

Another muscle group that is important to conceptualize is the brachioradialis muscle. The brachioradialis originates at the lateral supracondylar ridge of the humerus and inserts on the distal radius at the proximal aspect of the radial styloid process. Its primary action is elbow flexion and lies laterally crossing the elbow joint. The brachioradialis does not have much clinical application when it comes to musculoskeletal disorders so we will not talk much beyond its anatomic location and action.

CHAPTER 19 - THE ELBOW

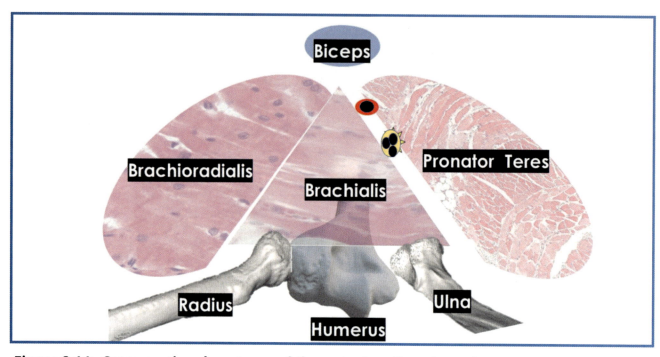

Figure 2.14: Cross sectional anatomy of the anterior elbow is analogous to a pyramid. The osseous structures form the base, the musculature form the middle portion and the biceps tendon is at the apex.

Figure 2.15: Anterior Elbow: The anterior triangle or pyramid

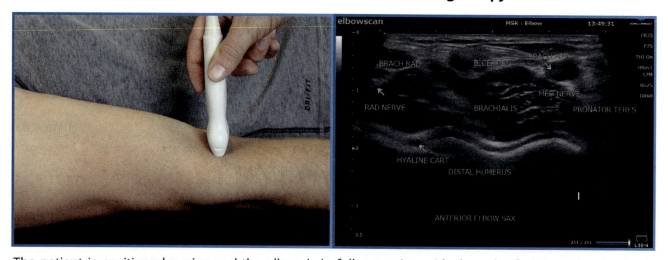

The patient is positioned supine and the elbow is in full extension with the palm facing up (supination). Place the probe in the short axis at the distal humerus and sweep proximally and distally. The brachial artery should be visualized superficially with the median nerve

CHAPTER 19 - THE ELBOW

Figure 2.16: Distal Brachialis Insertion

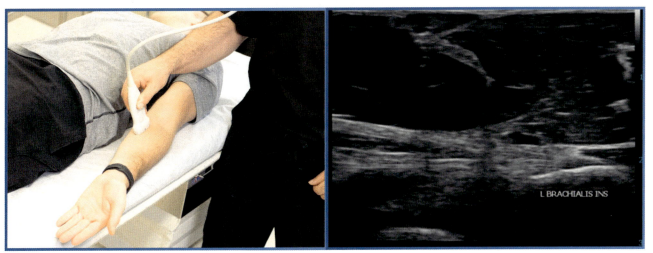

The brachialis is best viewed with the probe in the same plane as the distal biceps in the anterior window. To best visualize the brachialis insertion, the clinician should angle the distal end of the probe toward the proximal-medial ulnar tuberosity where the brachialis attaches.

The ultrasound image of the the brachialis has a very similar appearance to the biceps brachii at its insertion to the coronoid process and should be differentiated from the biceps anterior window by directing the distal end of the probe toward the ulna coronoid process instead of the radius.

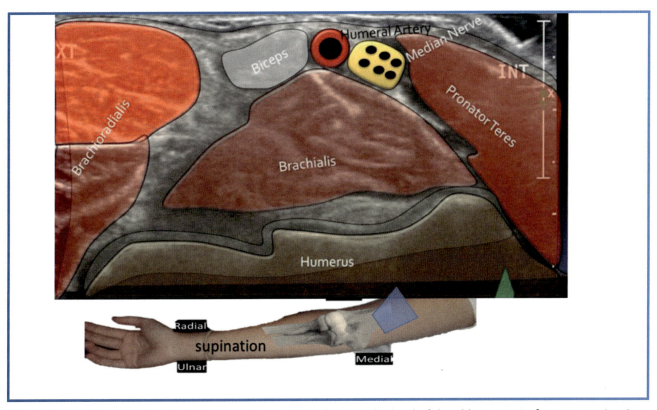

Illustration and Image: Short axis image of antecubital fossa at the level of distal humerus in forearm supination

A COMPLETE GUIDE TO REGENERATIVE MEDICINE ©

CHAPTER 19 - THE ELBOW

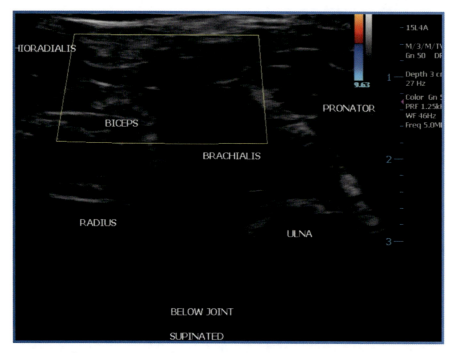

Image: Short axis image of antecubital fossa at the level of proximal radius and ulna in forearm supination

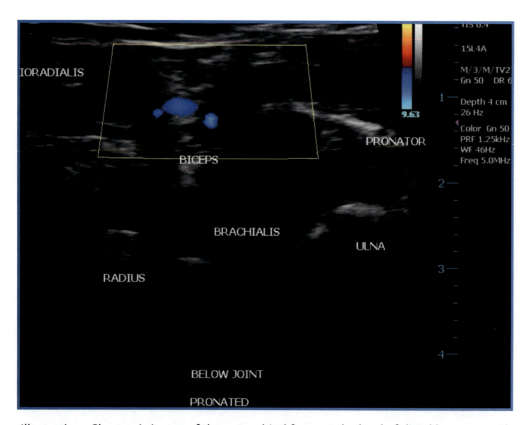

Illustration: Short axis image of the antecubital fossa at the level of distal humerus with forearm in pronation

EXOSOMES, PRP, AND STEM CELLS IN MUSCULOSKELETAL MEDICINE ©

Similar to brachioradialis, the supinator is another muscle group that needs to be conceptualized from an anatomic and sono-anatomy perspective (Figure 2.15). There are two heads of the supinator muscle, superficial and deep. The origin of the supinator can be found in multiple locations: lateral epicondyle, supinator crest, radial collateral ligament and the annular ligament. The superficial fibers wrap around the upper portion of the radius and insert onto the lateral edge of the radial tuberosity and the oblique line of the radius. The superficial fibers can insert as far distal as the insertion of the pronator teres. The deep fibers originate and form a membranous-like fascia that encompass the neck of the radius above the tuberosity and attaches posterior-medially; the majority the deep layer supinator inserts into the dorsal and lateral surfaces of the body of the radius, midway between the oblique line and the head of the bone. Due to its location adjacent to the lateral epicondyle, biceps brachii insertion and the brachialis insertion it is important to understand the supinator. The most common clinical scenario where the supinator is involved are cases of "supinator syndrome" where the radial nerve becomes impinged or entrapped at its entrance through the Arcade of Frohse prior to "splitting" the superficial and deep heads of the supinator.

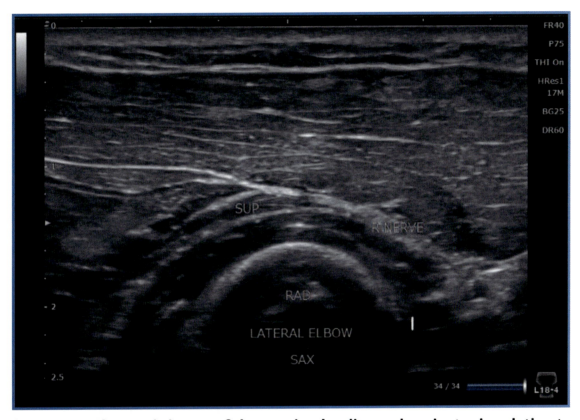

Figure 2.17: Short axis image of the proximal radius and supinator in relation to the radial nerve which splits the deep and superficial heads, is also visualized in short axis (SUP=Supinator, RAD=Radius, R Nerve=Radial Nerve)

Triceps/Posterior Elbow

The triceps has three heads located on the posterior aspect of the elbow/humerus and functions as the primary extensor of the elbow. The long head originates from the inferior aspect of the infraglenoid tubercle of the scapula, the medial head from the posterior surface of the humerus (inferior to radial groove) and the lateral head from the posterior surface of the humerus (superior to radial groove). The three three heads converge into an aponeurosis inserting onto the olecranon forming the triceps brachii insertion proper (Figure 2.16 and 2.17).

Injuries to the triceps brachii typically occur at the tendon insertion from mechanisms involving rapid eccentric force, or contusion. Occasionally there may be an avulsion fracture of the olecranon with a rupture of the superficial portion of the tendon attachment so if a calcification is visualized, don't assume this is an enthesophyte from a rheumatologic disorder. Look at the contralateral side and you can always get an MRI to see if there is a tear. With large ruptures, the superficial aspect of the tendon usually tears first. These cases typically involve distal triceps tendon insertion, typically partial thickness, where the superficial layer is torn with the long and lateral head. The deeper layers are usually intact. In many instances, the medial head remains intact while the lateral head usually tears 1-2 cm superficially. Injections to the tendon with orthobiologics (either PRP or stem cell) should start with the patient in supine or seated comfortably with the affected elbow flexed and resting on their abdomen (Figure 2.18). The triceps tendon is visualized in the long axis with the needle moving from proximal to distal in plane with the probe (Figure 2.19).

Figure 2.18: Distal Triceps Brachii Insertion Long Axis

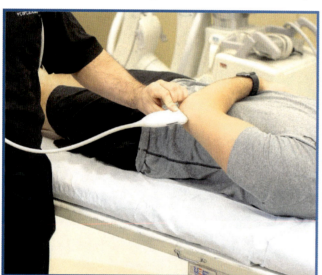
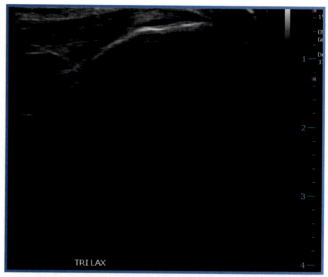
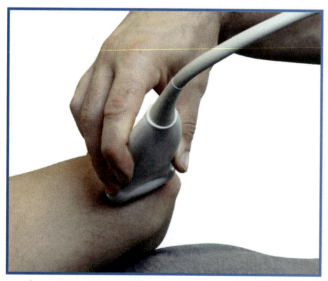
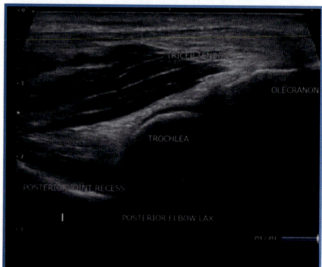

The patient is positioned in supine with the elbow in slight flexion resting across their abdomen. The probe is placed in parallel or long axis to the triceps muscle-tendon complex.

The long axis ultrasound image shows the triceps myotendon junction most superficial as well as the distal insertion. Deep to the triceps myotendon junction, the posterior fat pad/olecranon fossa are visualized

Figure 2.19: Distal Triceps Brachii Insertion Short Axis

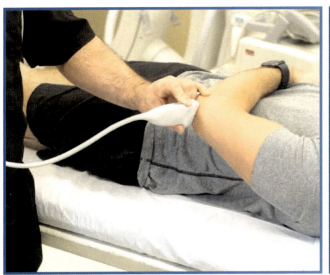
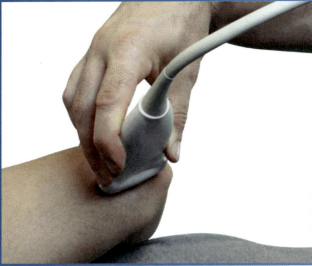

The patient is positioned in supine with elbow in flexion resting across their torso. The probe is positioned slightly proximal to the distal triceps insertion. The probe is placed in the short axis, perpendicular to the distal humerus and triceps muscle.

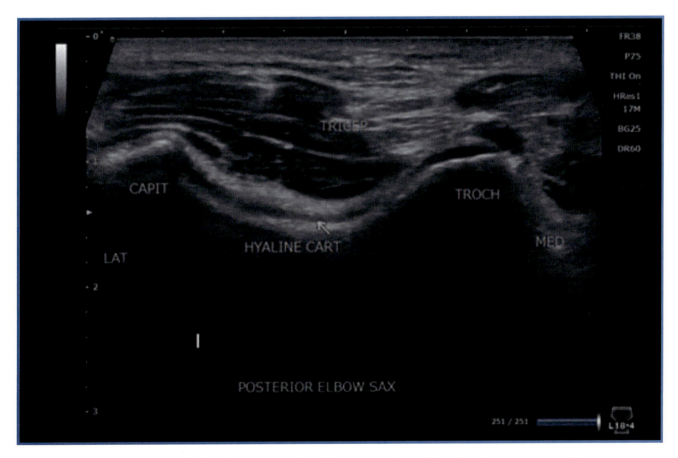

The ultrasound picture should display the medial and lateral portion of the distal humerus as well as triceps myotendon junction. This image is a good window to visualize the hyaline cartilage of the distal humerus

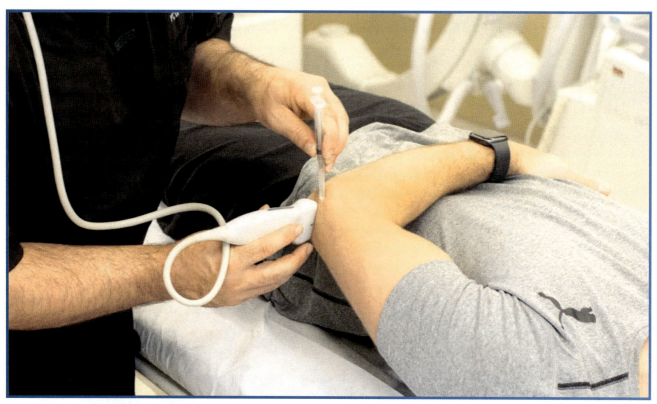

Figure 2.20: Ultrasound guided injection technique to the distal triceps. The patient is positioned supine with the elbow flexed and resting on the abdomen. The distal tendon is visualized in the short axis and the needle is moved lateral to medial, in-plane with the probe.

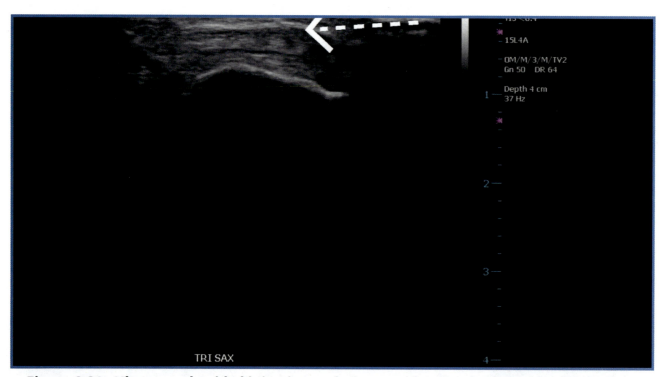

Figure 2.21: Ultrasound guided injection technique to the distal triceps brachii tendon. The tendon is visualized in the short axis and the needle is moved lateral to medial, in-plane with the probe.

CHAPTER 19 - THE ELBOW

Lateral Elbow

At the lateral epicondyle, the muscle-tendon attachments to the bony landmark are all named for their movement pattern: the extensor carpi radialis, the extensor digitorum, the extensor digitorum minimi, and the extensor carpi ulnaris. The ultrasound appearance of the lateral epicondyle is analogous to a ski slope with the proximal end being the top of the slope and the radio-capitellar joint being the bottom. The ultrasound image of the common extensor tendon itself should be hyperechoic, fibrillar/linear and fairly homogeneous in terms of echotexture and shape (Figure 2.20). The common extensor tendon shares roughly 50% of the bony footprint with the radial collateral ligament (Jacobsen et al., 2014) (Figure 2.21 and 2.22). This lateral epicondylar region is vulnerable to chronic strain and tendinopathic formation and patients who suffer epicondylalgia will often complain of pain with daily activities such as reaching with the elbow extended for a cup of water, opening a heavy door, and operating a keyboard and/or mouse. Injection to this area should be performed with the patient in supine with arm flexed and palm resting by their side or on the abdomen (2.23). The provider should visualize the common extensor tendon in the long axis and move the needle from distal to proximal in plane with the probe (2.24).

Figure 2.22: Lateral Epicondyle/Longitudinal/LAX

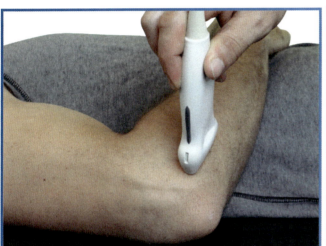

Patient is positioned in supine or seated with elbow flexed 45-90 degrees. The probe is placed in-plane or long axis to the extensor group of muscles on the forearm and parallel with the radius and lateral epicondyle.

The ultrasound image shows a hyperechoic "ski slope" at the common extensor tendon origin and also where the radial collateral ligament attaches. The common extensor tendon is hyperechoic/fibrillar at the tendon-bone interface. Appreciate the common shared footprint of the common extensor tendon and the radial collateral ligament (CET=Common Extensor Tendon, RCL=Radial Collateral Ligament, RAD Head=Radial Head, Annular LIG=Annular Ligament)

CHAPTER 19 - THE ELBOW

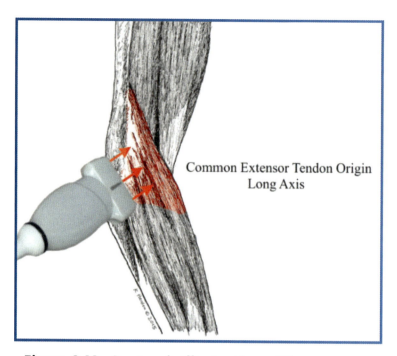

Figure 2.23: Anatomic Illustration of the common extensor tendon in long axis

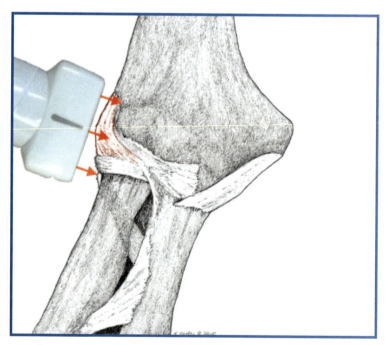

Figure 2.24: Anatomic illustration of the radial collateral ligament in long axis

CHAPTER 19 - THE ELBOW

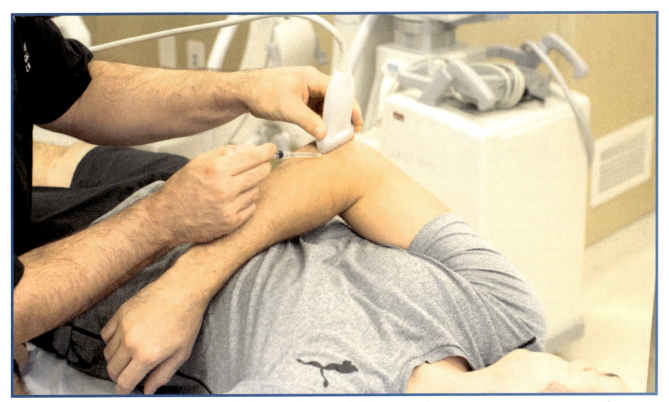

Figure 2.25: Ultrasound guided injection technique to the common extensor tendon. The patient is comfortably positioned supine with the elbow flexed and resting over the abdomen. The tendon is visualized in the long axis and the needle is moved distal to proximal, in-plane with the probe.

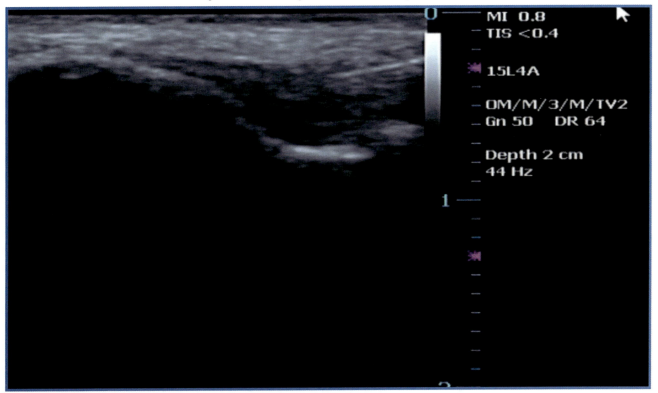

Figure 2.26: Ultrasound image of common extensor tendon in long axis with the needle moving distal to proximal in-plane with the probe. Note how the image of the tendon and lateral epicondyle were shifted to bring the tendon closer to the needle

CHAPTER 19 - THE ELBOW

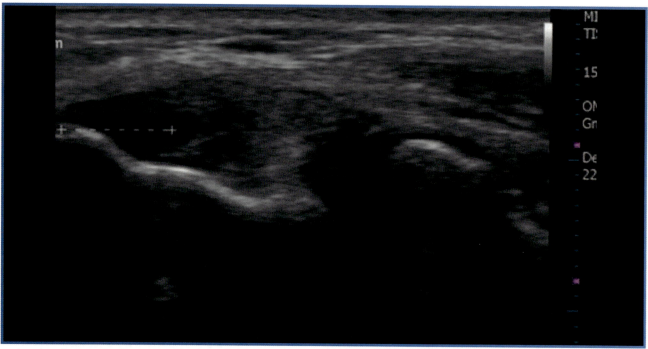

Image: long axis ultrasound image of the common extensor tendinopathy. The caliper markings indicate the hypoechoic region of tendinopathic formation.

Medial Elbow

All flexors of the forearm/wrist attach to the medial epicondylar region. The flexor carpi radialis, the flexor carpi ulnaris, the flexor digitorum superficialis, and the pronator teres form the common flexor tendon attachment at the medial epicondyle (Figure 2.25 and 2.26).

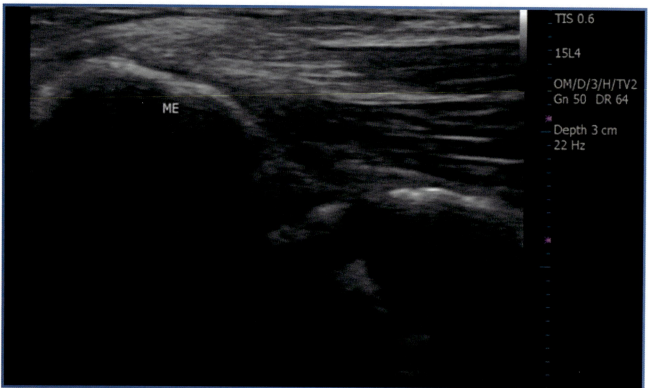

Figure 2.27: Long axis image of the common flexor tendon at the medial epicondyle (ME). The proximal tendon is visualized as a parrots beak attaching to the bony landmark on the upper left.

CHAPTER 19 - THE ELBOW

Figure 2.28: Medial Epicondyle: Longitudinal/LAX

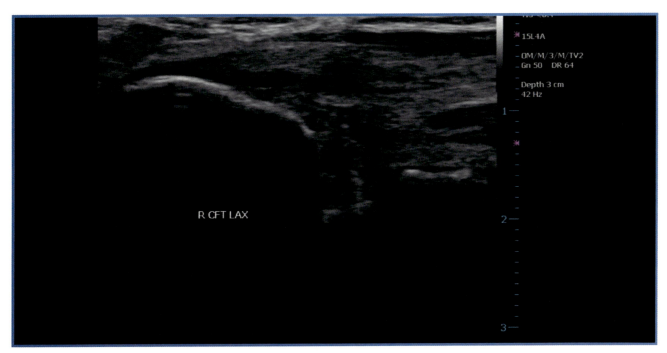

The patient is positioned in supine or on the affected side of the elbow with the elbow in full extension. The probe is placed in longitudinally/long axis to the wrist flexor muscle groups and parallel to the medial epicondyle and the ulna. The ultrasound image displays a hyperechoic/fibrillar "parrot's beak" appearance at the common flexor origin. (ME=Medial Epicondyle)

The medial epicondyle has a ski-slope appearance similar to the lateral epicondyle but; in contrast to the lateral epicondyle, does not share a footprint with the ulnar collateral ligament (Figure 2.26). Normal appearance of the common flexor tendon origin is similar to the common extensor tendon. The fibers should be linear, hyperechoic and relatively homogeneous in its shape. Common characteristics of common flexor tendinopathy are hypoechoic clefting (Figure 2.27), thickened, heterogeneous tendon shape pattern as well as the occasional enthesophyte formation at the proximal tendon-bone attachment site. Posterior to the medial epicondyle, the ulnar nerve travels through the osseous cubital tunnel consisting of the olecranon and medial epicondyle (Figure 2.28 and 2.29).

Figure 2.28: Long axis ultrasound image of common flexor tendinopathy as evidenced with tendon thickening and longitudinal hypoechoic clefting through the tendon midsubstance

Figure 2.29: Ulnar Nerve: Transverse/SAX

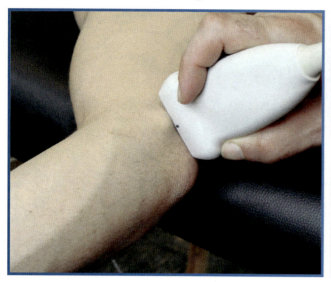
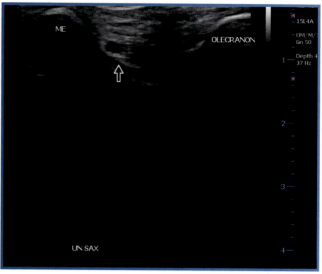

With the patient supine, slightly abduct the shoulder and place the elbow in 90° flexion and external rotation. Palpate the medial epicondyle and place the probe in the short axis just inferior to it over the cubital tunnel. The ulnar nerve is visualized in the cubital tunnel as a hyperechoic oval structure between the hyperechoic medial epicondyle and olecranon. Move the probe distally to examine the cubital tunnel retinaculum that can be seen superficially as a hyperechoic band overlying the medial epicondyle and olecranon. The medial head of the triceps tendon can be visualized overlying the olecranon as well.

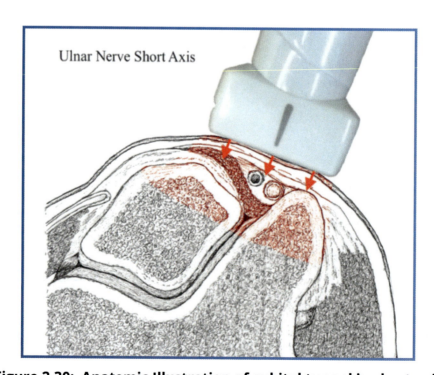

Figure 2.30: Anatomic Illustration of cubital tunnel in short axis

When delivering orthobiologics to the medial epicondyle, we encourage providers to visualize the structure in the long axis and move the needle distal to proximal, in-plane with the probe. The patient should be comfortably supine or side lying on the affected side and the same thing is true for the lateral epicondyle (Figure 2.30). We advise both the common flexor and extensor tendon be visualized in long axis, moving the needle distal to proximal in plane with the probe (Figure 2.31). This is very important because in both instances the provider will be able to visualize the apex of the tendon origin and it also becomes easier to fan out the PRP or stem cells. This is also the same approach when performing microtenotomy and fenestration of the diseased tendon fibers. Micro-tenotomy and fenestration techniques have demonstrated positive outcomes in the medial and lateral epicondylar region (along with other tendons) and are an excellent adjunct to orthobiologics because the healthy inflammation cascade it generates helps to synergistically heal the diseased tissues (Jacobsen et al., 2016).

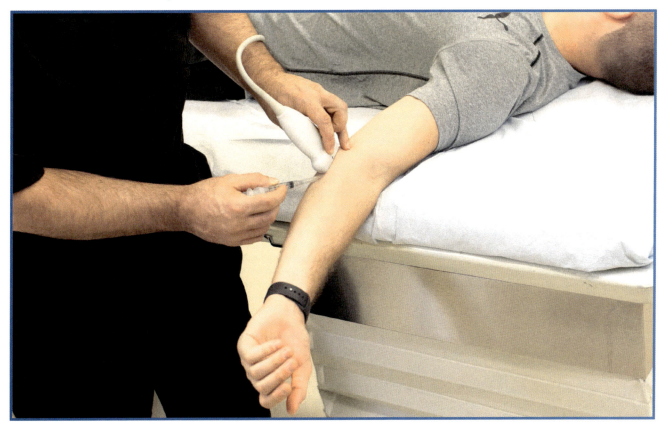

Figure 2.31: Ultrasound guided injection technique to the medial epicondyle and common flexor tendon. The patient is positioned supine with the elbow in full extension while the needle is moved distal to proximal, in-plane with the probe.

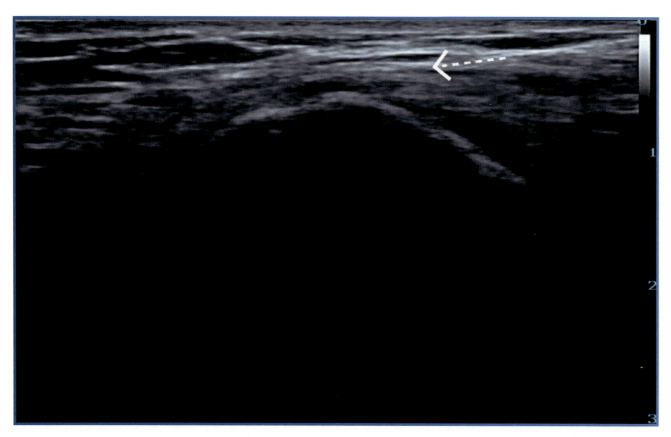

Figure 2.32: Long axis image of the common flexor tendon and medial epicondyle. The needle is visualized moving from distal to proximal in-plane with the probe

Injuries to the medial elbow ligaments are fairly common and are usually found in throwing athletes, competitive strength athletes or those in mixed martial arts and wrestling. The ulnar collateral ligamentous complex connects the medial epicondyle to the sublime tubercle of the ulna and is the primary passive restraint against excessive elbow valgus stress (figure 2.32). When performing this exam with ultrasound, the elbow is in 30-40 degrees of flexion with a slight valgus stress which places the structure on a stretch making the ligament appear more echogenic underneath the transducer (Figure 2.33). There are three portions of the UCL – the anterior band, the oblique band, and the posterior band. The anterior band of the UCL is the main stabilizer of elbow valgus stressors and, for the purposes of this book, is what we will identify with musculoskeletal ultrasound.

When injecting the ulnar collateral ligament we advise the provider to visualize the anterior band in the long axis and move the needle distal to proximal in plane with the probe while the patient is either in supine or side lying on the affected extremity with elbow in slight flexion (Figure 2.34). The needle is moved distal to proximal, in-plane with the probe (Figure 2.35).

CHAPTER 19 - THE ELBOW

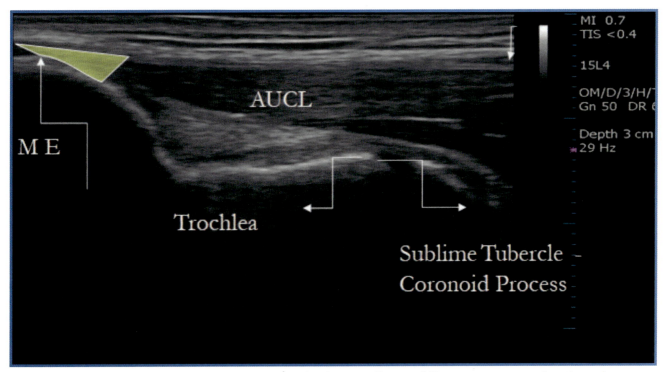

Figure 2.33: Long axis image of a normal ulnar collateral ligament. Bony landmarks are the medial epicondyle on the left and sublime tubercle of ulna on the right (ME-Medial Epicondyle, Yellow=Common flexor tendon origin, AUCL=Anterior Band Ulnar Collateral Ligament).

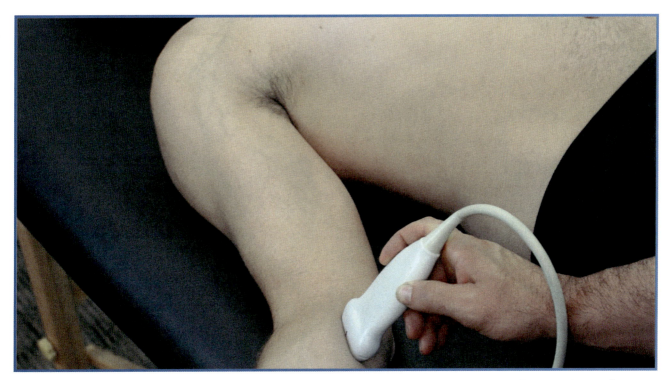

Figure 2.34: Ulnar collateral ligament visualization. The probe is in long axis to the ligament and the patient position is supine or side lying on the ipsilateral side

CHAPTER 19 - THE ELBOW

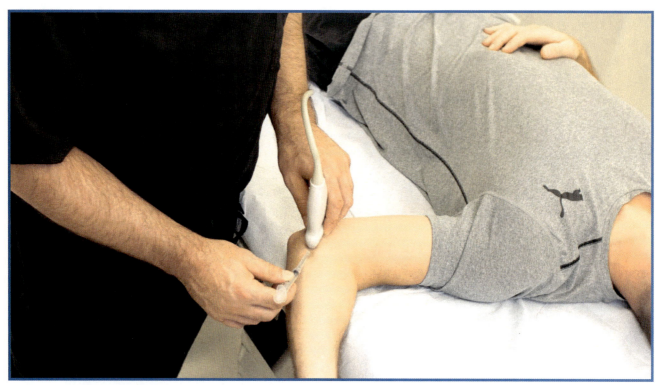

Figure 2.35: Ultrasound guided injection technique to the ulnar collateral ligament. The patient is positioned supine with the shoulder abducted slightly and the elbow flexed roughly 30-40 degrees. The probe is aligned in the long axis to the ligament and the needle is moved distal to proximal, in-plane with the probe.

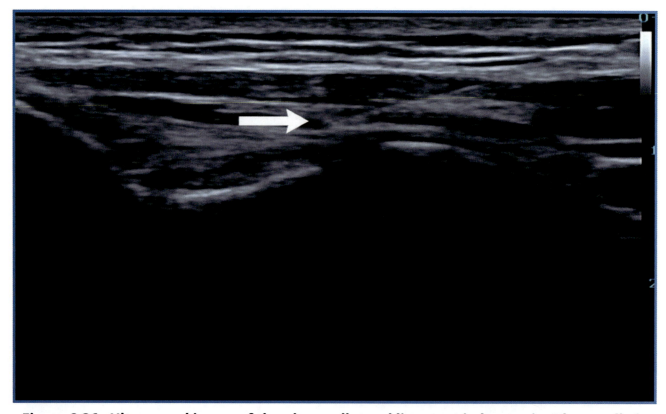

Figure 2.36: Ultrasound image of the ulnar collateral ligament in long axis. The needle is visualized moving distal to proximal in-plane with the probe.

CHAPTER 19 - THE ELBOW

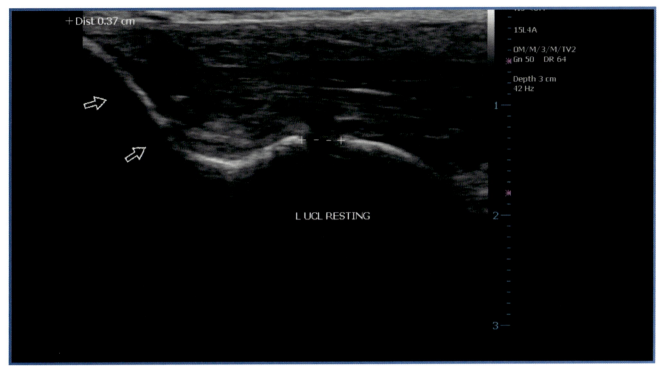

Image: Long axis ultrasound image of a partial tear in the ulnar collateral ligament. The elbow is in a rested position with caliper measurements measuring the joint space width. The arrows are pointing to the irregular, hypoechoic ligament-bone interface at the humeral attachment.

Sample Dictations:

The procedure and potential complications were discussed with the patient. After written and verbal consent were obtained, the patient was placed in the seated position. A tourniquet was placed on the [RIGHT] arm and the area was surveyed for large palpable veins. The antecubital area was prepped and draped in the usual sterile fashion using alcohol. Using an 20G needle, approximately [ ] ccs of blood was drawn from the patient and transferred to a specially prepared PRP tube containing anticoagulants. After the needle was removed, and a sterile bandage was placed over the entry site, the tube was vertically rotated back and forth five times.

The tube was placed in a centrifuge with an opposing counter-weight. After five minutes, the tube was removed and inspected. There was a visible gel, a buffy coat, and a golden liquid layer of PRP. The tube was vertically rotated back and forth five times. Afterwards, the PRP and buffy coat were gently extracted and transferred to a 10 cc syringe. The syringe was attached to a 22G 1.5" needle.

[Patient positioning as described above depending on the type of injection and approach]

The elbow was prepped and draped in the usual sterile manner using three coats of betadine. The area of interest was identified using sonography. With the probe held in place, a ½ a cc of 1% lidocaine was used to create a wheel at the entry site alongside the probe. The needle guidance software package was turned on. After a moment, with the probe held in place, the needle and syringe containing the PRP was advanced through the skin and the deeper tissues towards the target area. Under ultrasound guidance, the PRP was injected. The final image was recorded. The probe was moved, the needle was removed and a sterile gauze was held over the injection site with gentle pressure. A sterile bandage was applied. The patient was repositioned for comfort. The patient tolerated the procedure well with no apparent complications.

References:

Jacobsen J. Fundamentals of Musculoskeletal Ultrasound (3rd edition). Page 75. Elsevier, Sep 2017.

Sofka CM, Adler RS. Sonography of cubital bursitis. AJR Am J Roentgenol. 2004;183 (1): 51-3. doi:10.2214/ajr.183.1.1830051

Jacobson et al, Radial Collateral Ligament of the Elbow: Sonographic Characterization with Cadaveric Dissection Correlation and Magnetic Resonance Arthrography. J Ultrasound, Med. 2014;33:1041-1048

Jon A. Jacobson et al., Ultrasound Guided Percutaneous Tenotomy. Seminar in Musculoskeletal Radiology. 2016; 20(05): 414-421

CHAPTER 20 The Hand and Wrist

Colin Rigney, Pradeep Albert & Devi Nampiaparampil

> **CHAPTER PREVIEW**
>
> In this chapter we will cover sonoanatomy of the hand/wrist complex as well as patient and probe positions for proper evaluation. Additionally, the chapter will include common pictorial examples and explanations of pathology found with ultrasound as well as basic ultrasound-guided injection techniques.

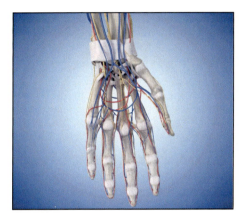

Patient Selection for Injection:
The type of procedure performed depends on the patient's clinical signs and symptoms.

For carpal tunnel injection:
Numbness, tingling and pain along the palmar surface of the hand

For De Quervain's tenosynovitis:
Pain in thumb with abduction and extension

For first metacarpal tunnel injection:
Pain with movements of the thumb

Small joints of the hand:
Stiffness and pain

Contraindications to Injection:
Systemic infection
Infection or rash over the puncture site
Coagulopathy (International Normalized Ratio [INR] > 1.3 or platelets < 50,000/ mm3)
Inability to reach target site because of prior surgery or scar tissue

Equipment and Supplies:
Alcohol swabs
Tourniquet
18G or 20G needle for blood draw
Tubing
PRP Kit
Gauze
Betadine or Chlorhexidine
Sterile drapes
Sterile gloves
Sterile ultrasound gel
Tuberculin syringe with needle (optional for local anesthetic in the skin)
Syringes
Bandaid
Positioning aids
Imaging Requirements for Procedure:
Ultrasound with linear high frequency probe

A COMPLETE GUIDE TO REGENERATIVE MEDICINE ©

Precautions:
1% lidocaine can be used for a skin wheal; avoid injecting lidocaine into the deep tissues or mixing it with the PRP

Potential Complications:
Bleeding
Infection
Post-procedural pain
Nerve injury
Risk of pneumothorax for scapulo-thoracic procedures
Vasovagal reactions and ataxia

Post-Procedure Care/ Follow-Up
After the procedure, the patient is observed and questioned nausea and lightheadedness. If there are no signs of a vasovagal reaction, the patient can sit and then stand. The affected area can be actively mobilized in a gentle fashion to spread the PRP.

If a procedural complication occurs, the physician and/ or staff should observe the patient until the symptom resolves. If the patient is vasovagal, consider giving them a snack and some fluids.

Hand/Wrist Anatomy

The wrist and fingers are combined in this chapter. The wrist is a complex joint with numerous bones and tendons with each having its own function (Figure 3.1). We will cover this in an overview so that the most commonly encountered musculoskeletal disorders of the hand/wrist complex will be addressed.

The most clinically relevant musculoskeletal disorders of the hand/wrist complex are found in the triangular fibrocartilage complex (TFCC), trapezium-first metacarpal osteoarthritis, the extensor tendons, the extensor carpi ulnaris, the carpal tunnel and the first extensor compartment (Dequervain's tenosynovitis). We will also include stenosing tenosynovitis of the A1 pulley (annular ligament) system (Figure 3.2). The triangular fibrocartilage complex has high specificity but low sensitivity in visibility of pathology with musculoskeletal ultrasound, and for this reason, if there is suspicion for a cartilage-complex tear with MSK ultrasound the provider can always order an MRI for confirmation.

The osseous anatomy of the wrist comprises the radius, ulna and the proximal carpal row, scaphoid, lunate, the triquetrum and the pisiform. The distal carpal row comprises the trapezium, trapezoid, capitate and the hamate.

Dorsal tendon compartments:

EPB = Extensor Pollicis Brevis
APL = Abductor Pollicis Longus
ECRL= Extensor Carpi Radialis Longus
ECRB = Extensor Carpi Radialis Brevis
EPL = Extensor Pollicis Longus
EIP = Extensor Indicis Proprius
EDC = Extensor Digitorum Communis
EDM = Extensor Digiti Minimi
ECU = Extensor Carpi Ulnaris

CHAPTER 20 - THE HAND AND WRIST

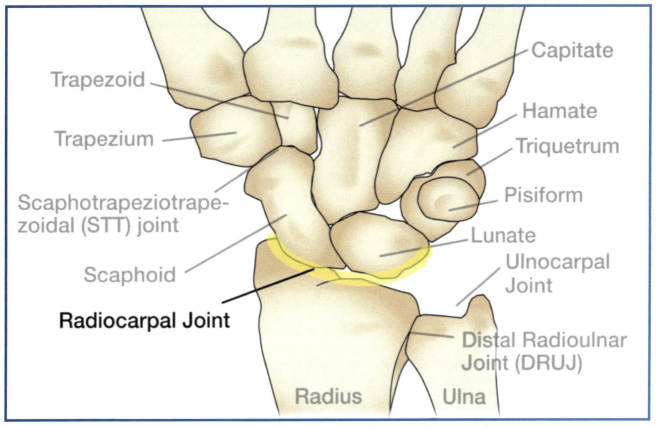

Figure 3.1: Osseous anatomy of the wrist complex

Below is an axial CT image of the wrist detailing the volar/dorsal anatomy of the carpal tunnel and dorsal tendon compartments as well as a coronal T1 MRI detailing the osseous anatomy and triangular fibrocartilage complex (Figure 3.3 and 3.4). These are useful structures to remember as we dig in further.

Compartment	Tendon	Pathology
1	EPB APL	De Quervain's tenosynovitis
2	ECRL ECRB	Intersection syndrome
3	EPL	Traumatic rupture with distal radius f Drummers wrist,
4	EIP EDC Posterior interosseous nerve	Extensor tenosynovitis
5	EDM	Rheumatoid Arthritis
6	ECU	*Snapping ECU, Tenosynovitis, Split Tears*

Figure 3.2: Helpful table to remember the dorsal tendon compartment contents and most common presentation of musculoskeletal disorders in each region

CHAPTER 20 - THE HAND AND WRIST

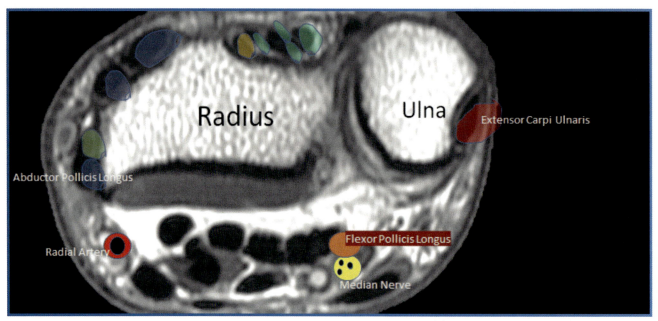

Figure 3.3: Axial CT of the wrist complex volar and dorsal structures

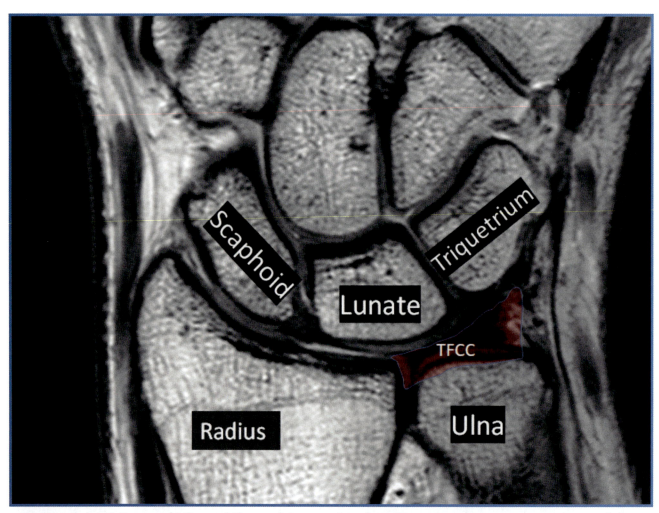

Figure 3.4: T1 Coronal View of the wrist complex detailing the osseous anatomy and the triangular fibrocartilage complex (TFCC)

CHAPTER 20 - THE HAND AND WRIST

Volar/Carpal Tunnel Structures

The carpal tunnel comprises the flexor tendons superficialis and profundus as well as the flexor pollicis longus tendon and the median nerve (Figure 3.5 and 3.6). The flexor carpi radialis tendon is superficial and anatomically outside of the carpal tunnel and located superficial and adjacent to the scaphoid.

The median nerve can be easily identified separate from the rest of the carpal tunnel contents by instructing the patient to "wiggle your fingers."

This can be done either actively or passively. When performed correctly, the flexor superficialis, profundus and pollicis longus tendon will contract and the median nerve will stay static and be "bounced around" by the tendons that are moving. Or using this maneuver in the long axis, the tendons will be seen gliding and the median nerve will not (Figure 3.7). The median nerve is also the most superficial structure within the tunnel. Sonographic characteristics of median nerve inflammation consistent with carpal tunnel syndrome are the following (Ziswiler et al., 2005) (Figure 3.8):

- Median nerve hypoechogenicity
- Circumferential measurement at level of Scaphoid-pisiform: >12mm² with >15mm² being definitive
- Bulging of carpal tunnel and transverse ligament
- Impingement of median nerve visualized in long axis

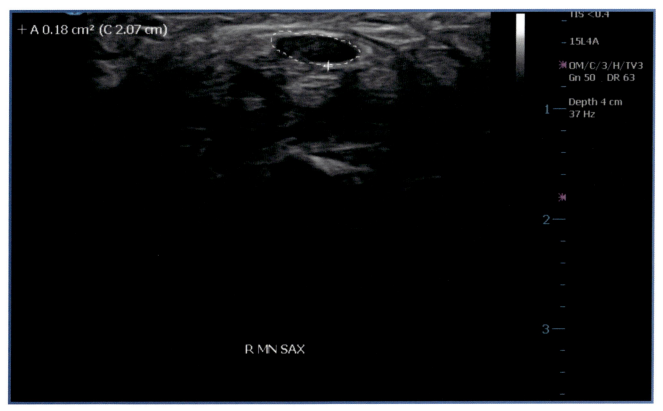

Figure 3.5: Short axis ultrasound image of median nerve swelling in the carpal tunnel as evidenced by the enlarged circumferential measurement of 18mm², hypoechoic nerve swelling and bulging of the transverse ligament

When injecting the carpal tunnel, the patient is positioned in seated or supine with the palm facing up (Figure 3.9). The carpal tunnel should be visualized in the short axis. The needle approach is ulnar to radial in the long axis with the probe. The ulnar to radial approach is the preferred method because it allows for hydrodissection both superficial and deep to the median nerve in the attempt to "free" it up (Figure 3.10). Hydrodissection uses an ultrasound-guided injection of medication or sterile saline to create a perineural fluid plane between the nerve and surrounding tissues and consequently improve the nerve mobility and has been shown to decrease gliding resistance against the nerve from adjacent structures in the carpal tunnel (Housner et al., 2009).

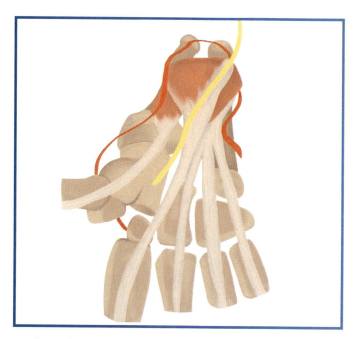

Figure 3.6: The Ventral Surface of the Bones of the Right Hand; Looking at the Median Nerve

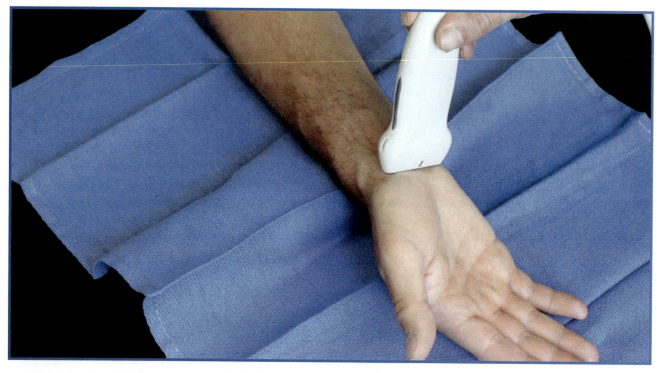

Figure 3.7: Ultrasound probe position to evaluate the volar wrist/carpal tunnel in short axis. The patient should be positioned comfortably in a seated position or supine

CHAPTER 20 - THE HAND AND WRIST

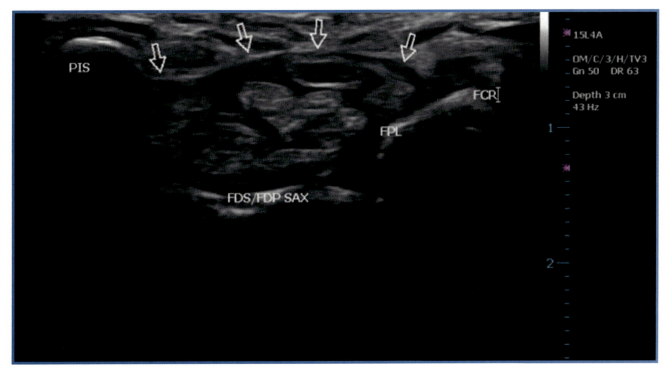

Figure 3.8: Cross Sectional Imaging of the median nerve in the carpal tunnel

The patient is positioned in seated or supine with the wrist in full supination. A gel bottle should be placed underneath the dorsal wrist to bring the volar structures closer to the probe. The probe should be placed at the volar aspect of the wrist at the level of the carpal bones, the pisiform and scaphoid make up the borders of the carpal tunnel. The median nerve is located beneath the flexor retinaculum; you can see the flexor pollicis longus which is deep to the median nerve if the patient wiggles their thumb this moves. The clinician takes a circumferential measurement of the median nerve at this level.

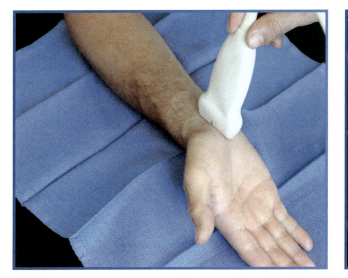
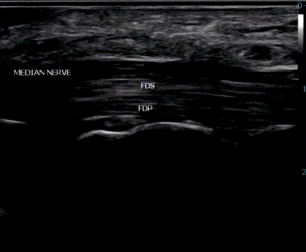

Figure 3.9: Median Nerve: Longitudinal/LAX

Place the probe longitudinally along the distal portion of the wrist. The median nerve courses medially through the transverse retinaculum of the wrist and is best visualized beyond the distal edge of the retinaculum. There can sometimes be anatomic variants to the median nerve such as a bifid nerve.

A COMPLETE GUIDE TO REGENERATIVE MEDICINE ©

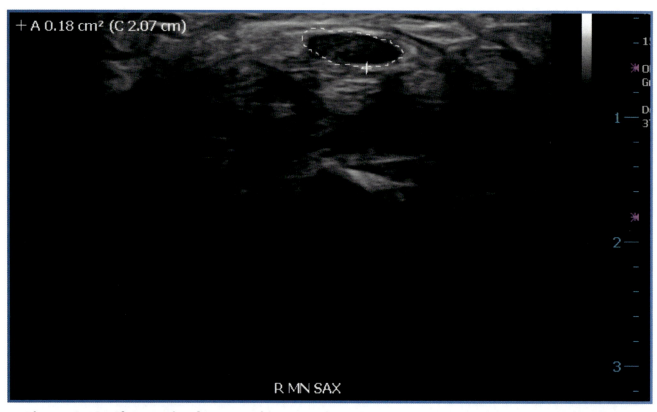

Figure 3.10: Short axis ultrasound image of median nerve swelling in the carpal tunnel as evidenced by the enlarged circumferential measurement of 18mm², hypoechoic nerve swelling and bulging of the transverse ligament

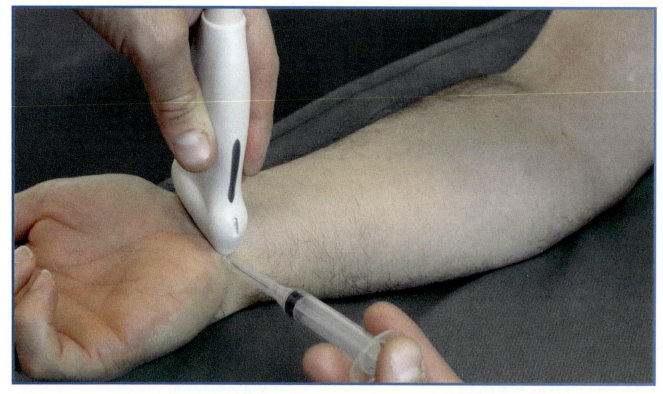

Figure 3.11: Ultrasound guided injection technique for the carpal tunnel. Needle is moved ulnar to radial, in-plane with the probe. The patient is positioned in supine or seated with a gel bottle placed under the wrist for better visualization

CHAPTER 20 - THE HAND AND WRIST

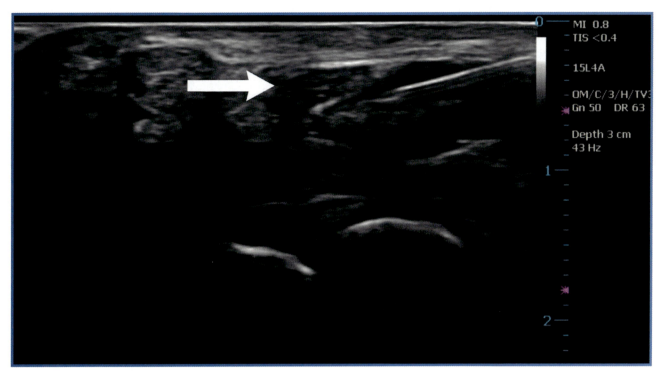

Figure 3.12: Short axis ultrasound image of median nerve swelling in the carpal tunnel as evidenced by the enlarged circumferential measurement of 18mm^2, hypoechoic nerve swelling and bulging of the transverse ligament

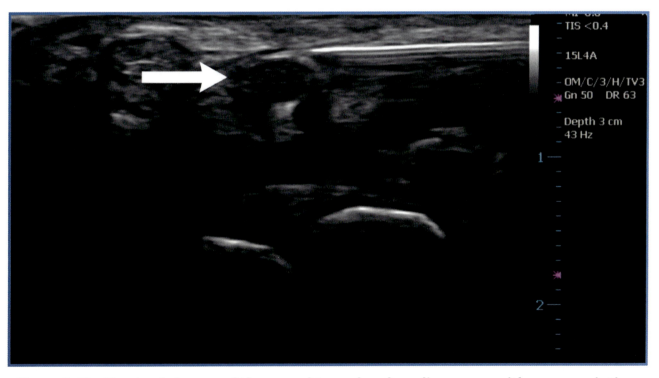

Figure 3.12: Short axis image of the carpal tunnel and median nerve with arrow pointing. The needle is moving from ulnar to radial (right to left) in-plane with the probe toward the superficial aspect of the carpal tunnel providing a hydrodissection of the nerve from the transverse carpal ligament.

Dorsal Wrist Structures

The distal radius intersects with the lunate and the scaphoid while the distal carpal row articulates with the metacarpals. There are six dorsal extensor tendon compartments. The first extensor compartment of the wrist is adjacent to the radius and it comprises the abductor pollicis longus and extensor pollicis brevis (Figure 3.11). The first dorsal tendon compartment is important because this is the site of DeQuervain's tenosynovitis with enlargement of the abductor pollicis longus and/or extensor pollicis brevis tendon.

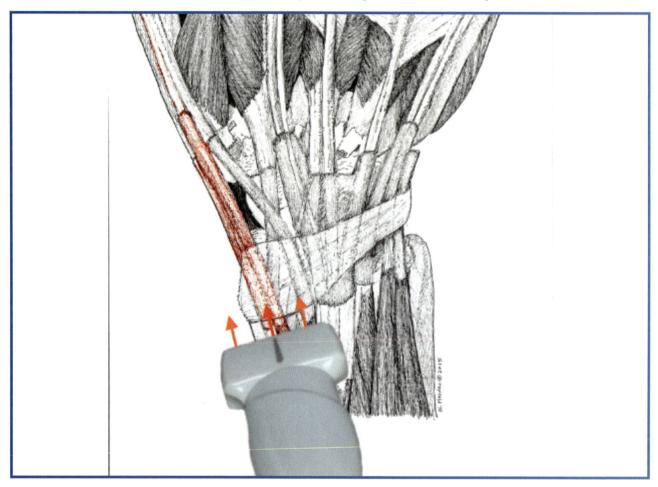

Figure 3.13: Pen and ink illustration of first dorsal wrist compartment in short axis

The second extensor compartment comprises the extensor carpi radialis longus and brevis tendons. The first and second extensor compartments overlap roughly 2-3cm proximal to Lister's tubercle. It is important to scan the region where the first and second compartments overlap in cases of radial sided wrist/forearm pain as this can be a sign of "intersection syndrome." Intersection syndrome is caused by friction of the first and second dorsal compartment structures against each other at the level they overlap proximal to the radial styloid. Lister's tubercle is a "home base" bony landmark that separates the third compartment (extensor pollicis longus tendon) from the second compartment (extensor carpi radialis brevis tendon and longus in the second extensor compartment) (Figure 3.12).

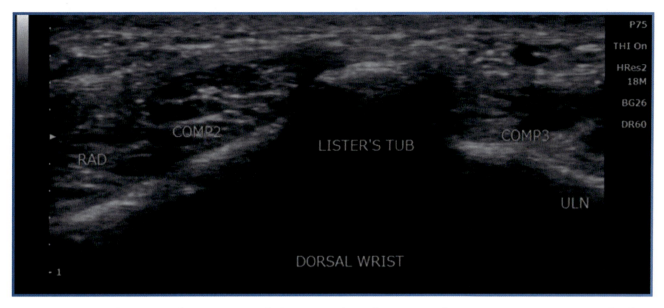

Figure 3.14: Ultrasound anatomy of Lister's tubercle separating compartments 2 and 3 in short axis (RAD=Radius, COMP2=Extensor Carpi Radialis Brevis and Longus, COMP3=Extensor Pollicis Longus, Lister's TUB=Lister's Tuberosity)

The third extensor compartment has one tendon and is composed of the extensor pollicis longus. Outside of possible injury and tearing secondary to a distal radius fracture or inflammatory arthritis, involvement of the extensor pollicis longus is not commonly seen in musculoskeletal disorders and will not be covered extensively outside of understanding its anatomic location. The fourth extensor tendon compartment is composed of the extensor indicis and extensor digitorum communis. The fifth extensor tendon compartment houses the extensor digiti minimi (Figure 3.13). Similar to the extensor pollicis longus, outside of rheumatoid arthritis and gout, the fourth and fifth compartment are not commonly involved in musculoskeletal disorders so we will not cover patho-anatomy to great extent.

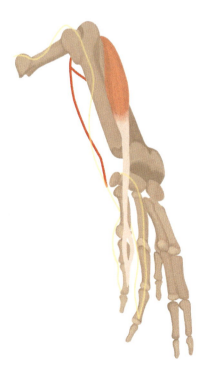

Figure 3.15: Fifth Compartment of the Wrist From Above: Looking From Pinky Towards the Wrist

Extensor Carpi Ulnaris and the Ulnar Wrist Structures

The sixth compartment adjacent to the ulna lies the extensor carpi ulnaris. The extensor carpi ulnaris is susceptible to injury, specifically in individuals participating in racquet sports, golf and high impact sports such as rugby and football (Evers et al., 2018). Sports or activities that create extensor carpi ulnaris tendon tears share similar features such as loading the wrist in vulnerable positions such as wrist flexion with supination or pronation or a sudden lateral force applied while the tendon is isometrically contracted (Evers et al., 2018). Extensor carpi ulnaris tenosynovitis is typically precipitated with microtrauma and instability secondary to repetitive motions as described above or possibly a singular incident where the wrist sustained a blow while in a vulnerable position (Campbell et al., 2013). Cases of isolated stenosing tenosynovitis of the extensor carpi ulnaris are uncommon and when they do, aren't typically sports related incidents (Hajj AA et al., 1986). Normal sonographic appearance of the extensor carpi ulnaris should be hyperechoic, linear and homogeneous in shape similar to the other dorsal compartment tendon structures.

Injection technique to the extensor carpi ulnaris can be performed with the patient seated with the wrist resting and directed slightly so the radius is closest to the table (Figure 3.14). The extensor carpi ulnaris is visualized in the long axis with the needle moving from distal to proximal, in-plane with the probe (Figure 3.15).

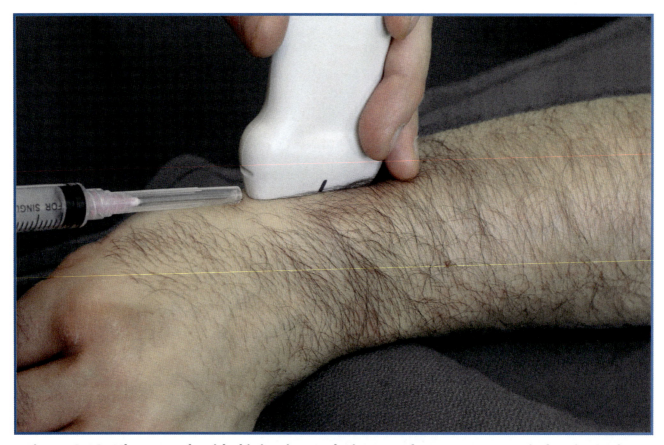

Figure 3.16: Ultrasound guided injection technique to the extensor carpi ulnaris tendon. The patient is positioned supine or seated with a gel bottle to place the wrist in slight radial deviation. The tendon is visualized in the long axis and the needle is moved distal to proximal, in-plane with the probe.

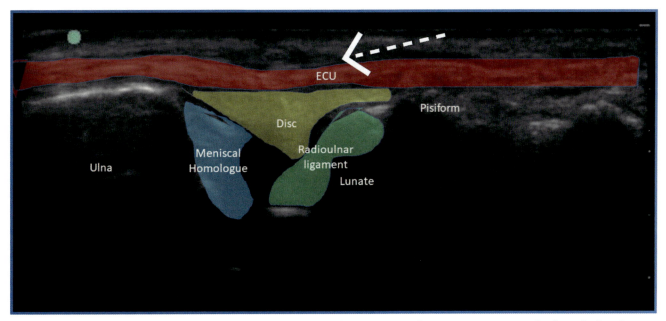

Figure 3.17: Ultrasound guided injection technique to the extensor carpi ulnaris in the long axis. The needle is moved distal to proximal, in-plane with the probe

Dequervain's Tenosynovitis

Dequervain's stenosing tenosynovitis is a common musculoskeletal condition that involves tendon entrapment in the first dorsal compartment of the wrist. With this condition thickening of the tendon sheaths around the abductor pollicis longus and extensor pollicis brevis develops where the tendons pass in through the fibro-osseous tunnel located along the radial styloid at the distal wrist (Satteson and Tannan. 2020) (Figure 3.16 and 3.17). The tendons in the first dorsal compartment (abductor pollicis longus and extensor pollicis brevis) are contained by a synovial sheath protecting them from adjacent structures that pass through an approximately 2 cm long fibrous tunnel passing over the radial styloid and under the transverse fibers of the extensor retinaculum, they are at risk for entrapment, particularly in the setting of acute trauma or repetitive motion (Ippolito et al., 2020). The condition is more common in females than males and typically occurs as a result of repetitive wrist straining with reaching, grasping and picking up items that involve radial or ulnar deviation.

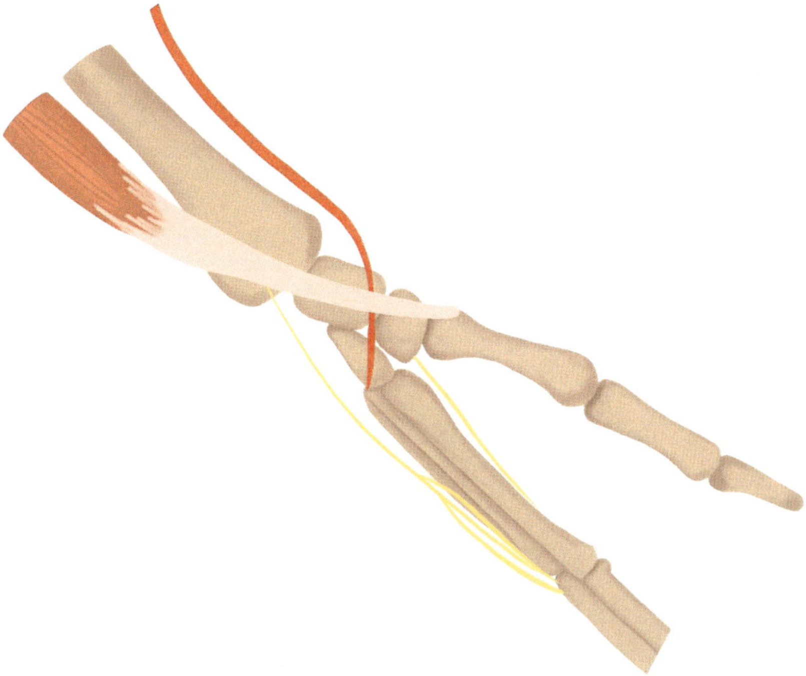

Figure 3.18: The Right Wrist Looking From the Thumb Towards the Pinky

It is also very commonly diagnosed in pregnant females or nursing mothers. Injection of PRP might be preferable in pregnant females to injecting steroid into this region (Chen et al., 2021). When performing injections in the first dorsal tendon compartment, remember its proximity to the radial artery (Figure 3.18-3.20). Subjacent to the abductor pollicis longus tendon is the scaphoid bone sitting right next to the radius and distally, where it becomes smaller. When injecting the first dorsal tendon compartment, the patient is in supine or comfortably seated with the radius/thumb facing upward (3.21-3.23). The compartment is visualized in the short axis and the needle is moved dorsal to volar in plane with the probe. Atypical appearance of the first dorsal compartment is hypoechoic thickening of the tendon sheath causing a "halo" surrounding the circumference of the tendon (Figure 3.24).

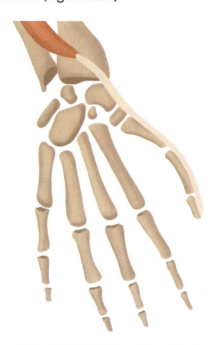

Figure 3.19: The Dorsal Surface of the Right Wrist; The Abductor Pollicis Brevis Tendon

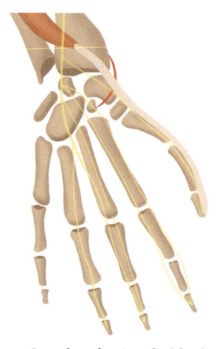

Figure 3.20: Radial Artery Crossing the Scaphoid; View From Above

CHAPTER 20 - THE HAND AND WRIST

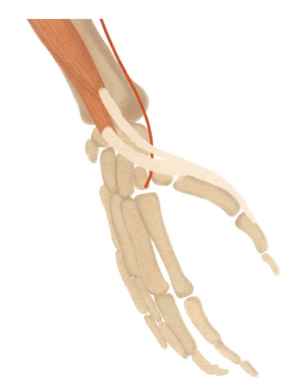

Figure 3.21: Right Hand: the Tendons Involved in DeQuervain's Tenosynovitis and their relation to the radial artery

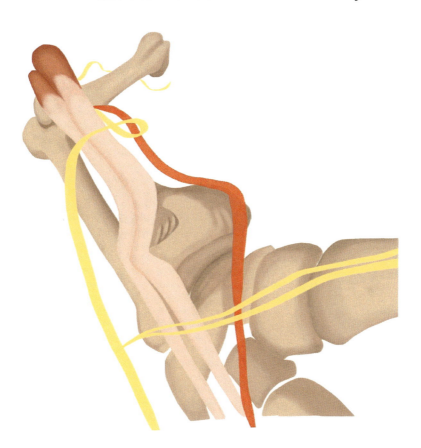

Figure 3.22: The Radial Artery Crossing the Scaphoid of the Right Wrist; Looking From Distal to Proximal

CHAPTER 20 - THE HAND AND WRIST

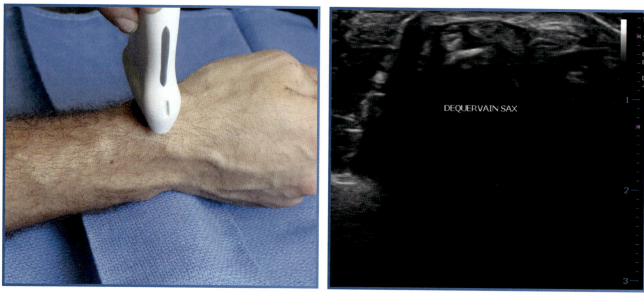

Figure 3.23: First Dorsal Tendon Compartment Transverse/SAX

To evaluate for DeQuervain tenosynovitis and properly assess the abductor pollicis longus and extensor pollicis brevis tendon. Place the probe across both of these tendons right on the styloid process of the radius. Note the bi-lobed appearance of the extensor pollicis brevis and abductor pollicis longus.

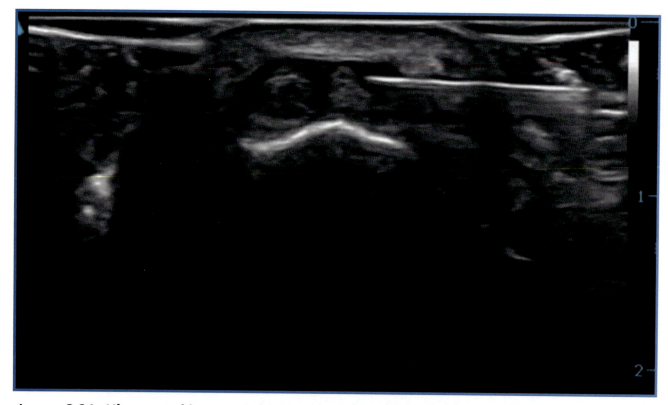

Image 3.24: Ultrasound image of the first dorsal compartment in short axis. The needle is moving dorsal to volar in-plane with the probe into the tendon sheath.

CHAPTER 20 - THE HAND AND WRIST

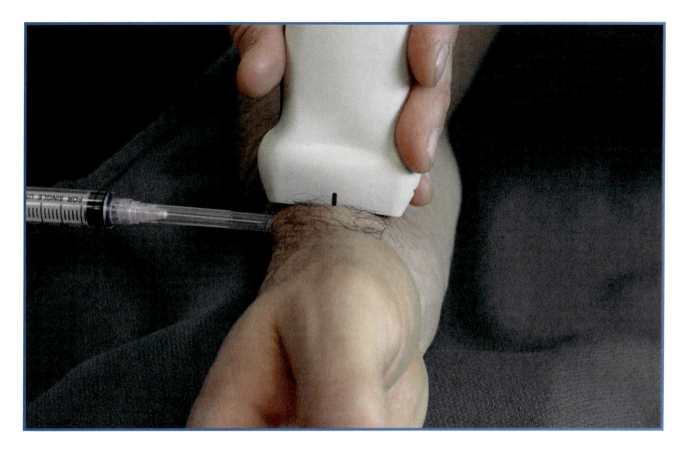

Figure 3.25: US Guided injection technique to the first dorsal compartment. Patient is positioned supine or seated with a gel bottle placed to get slight ulnar deviation. Structures are visualized in short axis and the needle is moving dorsal to volar, in-plane with the probe.

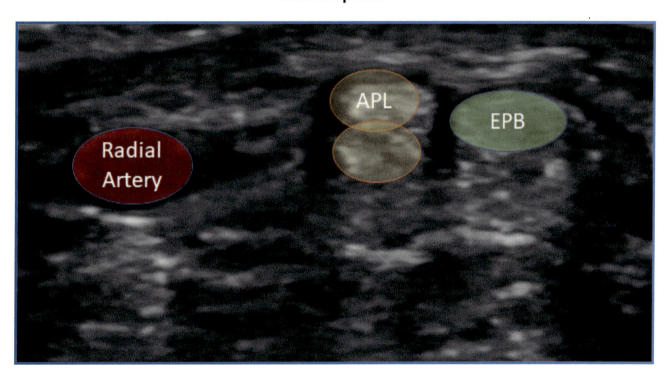

A COMPLETE GUIDE TO REGENERATIVE MEDICINE ©

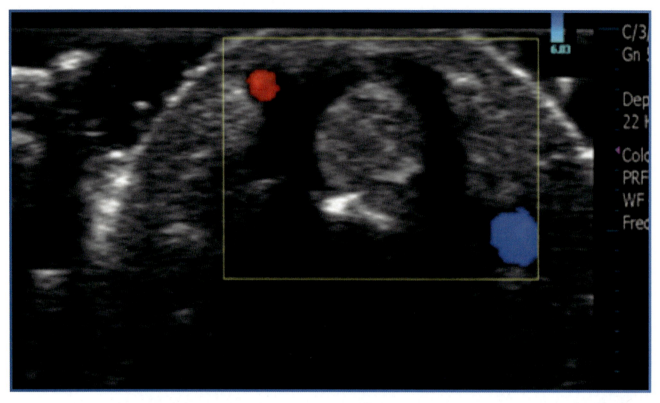

Figure 3.26: Short axis image of the first dorsal compartment presenting with Dequervain's syndrome as evidenced by the hypoechoic "halo" surrounding the tendon at the level of the radial styloid.

Radiocarpal Joints and Carpal Rows

Evaluation of the radiocarpal bone intersections as well as the intercarpal intersections with diagnostic ultrasound is necessary when preparing for intervention into the region. Clinically, the dorsal radio-lunate intersection and the intercarpal joints are a very common location for ganglion cysts to occur (Squab et al., 2014). Ganglions in this region usually are found directly over the proximal carpal row and occasionally the distal row, though they appear anywhere between the long thumb extensor laterally and the common finger extensors medially (Angelides et al., 1993). The main body of the cyst is tethered to the wrist capsule by a pedicle and this pedicle often penetrates the capsule and enters the scapholunate ligament creating a pathway or "stalk" of communication, this was found to be true in the vast majority of cases reported by Angelides and Wallace (Angelides and Wallace. 1976). Historical management of ganglion cysts in the dorsal wrist has typically been somewhat successful with aspiration and cortisone injection with the expectation that up to 80% of patients see a temporary benefit (Clay and Clement. 1988). However, with the advancement of musculoskeletal ultrasound training and resolution as well as the application and science of orthobiologics, PRP can be a safer alternative to cortisone because it does not carry risk of connective tissue weakening. In most non-surgical interventions of dorsal wrist ganglia, the stalk of the ganglia is still communicated with the potential space and runs the risk of reappearing. When preparing for an injection to the radial-scaphoid, lunate-scaphoid space, or to the ganglion itself. Place the wrist in flexion with bolster underneath the wrist and ulnar or radial deviation to slightly gap the joint (Figure 3.25 and 3.26). To inject here, visualize the radius and the scaphoid or lunate in the long axis; the needle will be moved distal to proximal, in-plane with the probe (3.27 and 3.28).

CHAPTER 20 - THE HAND AND WRIST

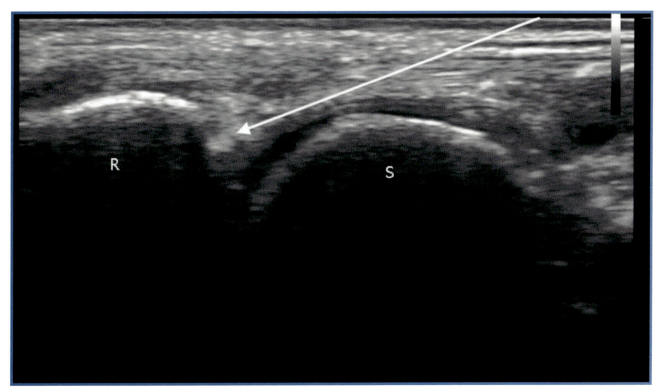

Figure 3.27: Ultrasound guided injection technique: Long axis ultrasound image of the radioscaphoid joint. The needle is moved distal to proximal, in-plane with the probe (R=Radius, S=Scaphoid)

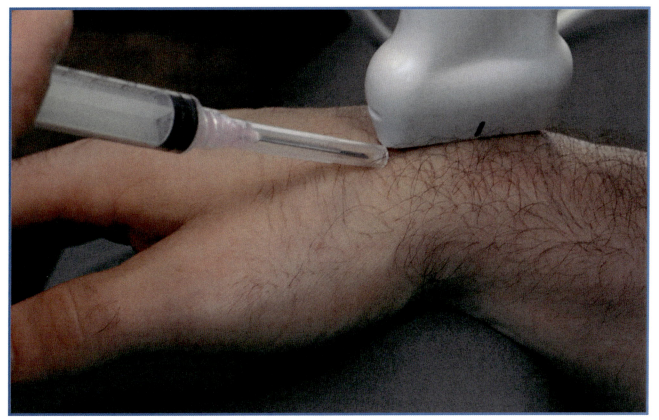

Photo 3.28: Ultrasound guided injection technique to the radiocarpal joint intersection. The patient is positioned in supine or seated. The joint structures are visualized in the long axis and the needle is moved distal to proximal, in-plane with the probe.

A COMPLETE GUIDE TO REGENERATIVE MEDICINE ©

CHAPTER 20 - THE HAND AND WRIST

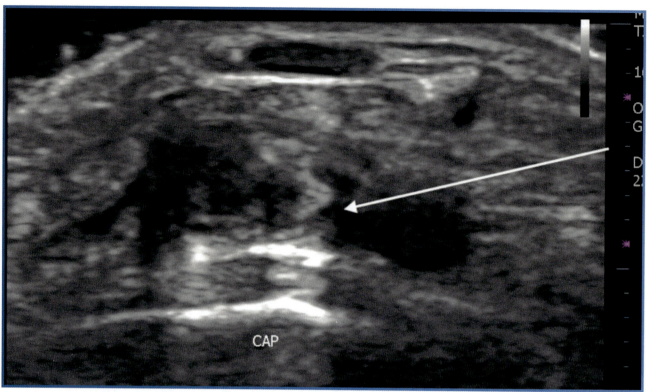

Image 3.29: Long axis image of ganglion cyst at the level of the capitate (CAP=Capitate). The mixed echo (hyper/hypoechoic) structure the needle trajectory is directed, is the ganglion cyst. The needle is moved distal to proximal, in-plane with the probe.

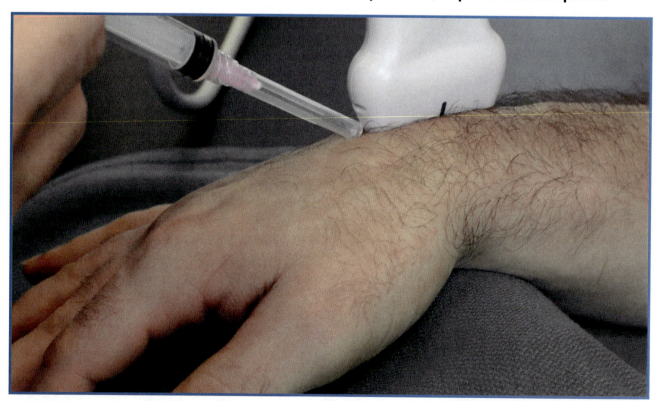

Photo 3.30: Ultrasound guided injection technique to the carpal joints for ganglion cyst. The patient is positioned supine or seated and the needle is moved distal to proximal, in-plane with the probe.

Triangular Fibrocartilage Complex

The triangular fibrocartilage (Figure 3.29) within the ulnar aspect of the wrist has multiple sites for needle access. Sonographically, the main anatomic landmark to evaluate for access is the distal radial-ulnar joint where the provider can inject the joint near the ulnar attachment of the cartilaginous complex (Figure 3.30). Be cautious about injecting into the fibrocartilage disc itself as this can cause tears of the triangular fibrocartilage. To avoid puncturing the cartilaginous disc, the provider can inject into the distal radio-ulnar joint using the technique described below (3.31 and 3.32). This technique "bathes" the triangular fibrocartilage complex and can infiltrate the cartilage disc through fissures in the tissue.

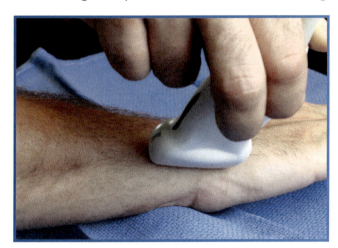 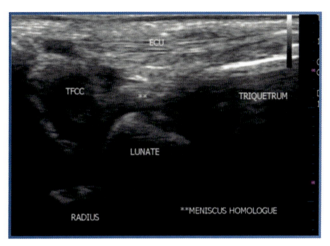

Figure 3.31: Triangular Fibrocartilage Complex: Longitudinal/Long Axis

Place the probe along the ulnar aspect of the wrist in the long axis to the distal ulna and extensor carpi ulnaris. Superficially the main structure is that of the collateral ligament. The TFC is the triangular structure deep to the extensor carpi ulnaris which is visible in long axis. (TFCC=Triangular Fibrocartilage Complex, **=Meniscal homologue/synovial tissue, ECU=Extensor carpi ulnaris which is visualized in long axis)

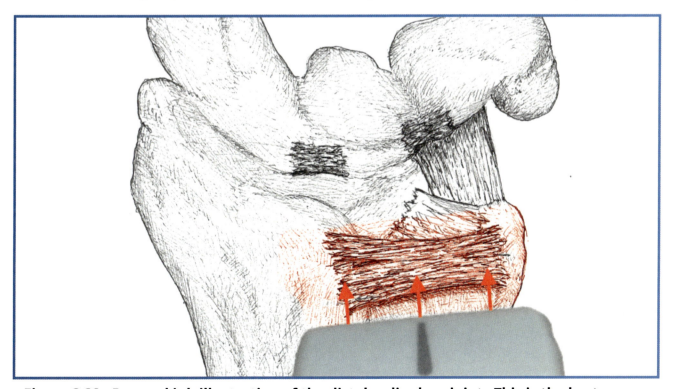

Figure 3.32: Pen and ink illustration of the distal radioulnar joint. This is the best access point for injection in cases of triangular fibrocartilage pathology

CHAPTER 20 - THE HAND AND WRIST

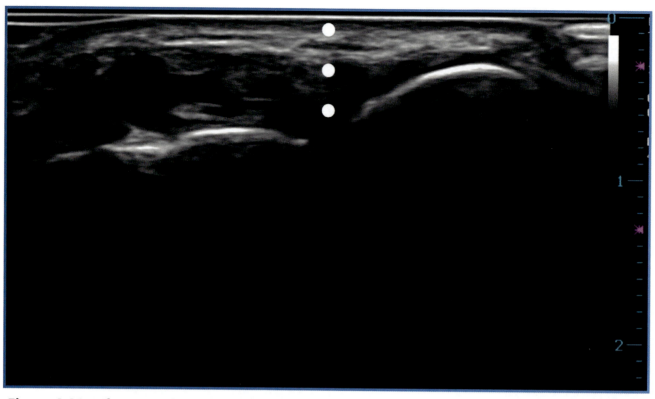

Figure 3.33: Ultrasound image of the distal radial-ulnar joint (radius on left, ulna on right). The needle is moving dorsal to volar out-of-plane with the probe. This technique provides access to the triangular fibrocartilage complex without going through the extensor tendons.

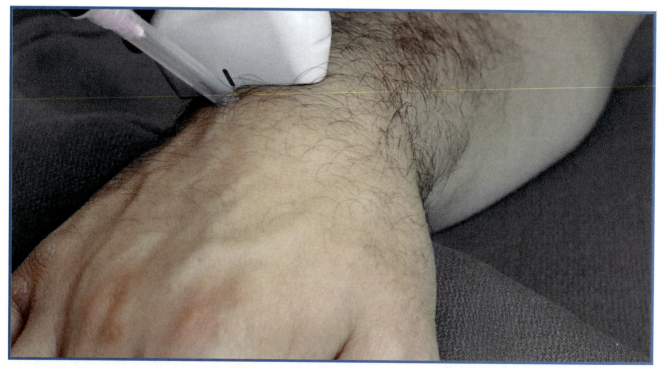

Figure 3.34: Ultrasound guided injection technique to the radioulnar joint. The patient is positioned in seated or supine with a gel bottle placed under the wrist crease to flex the joint. The needle is moved dorsal to volar, in-plane with the probe and is intended to treat triangular fibrocartilage pathology

CHAPTER 20 - THE HAND AND WRIST

Flexor Tendons/Annular Pulley System

Normal sonoanatomy of the flexor tendons, like elsewhere in the body, are hyperechoic when compared to skeletal muscles. The tendons and fibers are represented by a pattern of internal echoes (Figure 3.33). There are two flexor tendons in the fingers – the flexor digitorum superficialis which inserts at the base of the middle phalanx, and the flexor digitorum profundus, the deep tendon closest to the bone, which inserts onto the distal phalanx. The flexor digitorum superficialis attaches in two separate areas, it splits the profundus tendon and inserts onto the radial and ulnar base(s) of the middle phalanx. The flexor digitorum profundus has one attachment site onto the distal phalanx.

Figure 3.35: Annular Pulley System: Short and Long axis

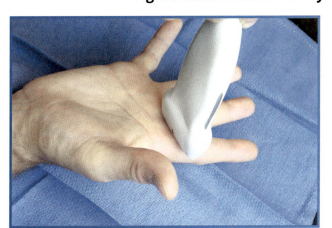
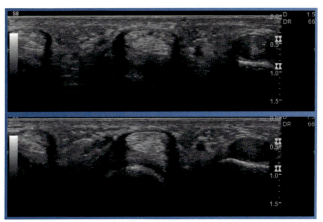
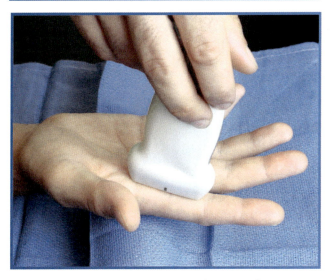
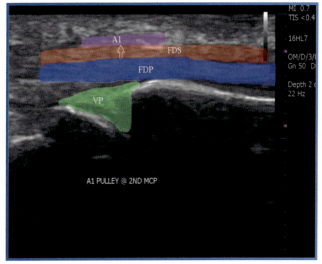

Probe position for long axis visualization of metacarpal-phalangeal joint and annular pulley. Patient is positioned supine or seated.

Top Right: Short axis ultrasound image of normal sonographic anatomy of the flexor digitorum profundus and superficialis.

Bottom Right: Ultrasound image of long axis metacarpal phalangeal joint. Purple=A1 pulley. Red=flexor digitorum superficialis. Blue=flexor digitorum profundus. Green=joint space of metacarpal phalangeal and volar plate

The annular pulleys are crucial to the function of the finger flexors and traverse over the tendons; they function as a retinaculum to keep flexor digitorum profundus and superficialis from subluxation or dislocation (Figure 3.34 and 3.35). Their normal sonographic appearance is that of being hypoechoic– visualized in short axis or long axis. When the patient flexes and extends the distal phalanx, the annular pulleys can be seen circumscribing or surrounding the flexor tendons.

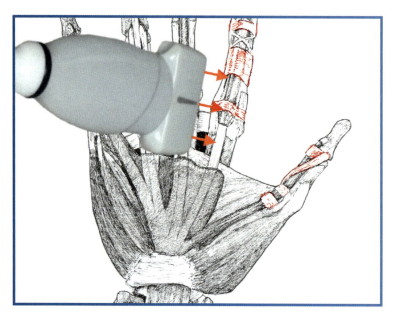

Figure 3.36: Pen and ink illustration of the annular pulley system

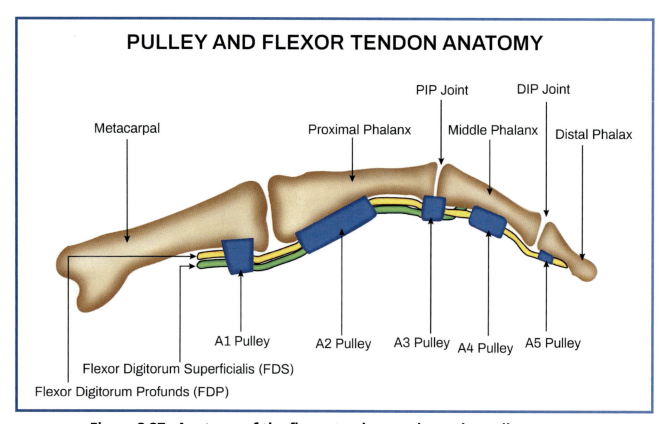

Figure 3.37: Anatomy of the flexor tendons and annular pulley system

CHAPTER 20 - THE HAND AND WRIST

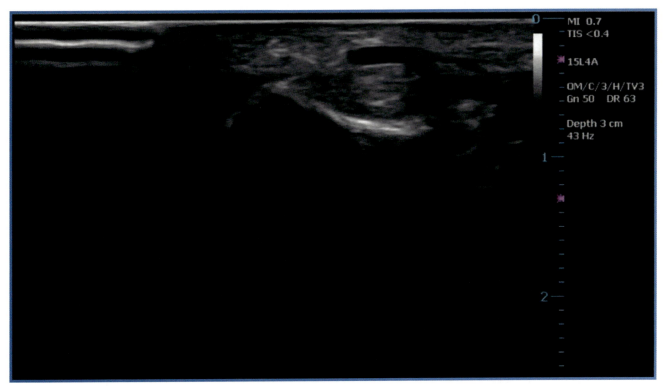

Figure 3.38: Short axis image of stenosing tenosynovitis of the flexor tendons in the finger. The hypoechoic structure directly superficial to the tendon signifies a ganglion and encroachment of the annular ligament and tendon sheath

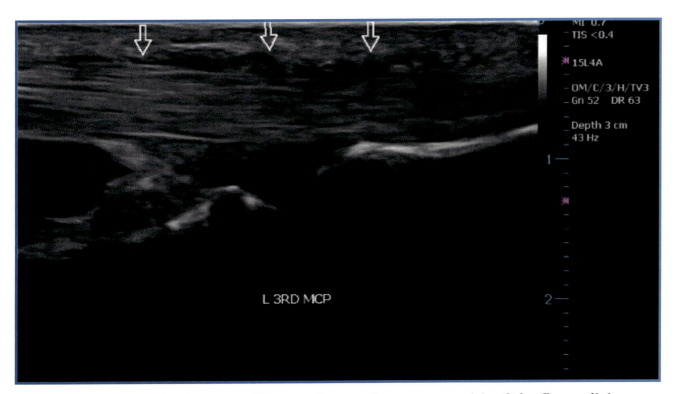

Figure 3.39: Long axis ultrasound image of stenosing tenosynovitis of the flexor digitorum profundus and superficialis at the level of the metacarpal phalangeal joint. The arrows are pointing to hypoechoic thickening of the annular ligaments

CHAPTER 20 - THE HAND AND WRIST

With stenosing tenosynovitis of the finger flexors, idiopathic tenosynovitis, and/or chronic rheumatoid arthritis, the fingers can get stuck in a bent position when moving into flexion and extension and there is often hypertrophy of the annular ligaments/annular pulley in this diagnosis. The provider can inject PRP into the A1 annular pulley and perform micro-fenestrations within the pulley and sometimes, this procedure is similar to an open "release" but can be performed percutaneously with ultrasound guidance. When delivering orthobiologics or fenestration of stenotic annular pulley systems, the patient is positioned in seated or supine with the palm facing upward. The needle is moved distal to proximal, in-plane with the probe (Figure 3.38 and 3.39). Be careful of patient sensibilities in this area due to the high density of nerve endings on the palmar surface of the hands and fingers. It should also be mentioned that providers should be careful not to cut or fenestrate A2 or A4 annular pulley(s) percutaneously unless fully aware of the potential risks.

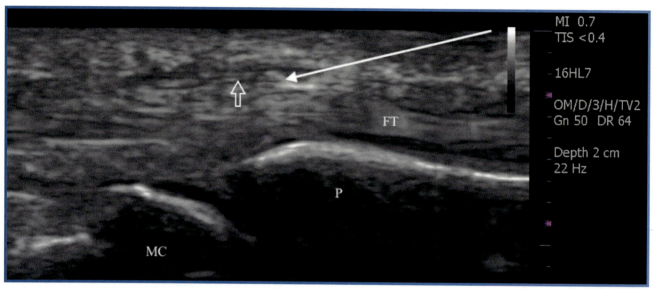

Figure 3.40: Long axis ultrasound image of the flexor tendons and sheath at the level of the A1 pulley at the metacarpal-phalangeal joint. The needle is visualized moving distal to proximal, in-plane with the probe (MC=metacarpal, P=phalange, FT=Flexor tendon, Arrow=A1 pulley location)

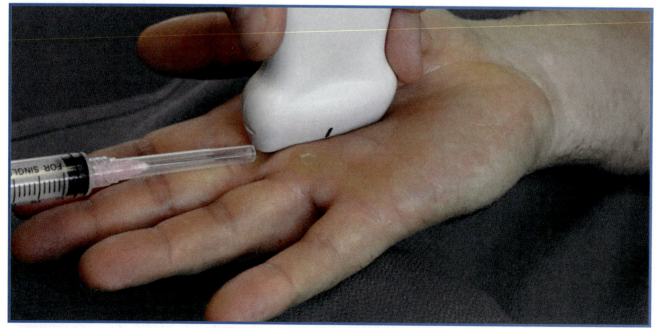

Figure 3.41: Ultrasound-guided injection technique for stenosing tenosynovitis "trigger finger" to the A1 pulley. Patient is positioned supine or seated. THe needle is moved distal to proximal, in-plane with the probe.

As with all percutaneous procedures, be careful to remember to screen for infection and other signs of diseases that may be a contraindication. If the patient has rheumatoid arthritis, the provider may opt to get an MRI prior to injection in order to screen for focal synovitis or evidence of proliferation as this combined with the ultrasound study can give the provider a firm diagnostic starting point. In the hands of a seasoned operator, musculoskeletal ultrasound is a very sensitive tool to evaluate focal synovitis as well as synovial hypertrophy, bony erosions and other soft tissue changes to the region in the hand/wrist complex (Tersely et al., 2017). Due to the high degree of technical skill required to both perform and assess musculoskeletal ultrasound imaging for signs consistent with rheumatoid arthritis, the MRI can be a fallback option as an imaging modality if the user isn't comfortable with grading the sono-anatomy.

First Carpal-Metacarpal Joint

Small joint injections with PRP and stem cells are excellent for pain, especially for first carpal-metacarpal joint pain (CMC). The first CMC joint is the most commonly affected joint in the hand for osteoarthritis and is an excellent location to deliver orthobiologics in cases where appropriate. The first carpal-metacarpal joint is a saddle joint with a range of motion to perform tasks that are unique to humans and range from gross motor to fine movements (ie: grasping and pinching). Normal sonographic appearance of the first carpal-metacarpal joint is highlighted by crisp, uninterrupted cortical outlines with the joint space resembling a homogeneous V-shaped interface (Figure 3.40).

Figure 3.42: 1st Carpal-Metacarpal Joint: Longitudinal

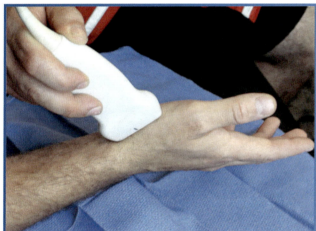
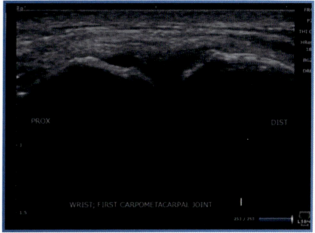

Position the patient supine or seated with the wrist in neutral over a gel bottle to encourage joint gapping. Place the probe along the long axis of the two tendons with the notch overlying the styloid process of the radius and sweep it slightly more distally to appreciate the first metacarpal joint.

Sonographic findings of first carpal-metacarpal joint arthropathy is marked with bony outgrowth at the joint interface, joint space narrowing and capsular tenting where joint material is extruded from the space (Figure 3.41).

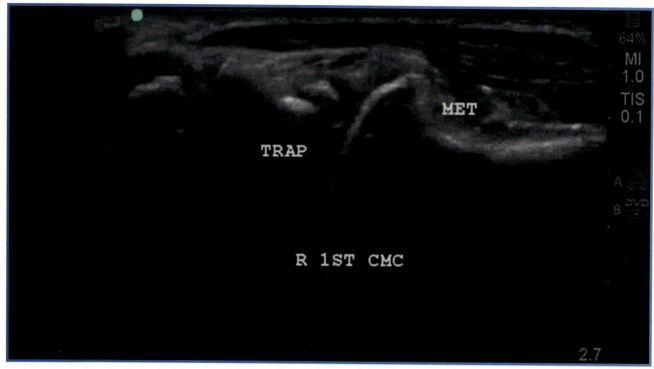

Figure 3.43: Long axis ultrasound image of first carpal-metacarpal arthritis. Observe the bony outgrowth at the metacarpal-trapezium intersection as well as joint space narrowing and capsular "tenting" (TRAP=Trapezium, MET=Metacarpal)

Gray's Anatomy describes the joint as an "articulation by reciprocal reception" that imparts arcs of motion in flexion-extension and abduction-adduction. Because of the joint's range of movement, it is prone to excess friction over time and subsequently, development of osteoarthritis. For the first CMC joint, we instruct to inject indirectly (or out-of-plane) intraarticularly at the base of the thumb which is the trapezium-metacarpal intersection with the needle moved in a radial to ulnar direction (3.42 and 3.43). Because the first carpometacarpal joint is such a small joint, we advise to inject approximately 1 cc of PRP using a 25G needle.

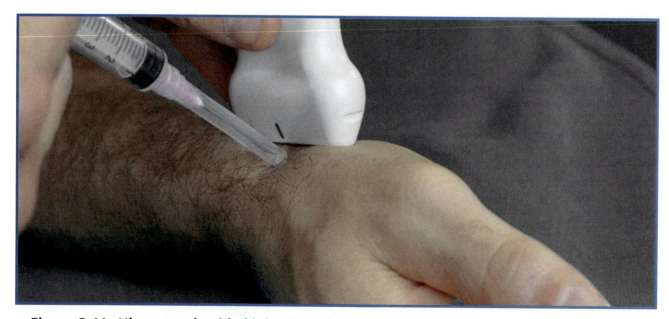

Figure 3.44: Ultrasound guided injection technique to the first carpal-metacarpal joint. The structure is visualized in long axis, the needle is moved dorsal to volar, out-of-plane with the probe

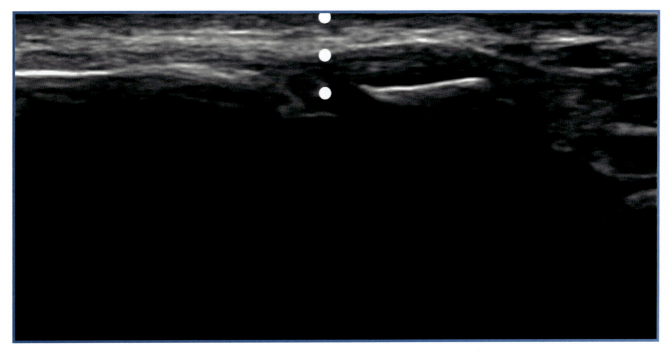

Figure 3.45: Ultrasound image of the first carpal-metacarpal joint in the long axis. The needle is moved in a radial to ulnar direction out-of-plane with the probe

The Ulnar Collateral Ligament of the Thumb

According to the American Academy of Orthopedic Surgeons, the ulnar collateral ligament (UCL) of the thumb is the most commonly injured ligament of the hand. It allows us to pinch and grasp objects.

Anatomically, the UCL is composed of a proper collateral ligament (PCL) and an accessory collateral ligament (Hung et al., 2020). The PCL originates from the dorsal third of the metacarpal head and inserts on the volar aspect of the proximal phalanx. The anterior cruciate ligament originates palmar to the PCL and runs continuously with the PCL to insert on the volar plate. The PCL is taut in flexion, while the anterior cruciate ligament is taut in extension. Both ligaments ensure the ulnar stability of the MCP joint. The Adductor pollicis inserts on the proximal phalanx, functioning as a dynamic stabilizer of the MCP joint (Ritting et al., 2010). It lies superficial to the UCL. Tears can be graded with musculoskeletal ultrasound OR MRI depending on the provider experience and preference. Treatment classifications of UCL tears are as follows (Kundu et al., 2012):

A "Stener Lesion" occurs when the aponeurotic band tears and avulses a fragment of the proximal phalanx and is typically pathognomonic with a high grade tear of the thumb UCL. It is also common to see isolated thumb UCL tears or sprains with an intact adductor pollicis aponeurosis. Since PRP and stem cells fall into "non-surgical management" and based on the classification system outlined above, we can deduct that the use of orthobiologics (PRP and Stem cell) of type I and II UCL tears as well as some type III tears have a good chance to respond positively.

- Type I: Minimally displaced/partial UCL tears usually heal with immobilization alone
- Type II: UCL tears that are displaced less than 3 mm can be healed with immobilization alone
- Type III: UCL tears that are displaced more than 3 mm will usually fail immobilization and most patients with require surgery
- Type IV: Stener lesion will require surgery in all cases

To proceed with the procedure into the thumb UCL, the patient should be positioned in seated or supine with the wrist in neutral with slight pronation. The ultrasound probe is positioned so that the relevant anatomy is visualized in the long axis and the needle is moved ulnar to radial out of plane with the probe to the affected portion of the ligament tear (Figure 3.45 and 3.46).

Figure 3.46: The Basal Joint/Thumb: Ulnar Collateral Ligament

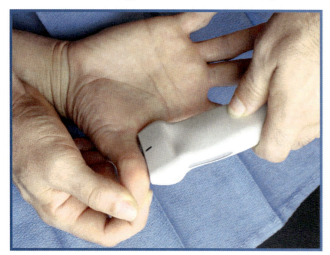
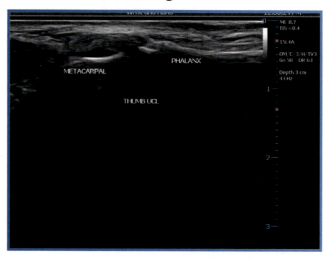
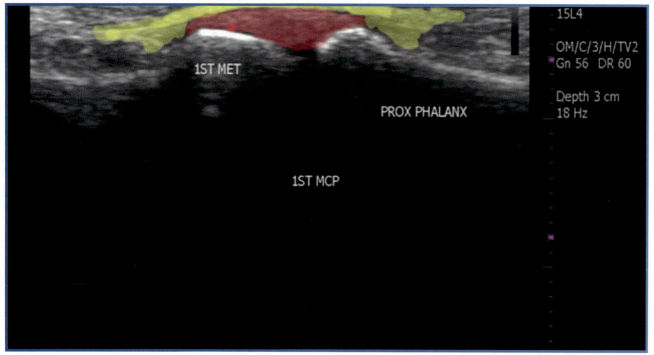

Patient is positioned supine or seated. Place the probe on the dorsal aspect of the hand along the second through fifth finger on the MCP to visualize the metacarpophalangeal joints.
Top Right: Sonoanatomy
Bottom: (Yellow=aponeurosis of the adductor pollicis and Red=ulnar collateral ligament of the thumb)

CHAPTER 20 - THE HAND AND WRIST

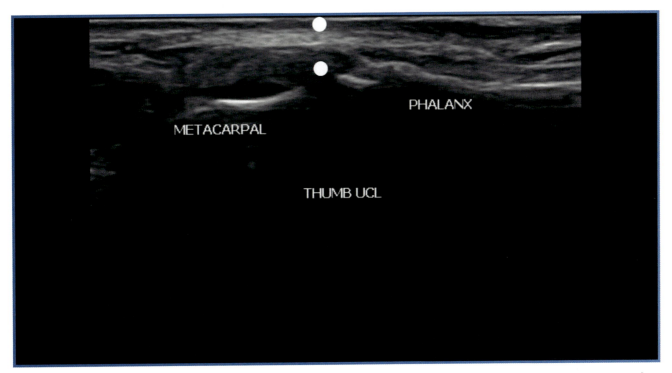

Figure 3.47: Ultrasound image of the thumb UCL in the long axis. The needle is moved ulnar to radial out-of-plane with the probe.

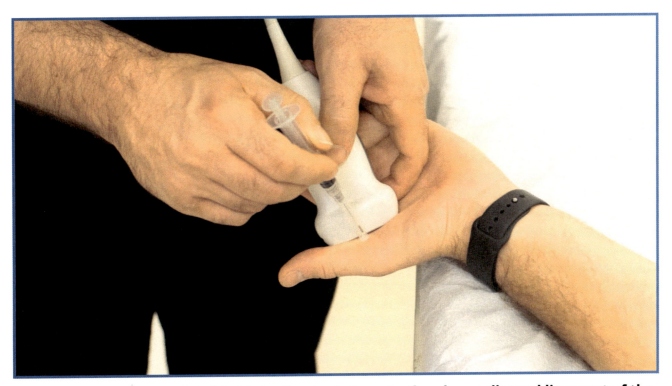

Figure 3.48: Ultrasound Guided injection technique to the ulnar collateral ligament of the thumb. The patient is positioned supine with the forearm/wrist supinated. The probe is positioned in the long axis and the needle is moved ulnar to radial, out-of-plane with the probe.

Sample Dictation/Note:

Sample Dictation for PRP:
The procedure and potential complications were discussed with the patient. After written and verbal consent were obtained, the patient was placed in the seated position. A tourniquet was placed on the right arm and the area was surveyed for large palpable veins. The antecubital area was prepped and draped in the usual sterile fashion using alcohol. Using an 20G needle, approximately [ ] ccs of blood was drawn from the patient and transferred to a specially prepared PRP tube containing anticoagulants. After the needle was removed, and a sterile bandage was placed over the entry site, the tube was vertically rotated back and forth five times.

The tube was placed in a centrifuge with an opposing counter-weight. After five minutes, the tube was removed and inspected. There was a visible gel, a buffy coat, and a golden liquid layer of PRP. The tube was vertically rotated back and forth five times. Afterwards, the PRP and buffy coat were gently extracted and transferred to a 10 cc syringe. The syringe was attached to a 22G 1.5" needle.

[Patient positioning as described above depending on the type of injection and approach]

The hand and wrist was prepped and draped in the usual sterile manner using three coats of betadine. The area of interest was identified using sonography. The area of interest was identified by the following landmarks: _____

With the probe held in place, a ½ a cc of 1% lidocaine was used to create a wheal at the entry site alongside the probe. The needle guidance software package was turned on. After a moment, with the probe held in place, the needle and syringe containing the PRP was advanced through the skin and the deeper tissues towards the target area. Under ultrasound guidance, the PRP was injected. The final image was recorded. The probe was moved, the needle was removed and a sterile gauze was held over the injection site with gentle pressure. A sterile bandage was applied. The patient was repositioned for comfort. The patient tolerated the procedure well with no apparent complications.

References:

Hans-Rudolf Ziswiler et al. (2005). Diagnostic value of sonography in patients with suspected carpal tunnel syndrome: A prospective study. Journal of Arthritis and Rheumatology, 52(1), 304-311.

Housner JA et al. (2009). Musculoskeletal sonography: evolving applications. Journal of Ultrasound in Medicine, 28(9), 1187.

Stefanie Evers, Andrew R. Thoreson, Jay Smith, Chunfeng Zhao, Jennifer R. Geske, and Peter C. Amadio. (2014). Diagnostic accuracy of magnetic resonance imaging, ultrasound and clinical evaluation in the diagnosis of De Quervain tenosynovitis. Iowa Orthopaedic Journal, 34, 184–190.

Campbell M, Kusne S, Renfree KJ, Vikram HR, Smilack JD, Seville MT, Orenstein R, Blair JE. (2015). Coccidioidal Tenosynovitis of the Hand and Wrist: Report of 9 Cases and Review of the Literature. Clinical Infectious Diseases, 61(10), 1514-20.

Hajj AA, Wood MB. (1986). Stenosing tenosynovitis of the extensor carpi ulnaris. The Journal of Hand Surgery, 11(4), 519–20.

Ippolito J.A., Hauser S., Patel J., Vosbikian M., and Ahmed I. Nonsurgical Treatment of De Quervain Tenosynovitis: A Prospective Randomized Trial. Hand 2020; 15(2): 215–219.

Chen et al. (2021). The diagnostic accuracy of ultrasonography in the detection of carpal tunnel syndrome: A meta-analysis. PLoS ONE, 16(4), e0250288.

Angelides A.C. Ganglions of the hand and wrist. Operative hand surgery, 3rd edition. New York: Churchill Livingstone. pp. 2157-2171.

Angelides A.C., Wallace P.F. The dorsal ganglion of the wrist: its pathogenesis, gross and microscopic anatomy, and surgical treatment. The Journal of Hand Surgery 1976; 1(3): 228-35.

Clay N.R., Clement D.A. The Treatment of Dorsal Wrist Ganglia by Radical Excision. Journal of Hand Surgery 1988; 13(2): 187-191.

Wu et al. (2018). Ultrasound-guided hydrodissection decreases gliding resistance of the median nerve within the carpal tunnel. Muscle & Nerve, 57(1), 25-32.

Campbell D., Campbell R., O'Connor P., and Hawkes R. Sports-related extensor carpi ulnaris pathology: a review of functional anatomy, sports injury and management. British Journal of Sports Medicine 2013; 47(17): 1105–1111.

Satteson E., and Tannan S.C. De Quervain Tenosynovitis. National Center for Biotechnology Information. Accessed on April 6, 2023, from https://www.ncbi.nlm.nih.gov/books/NBK442005/.

CHAPTER 21 The Hip

Colin Rigney, Pradeep Albert, Devi Nampiaparampil & Struan Coleman

CHAPTER PREVIEW

This chapter will cover sonoanatomy of the hip complex as well as patient and probe positions for proper evaluation. The chapter will also include common pictorial examples and explanations of sono-pathology found as well as basic ultrasound-guided injection techniques.

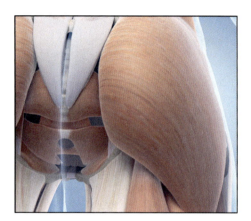

Patient Selection for Injection:
The type of procedure performed depends on the patient's clinical signs and symptoms.

Iliopsoas Bursitis:
Pain in the groin that is worse with hip flexion

Hamstring Injection:
Posterior gluteal pain radiating through the hamstring that is worse with knee flexion

Greater trochanteric Bursitis:
Pain laterally over the greater trochanter

Intra Articular Hip Injection:
Groin pain that is worse with weight bearing particularly rising from a chair

Contraindications to Injection:
Systemic infection
Infection or rash over the puncture site
Coagulopathy (International Normalized Ratio [INR] > 1.3 or platelets < 50,000/ mm3)
Inability to reach target site because of prior surgery or scar tissue

Equipment and Supplies:
Alcohol swabs
Tourniquet
18G or 20G needle for blood draw
Tubing
PRP Kit
Gauze
Betadine or Chlorhexidine
Sterile drapes
Sterile gloves
Sterile ultrasound gel
Tuberculin syringe with needle (optional for local anesthetic in the skin)
Syringes
Bandaid
Positioning aids
Imaging Requirements for Procedure:
Ultrasound with linear high frequency probe

Precautions:
1% lidocaine can be used for a skin wheal; avoid injecting lidocaine into the deep tissues or mixing it with the PRP

Potential Complications:
Bleeding
Infection
Post-procedural pain
Nerve injury
Risk of pneumothorax for scapulo-thoracic procedures
Vasovagal reactions and ataxia

Post-Procedure Care/ Follow-Up
After the procedure, the patient is observed and questioned nausea and lightheadedness. If there are no signs of a vasovagal reaction, the patient can sit and then stand. The affected area can be actively mobilized in a gentle fashion to spread the PRP.

If a procedural complication occurs, the physician and/ or staff should observe the patient until the symptom resolves. If the patient is vasovagal, consider giving them a snack and some fluids.

ANATOMY OF THE HIP

A low frequency curvilinear probe would be ideal for the hip because of the deep penetration.

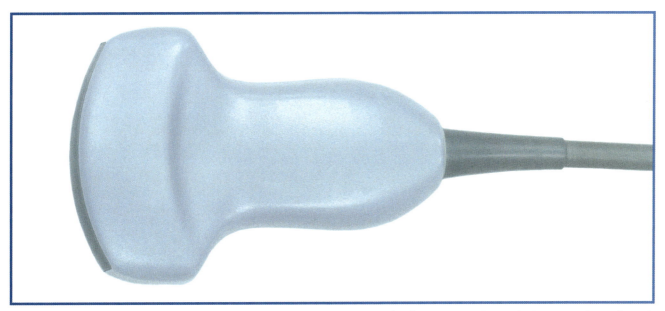

Historically, radiographs were the first studies used to image the hip. Later, CT and MRI were introduced. Ultrasound (US) has always had a relatively limited role in the evaluation of the intra articular hip joint structures due to the deep location of this joint. However, many hip diseases are well detectable with ultrasound, but before approaching such a study it is necessary to be thoroughly familiar with the normal anatomy and related ultrasound images (Molini et al., 2011).

The most visible portion of the hip labrum is the outer layer of the superior-anterior. Diagnostic ultrasound for musculoskeletal conditions is a point-of-care tool and is very dynamic in nature; the hip can be placed into special testing positions such as FADIR (flexion-adduction-internal rotation) to test for labral tears or FAI (femoral-acetabular impingement) and its dynamic capacity gives ultrasound an advantage over other static soft tissue imaging modalities but is also user and experience-dependent. The utilization of ultrasound to its full dynamic capacity often takes years of experience and training. In cases where intra-articular derangement is suspected, MRI often is the best option when ultrasound is inconclusive or not in the hands of an experienced operator.

Due to the deep anatomic location of the hip joint, there are limitations in appreciating the intra-articular structures as mentioned earlier. Even today with the advancements in ultrasound technology, it is impossible to rule out avascular necrosis, or stress fractures with ultrasound. The most common hip pathology visible with sonography are bursitis, tendinopathies, fluid, debris within the hip joint, and synovitis as well as specific labral tears with use of the dynamic component.

The hip joint is a ball and socket structure. The femoral head is convex and the acetabulum is concave to which it articulates.

There are five hip regions that we will organize the discussion into. These groups all cross the hip joint from different angles: the **lateral hip**, the **medial hip**, the **anterior hip**, the **posterior hip** and the **lateral rotator group**.

We will also discuss the hamstring origin at the Ischium; although these are not technically considered hip muscles but for completeness sake, they will be included in this chapter for they occupy the hip region.

The hip adductors and the lateral rotators are more difficult to image on sonographic evaluation because the level of technical skill to reliably evaluate must be very high. MRI evaluation can be an alternate imaging modality to evaluate these in case the user is not confident or experienced enough to evaluate with musculoskeletal ultrasound.

Let's dive into the anatomy.

The Lateral hip

The gluteal muscles (Gluteus maximus, medius and minimus) originate in various locations on the ilium and insert to the greater trochanter (Figure 4.1). The greater trochanteric region and the lateral hip is a common patient complaint and a common site to inject using ultrasound guidance. The lateral structures of the hip, such as the gluteus medius, gluteus minimus and tensor fascia latae all have attachments to and circa the greater trochanter. There are four facets of the greater trochanter – the anterior facet, lateral facet, the posterior facet, and the superior-posterior facet (Acronym: ALPS like the mountain to remember the facets) (Figure 4.2).

CHAPTER 21 - THE HIP

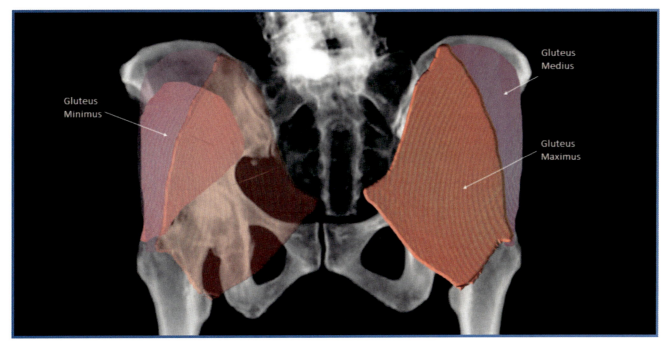

Figure 4.1: Radiographic illustration of gluteal muscle origins

The gluteus minimus has one insertion to the anterior facet of the greater trochanter. The gluteus medius has two insertion points to the greater trochanter: anterior band and posterior. The anterior band insertion of the gluteus medius attaches to the lateral facet and a posterior band gluteus medius attaches to the superior-posterior facet of the greater trochanter. The posterior facet of the greater trochanter is a bare facet where there is no tendon attachment but is the prime location where the largest peribursal fat layer of the sub gluteus maximus bursa is best identified with musculoskeletal ultrasound.

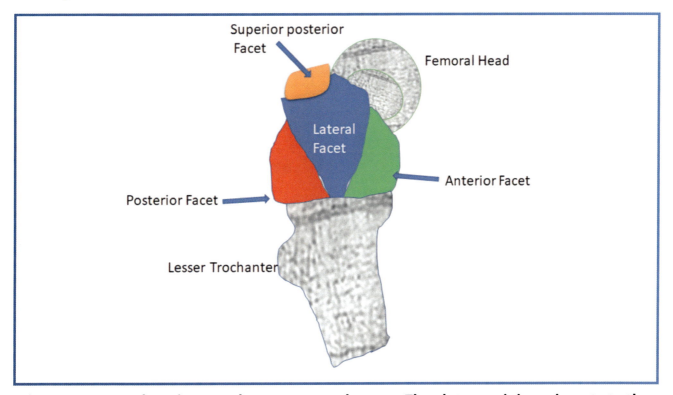

Figure 4.2: Facet locations on the greater trochanter. The gluteus minimus inserts to the anterior facet. The anterior band gluteus medius inserts to the lateral facet. The posterior band gluteus medius inserts to the superior-posterior facet.

A COMPLETE GUIDE TO REGENERATIVE MEDICINE ©

CHAPTER 21 - THE HIP

The normal sonographic appearance of the trochanteric attachments of the gluteal tendons, gluteus minimus and medius are similar to that of most other tendons in the body. They should appear homogeneous, hyperechoic, and have a smooth, uninterrupted cortical surface at the tendon-bone interface (Figure 4.3-4.6). Something that could be helpful to remember when evaluating the region is that the long axis insertions of these tendons are very similar to that of the rotator cuff in the shoulder. The fact that the gluteus minimus and medius also function like the rotator cuff of the hip can serve as another layer of knowledge when educating your patients regarding their pathology here.

Figure 4.3: Gluteus Minimus Tendon: Anterior Trochanteric Facet Longitudinal/LAX

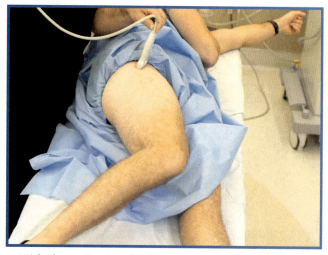
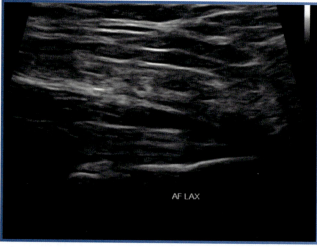

With the patient in the lateral decubitus position, place the probe in a longitudinal orientation across the anterior portion of the greater trochanter. The gluteus minimus tendon can be appreciated as a linear, hyperechoic structure that inserts onto the anterior facet of the greater trochanter. This muscle combines with the gluteus medius to abduct and internally rotate the hip. The iliotibial band is visible as the linear, hyperechoic structure moving right to left above the bird's beak tendon insertion.

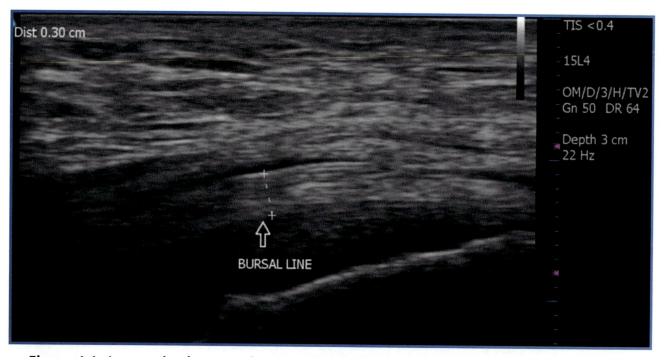

Figure 4.4: Long axis ultrasound image of the gluteus medius. The arrow and calipers marcate the normal sono-anatomy and location of the sub-gluteus maximus bursa (Greater Trochanteric Bursa)

Figure 4.5: Gluteus Medius Tendon Anterior Band: Lateral Facet Longitudinal/LAX

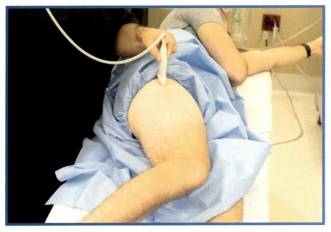
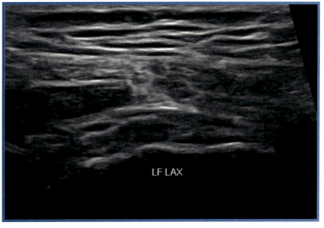

The patient is positioned in the lateral decubitus position, the probe is placed in a longitudinal orientation across the greater trochanter and translated over the lateral facet of the greater tuberosity to locate the gluteus medius tendon. The gluteus medius is slightly more posterior in relation to the gluteus minimus. The iliotibial band is viewed as the linear, hyperechoic structure lying superficial to the gluteus medius in the long axis. The proximal end of the probe is focused more to align with the coronal plane of the body.

Figure 4.6: Gluteus Medius Tendon Posterior Band: Superior Posterior Facet LAX

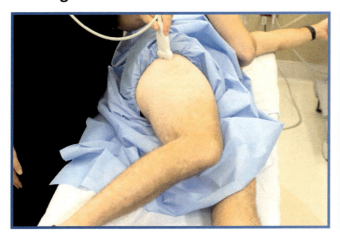
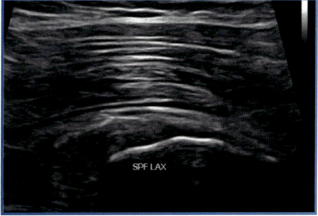

With the patient in lateral decubitus position, place the probe in a longitudinal orientation across the posterior-superior aspect of the greater trochanter and direct the proximal end of the probe posteriorly. The proximal end of the probe is angled to face more posteriorly to align with the posterior fibers of the gluteus medius.

The greater trochanteric bursa is **not** ONE bursa!

There are multiple bursae in the trochanteric region. In fact, it has been hypothesized that the features of the multiple bursae found in the trochanteric region are acquired over a lifetime as a consequence of excessive friction between the greater trochanter and the gluteus maximus as it inserts into the fascia latae (Dunn et al., 2004). The subgluteus maximus bursa, known as the Greater Trochanteric Bursa, is the largest bursa in the region and lies superficial to the gluteus minimus and medius tendons. There is also the sub-gluteus minimus and subgluteus medius bursa which both lie deep to the gluteus minimus and medius insertions to their respective places on the trochanter facets (Dunn et al., 2004) (Figures 4.7 and 4.8). Occasionally these bursae can become inflamed and impinged by the gluteus minimus and medius against the bony interface of the tendon attachment.

CHAPTER 21 - THE HIP

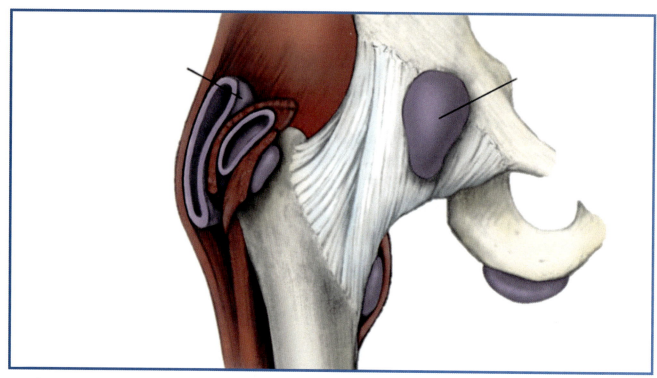

Figure 4.7: Cross sectional illustration of the trochanteric bursae and iliopsoas bursa

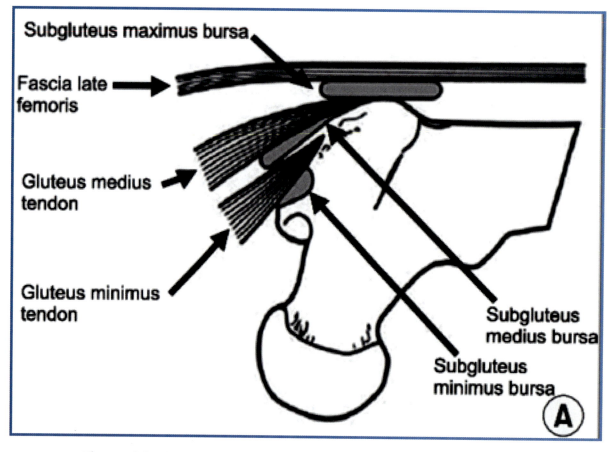

Figure 4.8: Cross sectional illustration of the trochanteric bursae

In an ultrasound evaluation of the gluteal insertions, first identify the "peak" of the greater trochanter. The "peak" or "apex" of the greater trochanter represents the dividing line between the anterior and lateral-posterior facets where gluteus medius and minimus insertions are located (Figure 4.9). To best identify anatomic landmarks in the region, place the probe in the short axis to the proximal third of the thigh, at this level the femur is round and convex. From here slowly translate the probe proximally until the convex femur turns into a sharp "peak" (see image below). This is the region where the gluteal insertions are located and best evaluated. It is also here that the subgluteus maximus bursa (most commonly referred to as greater trochanteric bursa) is easily identified. For identification purposes in this region, the iliotibial band is located here at one of its origins to the tensor fascia latae and it lies superficial to the gluteal tendons as detailed in the long axis pictures below. From here, the iliotibial band can be followed as it moves distally along the lateral femur and inserts to the proximal tibia at Gerdy's tubercle.

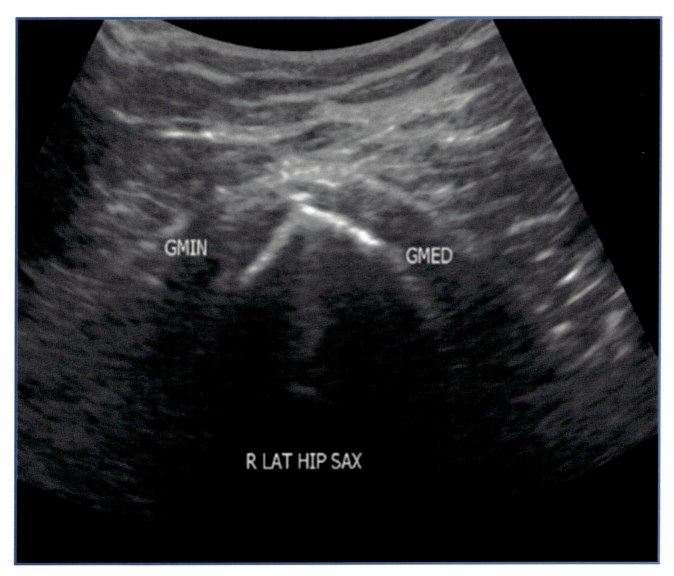

Figure 4.9: Short axis ultrasound image of the "peak" of the greater trochanter. From here, it is easier to orient and focus on isolating gluteus minimus and medius tendon insertions with diagnostic ultrasound. (GMIN=Anterior, GMED=Posterior)

CHAPTER 21 - THE HIP

When performing an injection to the trochanteric region (gluteus minimus, medius or trochanteric bursa), the patient is in lateral decubitus with the affected side facing upward. The transducer is in short axis to the structures gluteus medius or minimus and the needle is moved posterior to anterior in plane with the probe (Figure 4.10-4.12).

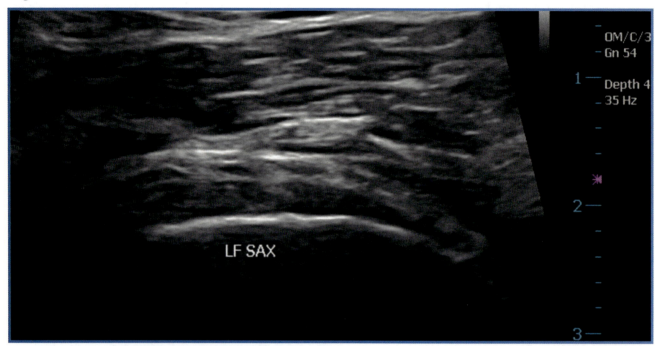

Figure 4.10: Short axis ultrasound image of the lateral facet and gluteus medius anterior band attachment. The trochanteric bursa is located as the hyperechoic region just superficial to the tendon (LF=Lateral Facet of Gluteus medius anterior band insertion).

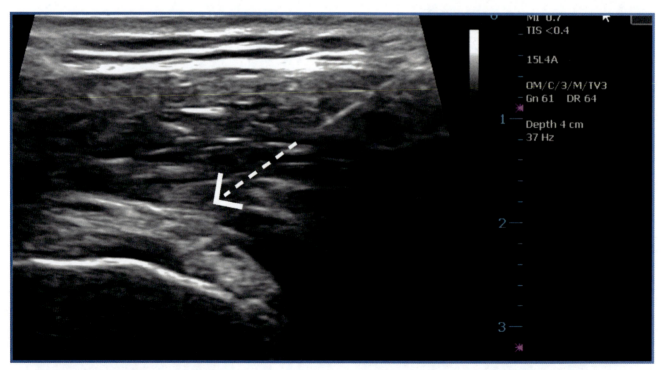

Figure 4.11: Short axis image of the gluteus medius tendon at the lateral facet. The needle is moving posterior to anterior in-plane with the probe. The arrow is pointing to the hyperechoic trochanteric bursal line. Advance the needle past the bursa for an intratendinous injection

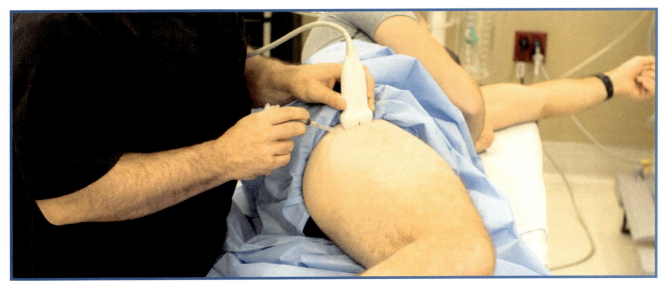

Figure 4.12: Ultrasound guided injection technique to the gluteus medius insertion. The patient is positioned comfortably in lateral decubitus, the structure is visualized in the short axis and the needle is moved posterior to anterior, in-plane with the probe.

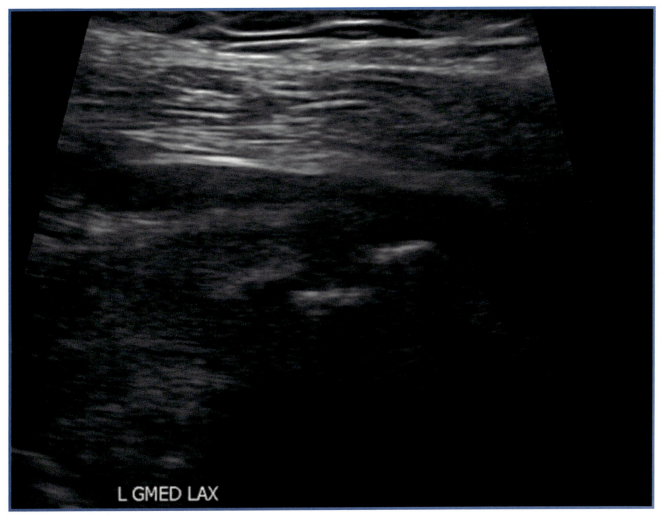

Figure 4.13: Long axis ultrasound image of a tear in the gluteus medius insertion as evidenced by the cortical step off deformity, discordance of tendon fibers as well as trochanteric bursal effusion occurring secondary to the chronic tear.

Anterior Hip Structures

In order to perform an ultrasound evaluation of the anterior hip structures, start by orienting the anatomy in a long axis view with the leg slightly abducted and rotated outward with the knee in resting position. This is the best position available to visualize the pertinent structures with musculoskeletal ultrasound (Figure 4.14).

The femoral-acetabular joint is a ball and socket structure. It is important for the provider to grasp a firm visualization on the femoral head-neck junction and the anterior hip capsule of the iliofemoral ligament and take a diameter measurement (Figure 4.15). A normal diameter long axis measurement of the anterior hip capsule is between 4-6mm (Jacobsen, 2017) in a resting position of hip neutral, slight abduction and slight external rotation (non-impingement position). Jon Jacobsen has described abnormal findings of the hip capsule in the non-impingement position outside of the normal range as an indirect sign of intra articular derangement. The femoral head should be smooth and convex with the visible portion of hyaline cartilage lining the femoral head also smooth and uninterrupted and should also have a convex and symmetrical relationship with the visible portion of the acetabulum and superior labrum (Jacobsen, 2017). Atypical sonographic findings of the hip joint include (Bianchi S. et al., 2007):

- Joint effusion evaluated at the femoral head-neck junction
- Loss of femoral head convexity
- Bony outgrowth at the visible portion of the acetabulum

To optimally image the anterior hip joint in preparation for a percutaneous procedure in the long axis, place the probe over the femoral-acetabular joint at the level of the inguinal crease. The patient is positioned supine and the leg slight abducted and externally rotated in the position consistent with the diagnostic views. The needle is moved from distal to proximal toward the femoral head junction in-plane with the probe. Keep the convexity of the femoral head in view; the needle should be angled toward the femoral head/neck junction and the anterior hip capsule of the iliofemoral ligament. When injecting the anterior hip capsule, the provider should see fluid filling and infiltrating the joint space.

Figure 4.14: Anterior Hip: Longitudinal/LAX Oblique

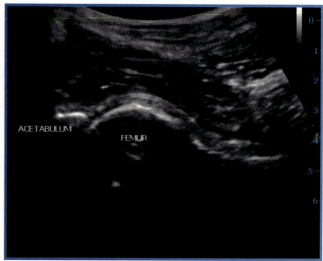

Patient is positioned supine with the probe placed longitudinally over the femoral-acetabular joint. The curvilinear probe enables better depth of penetration and wider field of view.

CHAPTER 21 - THE HIP

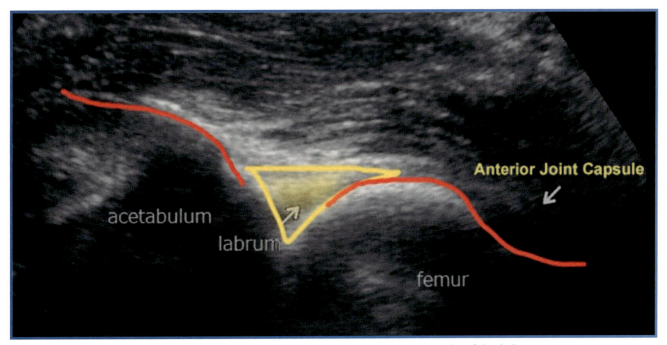

Figure 4.15: Normal long axis appearance of the anterior hip joint anatomy

To optimally image the anterior hip joint in preparation for a percutaneous procedure in the long axis, place the probe over the femoral-acetabular joint at the level of the inguinal crease. The patient is positioned supine and the leg slight abducted and externally rotated in the position consistent with the diagnostic views. The needle is moved from distal to proximal toward the femoral head junction in-plane with the probe. Keep the convexity of the femoral head in view; the needle should be angled toward the femoral head/neck junction and the anterior hip capsule of the iliofemoral ligament (Figure 4.16 and 4.17). When injecting the anterior hip capsule, the provider should see fluid filling and infiltrating the joint space. Ultrasound evidence of degenerative hip joint pathology is variable and it is difficult to grade joint space narrowing using ultrasound. Instead, we use indirect ultrasonographic signs of degenerative joint pathology such as interrupted cortical surface along the femoral head and acetabulum and the presence of paralabral cyst (Figure 4.18).

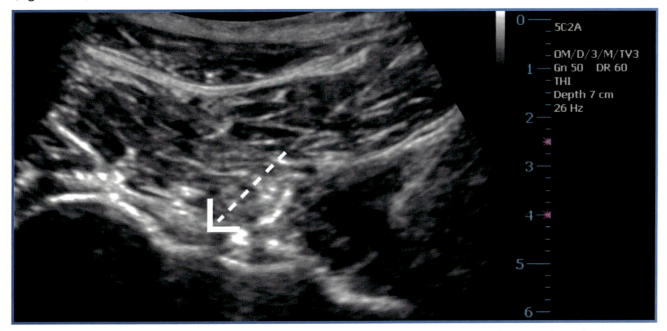

Figure 4.16: Ultrasound image of the femoral head-neck junction in long axis. The needle is visualized moving from proximal to distal in-plane with the probe.

A COMPLETE GUIDE TO REGENERATIVE MEDICINE ©

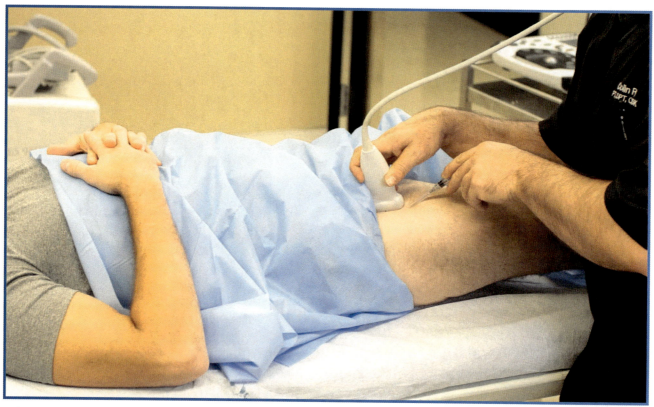

Figure 4.17: Ultrasound guided injection technique to the hip joint capsule via an anterior approach. The patient is positioned supine with the affected extremity in slight abduction. The needle is moving distal to proximal toward the femoral head neck junction, in-plane with the probe.

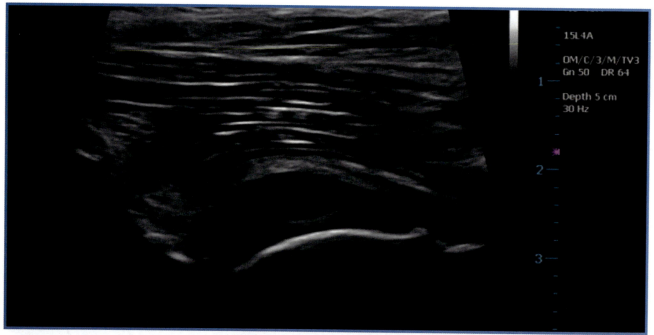

Figure 4.18: Long axis ultrasound image of the hip joint with paralabral cyst formation secondary to osteoarthritis. Also note the interruption of the cortical outline of the proximal femur (Left=Proximal, Right=Distal).

The iliacus and psoas major comprise the iliopsoas group in the anterior hip and can be a source of anterior hip pain. The psoas major is a large muscle that arises from lateral aspects of vertebrae L1-L5. The iliacus originates in the anterior iliac fossa and conjoins with the psoas major at the level of the ilioinguinal ligament forming the iliopsoas muscle-tendon and inserting to the lesser trochanter. The psoas and iliacus muscle groups are analogous to a filet mignon and are powerful force generators in hip flexion. Because of their attachments to the lumbar region and the ilium, the hip flexors, psoas and iliacus, can be involved in cases of low back pain when they become chronically shortened or "tight" over a period of time (Tufo, OMS IV et al., 2012). It is important to clinically correlate these muscle-tendon groups as well as identify with musculoskeletal ultrasound. To optimally visualize the iliopsoas insertion, the patient needs to be positioned in supine with the affected extremity in figure four position: hip flexion, abduction, and external rotation (Figure 4.19). This position places the iliopsoas tendon on a stretch and makes the tendon more echogenic and visible to ultrasound (4.20 and 4.21). For optimal resolution in using the dynamic capacity of ultrasound to its fullest extent, it is important to fix the distal end of the probe on the lesser trochanter and swivel the proximal end of the probe onto the iliopsoas tendon moving to the bony attachment. This allows the operator to clearly visualize the linear tendon fibers moving to and from the lesser trochanter attachment.

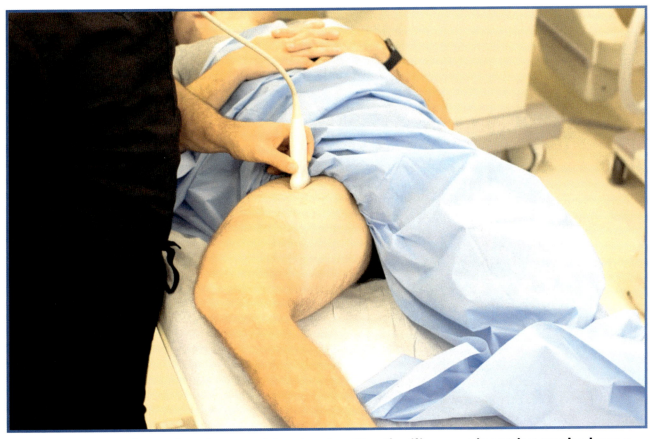

Figure 4.19: Probe and patient position to visualize the iliopsoas insertion to the lesser trochanter.

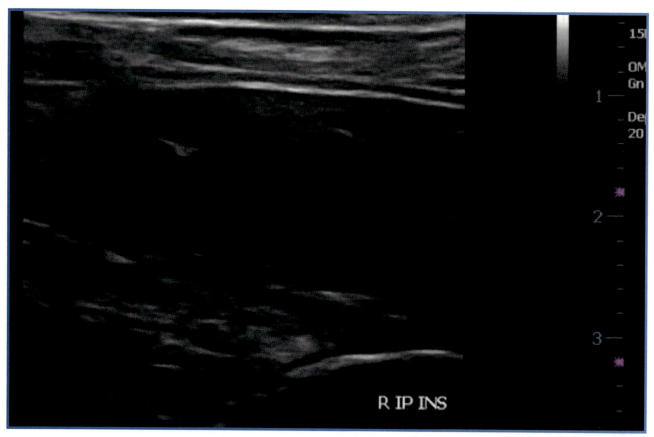

Figure 4.20: Ultrasound Image of Iliopsoas insertion in long axis to the lesser trochanter (IP=iliopsoas, INS=Insertion)

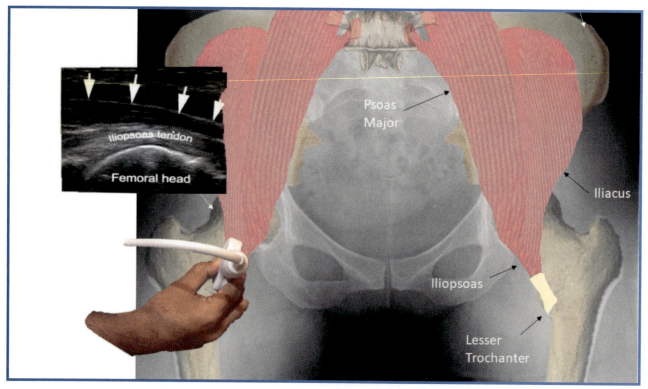

Figure 4.21: Iliopsoas insertion to lesser trochanter with ultrasound orientation in long axis

Hip and groin pain involving the iliopsoas presents a diagnostic and therapeutic challenge because the differential diagnosis can be very extensive, comprising intra-articular and extra-articular pathology and referred pain from lumbar spine, knee and elsewhere in the pelvis (Yeap PM and Robinson P. 2017). Given the numerous complexities of the hip region in musculoskeletal conditions, image-guided injections are useful both for the diagnostic workup and treatment (Pelsser et al., 2001). We know that diagnostic ultrasound is safer than most every other imaging modality because it does not carry the risks of ionizing radiation. The choice of ultrasound probe is important – use of a high-frequency (> 10 MHz) linear array transducer is recommended but lower-frequency curvilinear probes may be occasionally required to visualise deep structures in patients with a large body habitus. A preliminary diagnostic sonographic examination, including colour Doppler of the area to be punctured is necessary to define the relationship of adjacent neurovascular structures.

Healthy sonographic characteristics of the iliopsoas tendon is similar to other regions of the body. It should be linear, hyperechoic/fibrillar, symmetrically homogeneous in shape as well as have an uninterrupted tendon-bone interface without cortical irregularity. Atypical findings of iliopsoas tendinopathy include tendon thickening, hypoechoic clefting, heterogeneous/asymmetric shape and can be a source of extra articular snapping hip (Pelsser et al., 2001). To evaluate the snapping iliopsoas tendon, the transducer is placed just above the hip joint parallel to the public bone in the transverse-oblique plane oriented along the short axis of the iliopsoas tendon (Figure 4.21). The patient is asked to place the hip in the flexion-abduction-external rotation position (flexion, abduction, external rotation), and then return to full extension (neutral position) (Figure 4.22 and 4.23). While the hip is in the frog leg position, the iliopsoas tendon should be visualized laterally and rotates anteriorly to the iliopsoas muscle, and it slides back smoothly to the posteromedial side of the iliopsoas muscle when the hip is returned to neutral position. In the snapping iliopsoas tendon, an abrupt return of the tendon from the lateral-to-medial position is observed, combined with an audible snap sound (Pelsser et al., 2001; Hashimoto et al., 1997).

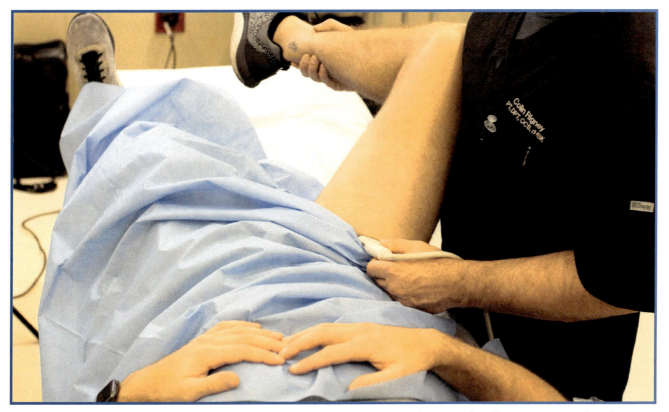

Figure 4.22: Snapping iliopsoas assessment start position. The iliopsoas tendon is visualized in the short axis along with the hip joint line in the short axis.

Figure 4.23: Psoas Major Tendon: SAX Snapping Hip Assessment Image Finish Position

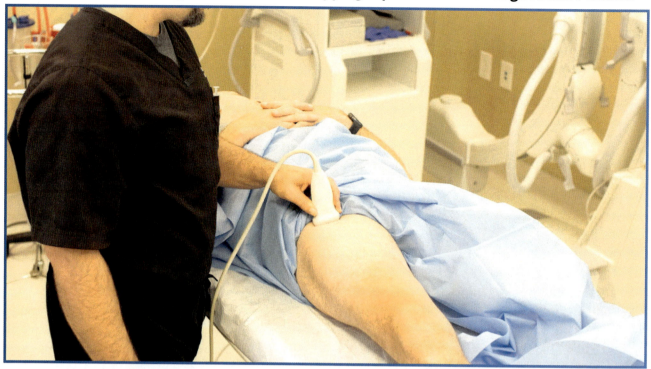
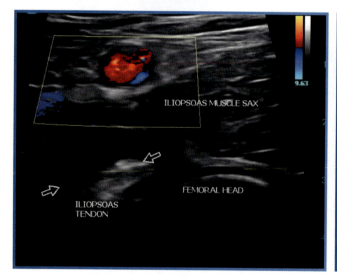
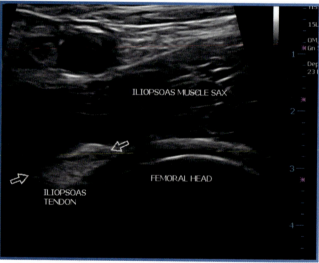

The hypoechoic iliopsoas muscle is superficial to the hyperechoic tendon. Arrows are focused on the iliopsoas tendon at the level of the femoral head/acetabulum to its medial position. This is where the operator should concurrently feel and visualize a "click" over the acetabulum.

CHAPTER 21 - THE HIP

Differential diagnosis considerations in the hip that may be of concern are injury and avulsion of the lesser trochanter apophysis which can happen in children. In cases where adults present with injury, edema, or avulsion of the lesser trochanter, the provider must assume it is a malignancy until proven otherwise. This is because tumoral spread/malignancy along the iliopsoas tendon goes through and attaches and goes from the deep iliac chain and travels along the tendon into the lesser trochanter.

In preparation for an injection to the iliopsoas insertion, the patient is positioned supine with the affected extremity in the frog modified FABER position (flexion-abduction-external rotation) (Figure 4.24). Identification of the distal insertion is paramount, it is important to fix the distal end of the probe on the lesser trochanter and swivel the proximal end of the probe onto the iliopsoas tendon moving to the bony attachment. The needle is moved from distal to proximal in-plane with the probe (Figure 4.25).

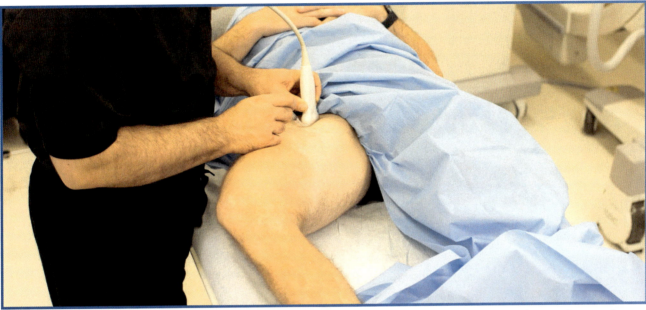

Figure 4.24: Ultrasound guided injection technique to the iliopsoas insertion. The patient is positioned supine in the figure 4 position (flexion-abduction-external rotation) and the needle is moved distal to proximal, in-plane with the probe.

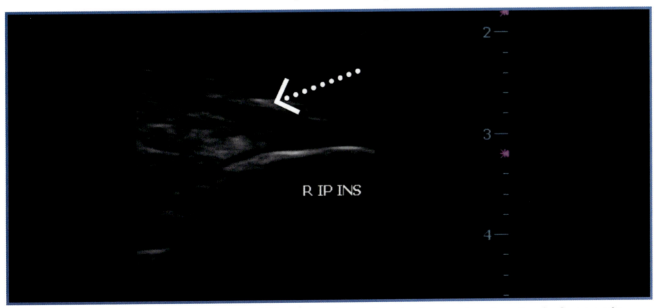

Figure 4.25: Ultrasound image of iliopsoas insertion to lesser trochanter in long axis (IP=iliopsoas, INS=insertion). The needle is moving distal to proximal in-plane with the probe.

CHAPTER 21 - THE HIP

The Medial Hip/Adductor muscles

The medial structures of concern are the adductors longus, brevis and magnus which all insert to the pubic region (Figure 4.26-4.28). The adductor longus inserts to the anterior pubic tubercle and shares a common aponeurosis with the distal rectus abdominis and pyramidalis muscle on the anterior surface of the pubic symphysis region (Figure 4.27). The adductor brevis inserts slightly posterior to the adductor longus on the pubic tubercle and the adductor magnus inserts on the posterior-medial surface of the ischium and lies closer to the hamstring conjoint tendon. Due to the fact this location is a very technically challenging piece of anatomy to reliably diagnostically visualize with a high level of accuracy, ultrasound guided procedures to this area is to be performed only in cases where the operator has the requisite training and experience in musculoskeletal ultrasound. When performing an injection to this region the patient is lying supine with the leg slightly abducted and externally rotated (FIgure 4.30). The needle will move distal to proximal in-plane with the probe (Figure 4.31).

Figure 4.26: Adductor Muscle Group Long Axis

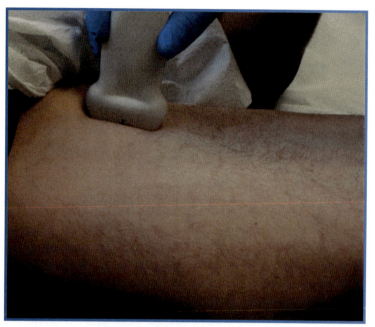
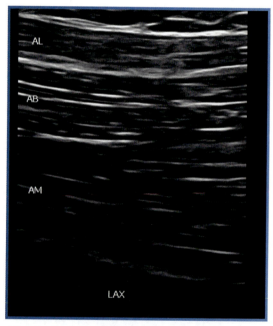

The patient is positioned in side lying or supine frog leg with affected hip abducted and slightly flexed at the hip. The probe is placed in the long axis or parallel with the adductor muscle grouping and can be followed to the pubic attachment.

Ultrasound image from superficial to deep in long axis is the adductor longus, adductor brevis and adductor magnus.

CHAPTER 21 - THE HIP

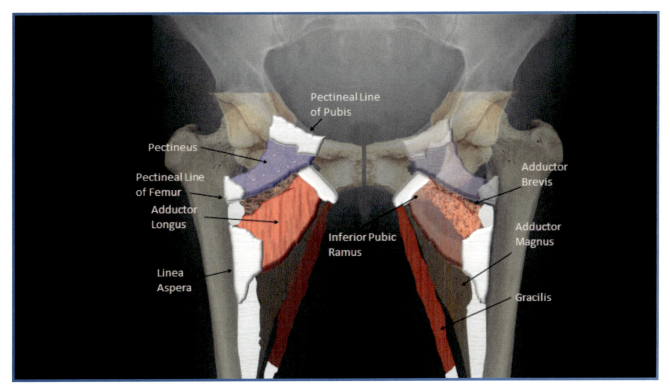

Figure 4.27: Radiologic illustration of the medial hip muscle complexes

Figure 4.28: Adductor Muscle Group Short Axis

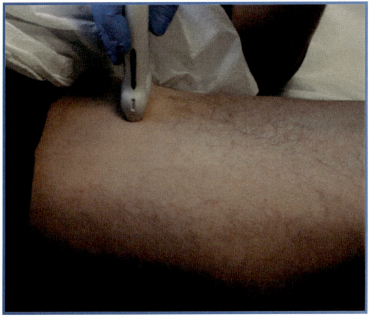

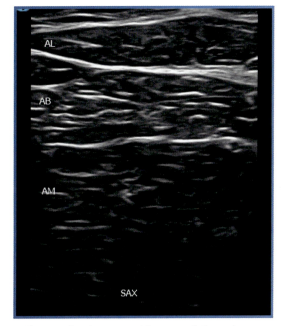

The patient is positioned in side lying or supine frog leg with affected hip abducted and slightly flexed at the hip. The probe is placed in the short axis or transverse with the adductor muscle grouping and can be followed to the pubic attachment.

Short axis ultrasound image of the adductor muscles from superficial to deep: adductor longus, adductor brevis and adductor magnus (AL=Adductor Longus, AB=Adductor Brevis, AM=Adductor Magnus).

A COMPLETE GUIDE TO REGENERATIVE MEDICINE ©

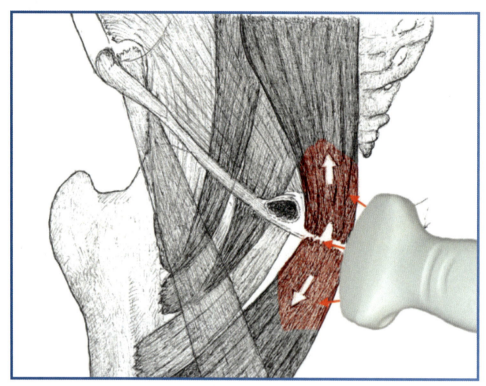

Figure 4.29: Long axis illustration of the conjoint tendon consisting of the distal rectus abdominis and adductor longus

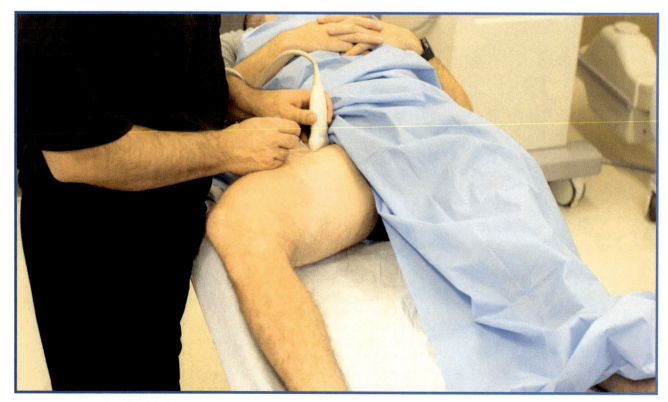

Figure 4.30: Ultrasound guided injection technique to the proximal attachment of the adductor longus. The patient is positioned comfortably supine with the affected leg in slight flexion and abduction. The needle is moved distal to proximal, in-plane with the probe.

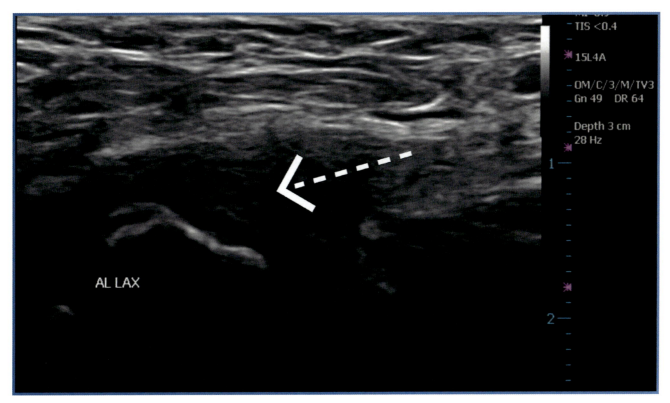

Figure 4.31: Ultrasound guided injection to the proximal adductor longus. The patient is positioned with the affected leg extended in slight abduction and external rotation while the needle is moved distal to proximal, in-plane with the probe.

Lateral Hip Rotator Group

The deep hip lateral rotators are a group of six muscles that stabilize the hip with the primary function being external rotation. From proximal to distal they consist of: piriformis, gemellus superior, obturator internus, gemellus inferior, obturator externus, and the quadratus femoris. From a clinical application standpoint, the main muscle covered in this text is the piriformis because this is the muscle that is most prone to disorder due to its close proximity to the sciatic nerve making it susceptible for thickening and impingement (Hopayian et al., 2010).

Henry Gray "Gray's Anatomy 15th ed." describes the piriformis originating from the anterior portion of the sacrum in three fleshy planes (middle three pieces of its own half and adjoining lateral mass, and medially between the anterior sacral foramina) as well as from the superior margin of the greater sciatic notch and to a lesser extent the sacroiliac joint capsule and the sacrotuberous ligament. The muscle passes out of the pelvis and fills the upper part of the greater sciatic foramen into the gluteal region. The piriformis exits the pelvis through the greater sciatic foramen and co-joins with the superior gemellus, inferior gemellus and obturator internus to insert on the apex of the greater trochanter of the femur.

Piriformis syndrome encompasses a constellation of symptoms, including buttock and leg pain and with ultrasound, can be a reliable diagnostic tool for clinical diagnosis of piriformis syndrome (Zhang et al., 2019). It has been described for 500 years, yet remains controversial in the literature and in clinical practice ((Jankovic et al., 2013; Santamente et al., 2015; Fishman and Shaefer. 2003). The primary sonographic characteristics found in patients with piriformis syndrome are atypical cross sectional thickness in short axis, increased diameter measurement in long axis and hypoechogenicity compared to the uninvolved side or other healthy patients (Zhang et al., 2019). Using these characteristics as a tool to objectively define the health of the piriformis and combined with a thorough physical exam and history, ultrasound can be an extremely useful tool in the point of care setting to help diagnose piriformis syndrome. As with all procedures described in this text and especially with the piriformis, to become a competently reliable interventionist with ultrasound one must be able to read and assess the sonographic characteristics of the tissue at hand prior to simply performing a procedure.

To reliably visualize the piriformis muscle with consistency, one must have a systematic protocol. The patient can be positioned prone with a pillow underneath the hips to place the hip rotators on a slight stretch. This will elicit a better image. To optimize reproducibility, piriformis localization is based on bony acoustic landmarks. The posterior superior iliac spine (PSIS) is scanned by initially palpating it and then placing the transducer horizontally across it. The gluteus maximus is the easiest muscle to identify because of its bulk and because it lies most superficially to every structure at this level. Starting at the PSIS in the short axis and keeping the gluteus maximus muscle (most superficial) clearly visualized, the operator should slowly translate the probe inferiorly until the muscles begin to appear deep to the gluteus maximus. The first muscle encountered with this maneuver will be the piriformis in the long axis. To help confirm that it truly is the piriformis, the operator can bend the affected knee to between 45-90 degrees and slowly internally-externally rotate the hip and the external rotator groups will move in sync with the movement pattern. If there is concern or question of which muscle is the piriformis, just recall that the piriformis is the most superior of the six (Figure 4.32 and 4.33). Another important anatomic structure to be mindful of when preparing for intervention to the deep hip rotator region is the sciatic nerve. The sciatic nerve passes just underneath the piriformis muscle in most of the population; however, there are anatomic variances to be aware of so careful "clearing" to identify the nerve location should be performed prior to any intervention (4.34).

When performing an ultrasound guided injection to the piriformis, the patient is prone with a pillow underneath the hips to place the external rotators on a slight stretch and bring them closer to the ultrasound probe. The muscle-tendon of the piriformis is visualized in long axis and the needle approach is lateral to medial in-plane with the probe (Figure 4.35 and 4.36).

Figure 4.32: Piriformis Muscle: Longitudinal/LAX

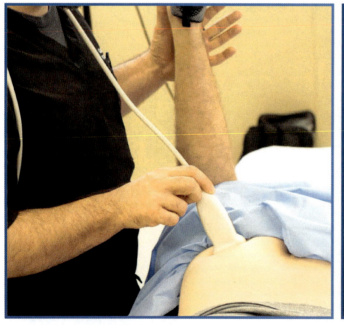
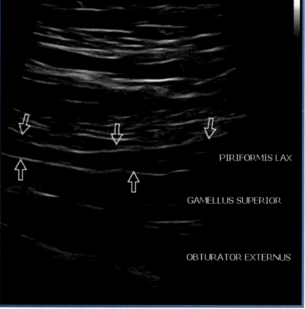

Patient is positioned prone with hips in slight flexion (place bolster underneath to put hip extensors on stretch). Place transducer longitudinal to the hip external rotators. Identify the gluteus maximus in short axis at the iliac fossa then slowly translate the transducer inferiorly until you see the distinct musculature of the deep hip external rotators underneath the gluteus maximus. The knee is placed in flexion so the operator can dynamically internally-externally rotate the hip for confirmation of the structure. The piriformis is the most superior muscle of the six deep hip external rotators and is best visualized at the sacral attachment. From here, the operator can scan toward the femoral attachment to visualize the length of the muscle and tendon.

CHAPTER 21 - THE HIP

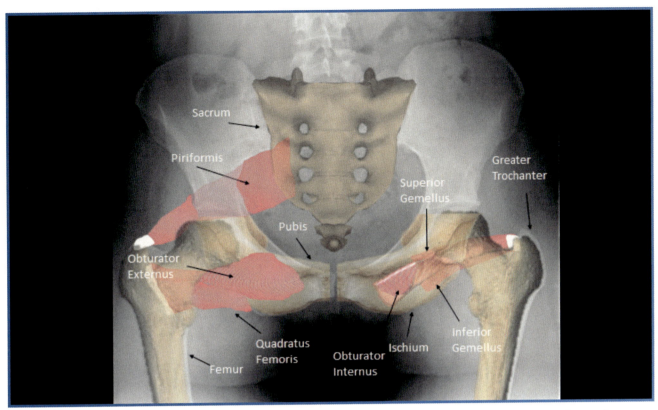

Figure 4.33: Radiologic illustration of the deep hip rotator anatomy. Note how the piriformis is located most superior of the six muscle groups

Figure 4.34: Piriformis Muscle & Sciatic Nerve: Longitudinal/LAX

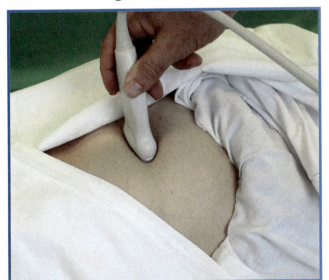
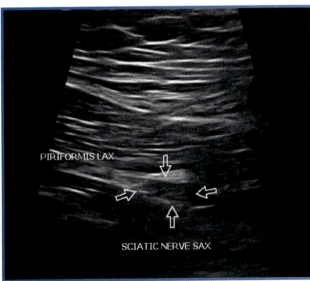

Patient is positioned prone with hips in slight flexion (place bolster underneath to put hip extensors on stretch). Place transducer longitudinal to the hip external rotators. First, identify the piriformis as described above. The sciatic nerve sits and exits just below the mid-portion of the piriformis muscle and is at this position where the operator can best view the nerve in the short axis.

A COMPLETE GUIDE TO REGENERATIVE MEDICINE ©

CHAPTER 21 - THE HIP

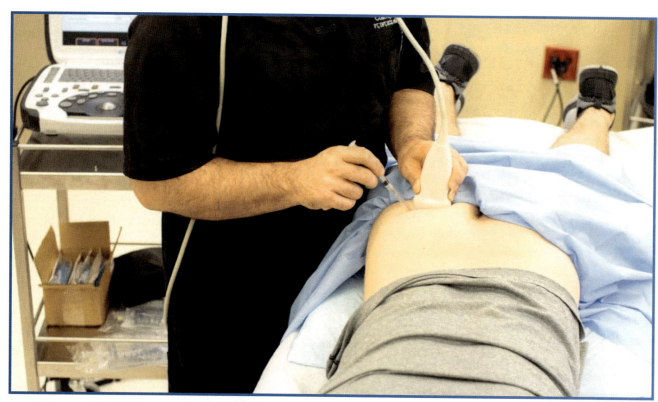

Figure 4.35: Ultrasound guided injection technique to the piriformis. The patient is positioned comfortably in prone with a pillow underneath the hips. The needle is moved lateral to medial, in-plane with the probe

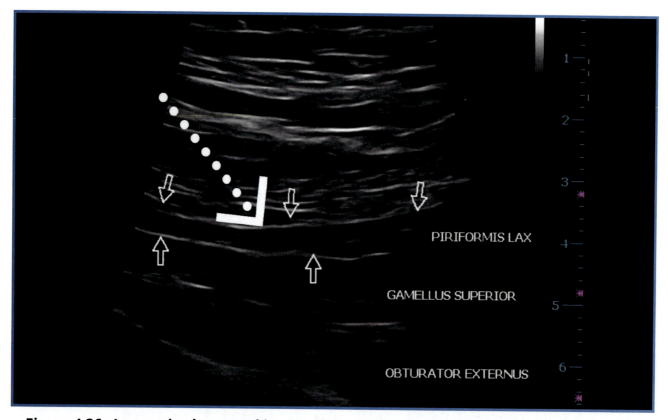

Figure 4.36: Long axis ultrasound image of the piriformis with the needle moving from lateral to medial in-plane with the probe

CHAPTER 21 - THE HIP

Posterior Hip/Hamstrings:

The hamstring tendons originate at the posterior aspect of the ischial tuberosity and consists of two common attachments; the semimembranosus and the conjoint tendon (Figure 4.37 and 4.38). The semimembranosus muscle originates from the ischial tuberosity deep and lateral to the conjoint tendon, it is a long tendon and as it moves distally, it becomes a membrane at the upper 3rd of the thigh before then forming into muscle again; hence the name semimembranosus. The semimembranosus inserts distally to the posterior aspect of the proximal tibia. The semitendinosus and the biceps femoris conjoint together at the ischial tuberosity; hence the name conjoint tendon. The biceps femoris inserts distally to the lateral and posterior aspect of the fibular head. Distally, the semitendinosus joins the sartorius and gracilis, forming the pes anserine group at the posterior-medial knee, inserting to the proximal third/anterior-medial aspect of the tibia.

Figure 4.37: Hamstring Tendon Origin: Semimembranosus Longitudinal/Long Axis

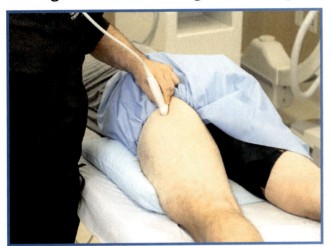
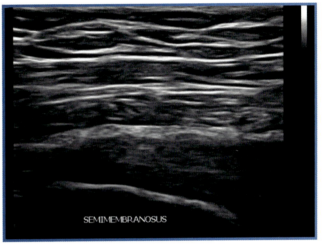

The patient is positioned prone with a pillow or bolster underneath the hips to place the hamstring origin on slight tension. The probe is positioned superior-laterally on the ischial tuberosity in long axis to best view the fibrillar origin of the semimembranosus

Figure 4.38: Hamstring Tendon Origin: Conjoint Tendon Longitudinal/Long Axis

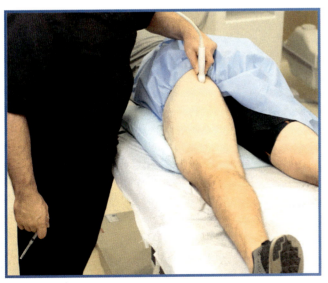
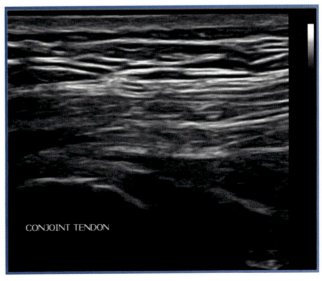

The patient is positioned prone with a pillow or bolster underneath the hips to place the hamstring origin on slight tension. The probe is positioned posterior-central on the ischial tuberosity in the long axis to best view the fibrillar origin of the conjoint tendon.

A COMPLETE GUIDE TO REGENERATIVE MEDICINE ©

Prior to detailing how to inject the proximal hamstring structures, it is necessary to describe the sonographic anatomy of the region. Percutaneous procedures to the high hamstring can be complex because the technical skill required to image the area is fairly difficult. When scanning the proximal hamstrings, it is important to adhere to a protocol-based system that is replicable. When examining the ischial tendon attachments, we advise to place the patient in prone with a pillow underneath the hips to place the structures on slight tension for optimal ultrasound visibility. We recommend the examination begin with longitudinal scanning at the level of the ischial tuberosity, which can be palpated, being a good anatomic landmark (Becciolini et al., 2019). To improve image quality, we suggest starting with a slight lateral approach on the ischial tuberosity and the patient should be informed that the transducer may have to be pressed hardly; this maneuver is also recommended in symptomatic patients to reproduce pain: so-called sonopalpation (Nasarian et al., 2008). The lateral aspect of the ischial tuberosity is where the semimembranosus can be identified with the conjoint tendon slightly medial to it. Located distal to the ischial tuberosity and lateral to the hamstring muscle complex tendon, the sciatic nerve, a fascicular and flattened structure, can be easily shown in short axis: it descends between and deep to the long head of the biceps femoris and the semitendinosus muscle, superficial to the adductor magnus muscle (Hung et al., 2016). The sciatic nerve enters deep to the gluteal region along the lower edges of the piriformis muscle. From here, at the proximal third of the thigh, the nerve goes down into the gluteus maximus muscle between the greater trochanter and the ischial tuberosity and adjacent to the hamstring muscles biceps femoris and semitendinosus in the posterior thigh, the adductor magnus is deep to the hamstring musculature and sciatic nerve (Figure 4.39).

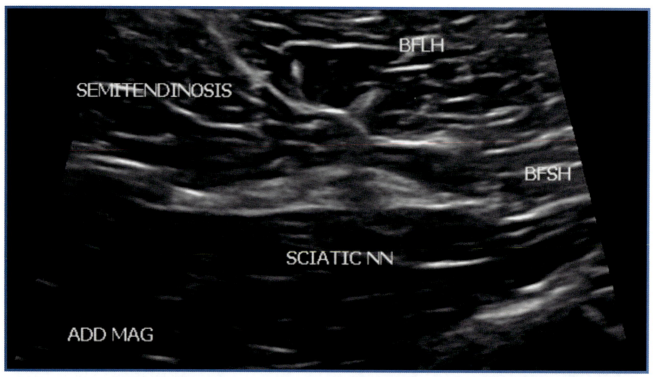

Figure 4.39: Short axis ultrasound image of the hamstring muscle groups in the proximal third of the thigh. The sciatic nerve is located superficial to the adductor magnus. BFLH=Biceps Femoris Long Head, BFSH=Biceps Femoris Short Head

Proximal hamstring injuries can occur acutely or from chronic overuse. Acute proximal hamstring injuries typically occur from a rapid, forced eccentric moment such as when someone does the splits, initiates a sudden change in direction in an athletic endeavor or slips on a child's toy in a dark room. Acute injuries are usually accompanied with a significant fluid collection as well as the occasional avulsion fracture of the ischium. Chronic proximal hamstring injuries usually occur in athletes (both competitive and recreational) athletes who have ignored the lingering problem over a period of time. Chronic hamstring tears usually present themselves in the form of tendinopathy from a "strain to failure" type of mechanism. Sonographic characteristics of proximal hamstring tendinopathy is similar to other regions in the body: thickened tendon with hypoechoic clefting and cortical irregularities at the tendon-bone interface (Figure 4.40).

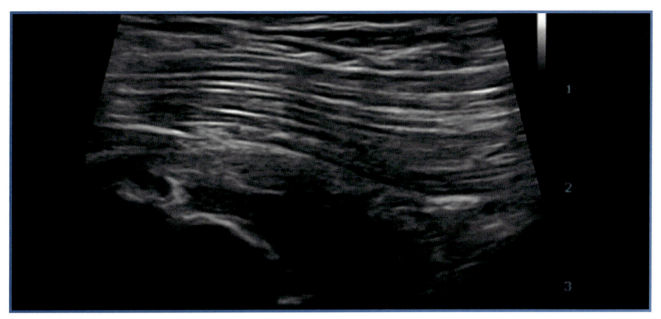

Figure 4.40: Long axis ultrasound image of semimembranosus tendinopathy evidenced by tendon thickening, hypoechoic clefting and cortical irregularity at the proximal attachment.

When performing ultrasound guided procedures to the proximal hamstring tendons we advise positioning the same as during examinations (prone with pillows underneath the hips to place the tendons on a slight stretch). The structures are visualized in the long axis and the needle should be moved from distal to proximal in-plane with the probe.

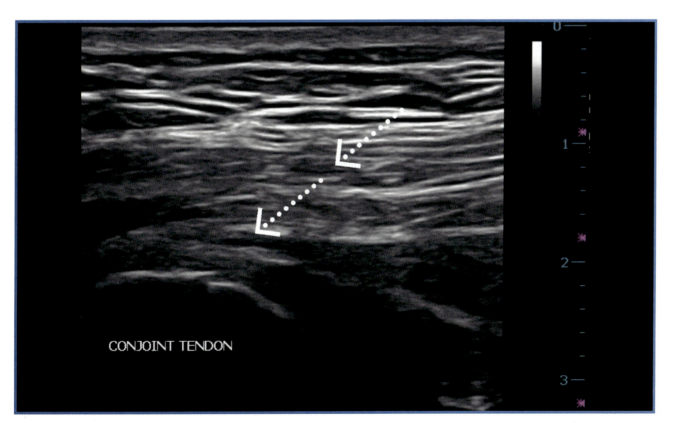

Figure 4.41: Long axis ultrasound image of the conjoint tendon attachment at the ischium. The needle is moved distal to proximal in-plane with the probe

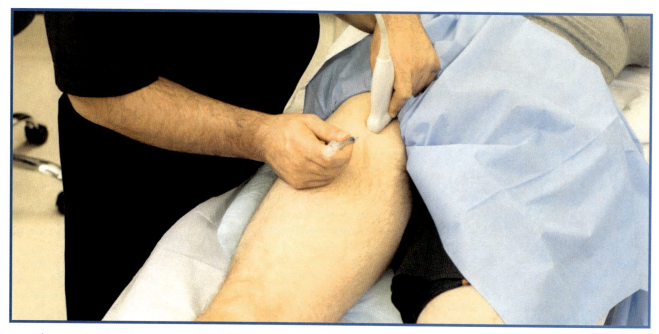

Figure 4.42: Ultrasound guided injection technique to the proximal hamstring origin. The patient is positioned comfortably in prone, with a pillow underneath the hips. The hamstrings are visualized in the long axis and the needle is moved distal to proximal, in-plane with the probe.

Sacroiliac Joint

Henry Gray (Gray's Anatomy 15th ed.) describes the sacroiliac articulation as an amphiarthrodial joint formed between the lateral surfaces of the sacrum and the ilium. The anterior or auricular portion of each surface is covered with a thin plate of cartilage, thicker on the sacrum than the ilium. These are in close contact with each other, and are united together by irregular patches of softer fibro-cartilage and by fine fibers of interosseous tissue at the upper and posterior portion (Gray et al., 1995) The joint is connected by a series of ligaments such as the anterior sacroiliac ligament, posterior sacroiliac ligament, the great or posterior sacro-sciatic ligament and the lesser or anterior sacro-sciatic ligament (Gray et al., 1995). There are 35 muscles that attach near or around the sacroiliac joint (Calvillo et al., 2000) making it a complex region to both diagnose and treat.

There is some variance in the literature regarding the pathomechanics and etiology of sacroiliac dysfunction but it can be generally described as a broad term referring to abnormal biomechanical dysfunction of the joint and common causes of sacroiliac dysfunction are trauma, hypermobility, degeneration, osteoarthritis and inflammation (Simopoulos et al., 2012). For the purposes of this book we'll cover some general aspects of sacroiliac dysfunction and how to address it with orthobiologics using ultrasound; however, the comprehensive examination and diagnosis of this region goes beyond the scope of this text so we'll collectively leave it to the practitioners and clinicians to come to their own conclusions in the decision to treat.

In contrast to many other body regions discussed in this book, the sacroiliac joint is not a very sensitive location to diagnose using ultrasound. The diagnosis of sacroiliitis is primarily a clinical decision made by the provider based upon the physical exam, history, radiographs and possibly MRI/CT.

Use of ultrasound for needle guidance into the sacroiliac joint is a very technically challenging procedure. There is much literature available stating that many ultrasound guided procedures to this region are not accurate. A recent cadaver study reported in the Physical Medicine and Rehabilitation Journal that only 1 in 20 injections using ultrasound were successful in getting into the sacroiliac joint (Zheng et al., 2019). In contrast with fluoroscopy and coupled with the fact that ultrasound cannot provide the requisite lateral view or arthrogram as contrast, the study suggests that the success rate of ultrasound guided sacroiliac joint injections are low in part due to the high operator dependency of the modality and that inherently variable skill of the user is likely a major cause of the widely variable success rates reported across the literature (Zheng et al., 2019).

With any technical skill, repetition is the key to being successful. To successfully inject the sacroiliac joint, the provider must be able to reliably find the joint space. The easiest way to do this is to palpate the posterior superior iliac spine (PSIS), place the probe in the short axis over the landmark and slowly translate the probe distally in the short axis while keeping the posterior ilium in view (Figure 4.43). The joint line will be found roughly 1-2cm distal from the palpation landmark of the PSIS.

When injecting the sacroiliac joint with ultrasound the needle is best visualized moving medially to lateral, in-plane with the probe (Figure 4.44 and 4.45).

Figure 4.43: Sacroiliac Joint Imaging: Transverse/SAX

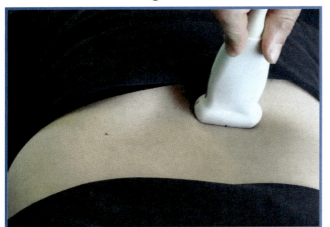
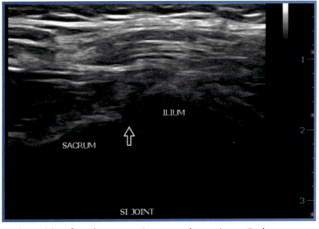

The patient is positioned prone with the bolster underneath ankles for decrease in neural tension. Palpate the posterior superior iliac spine and place the probe in the short axis over it. From here, translate the probe distal until the sacrum is visualized; here the space between the bony contours of the sacrum and ilium represents the posterior aspect of the SI joint. (Arrow is pointing to the joint space)

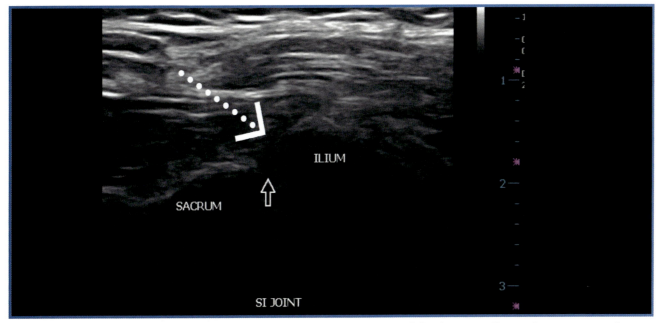

Figure 4.44: Ultrasound image of the sacroiliac joint with the needle trajectory moving medial to lateral in-plane with the probe

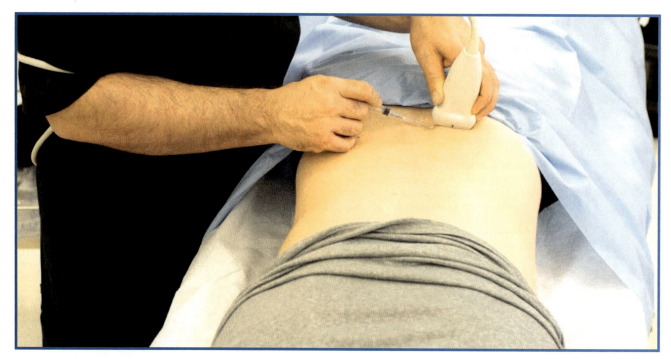

Figure 4.45: Ultrasound guided injection technique to the sacroiliac joint. The patient is positioned comfortably in prone, with a pillow underneath the hips. The joint is visualized in the long axis and the needle is moved medial to lateral, in-plane with the probe.

Based on Dr. Albert's clinical experience:
Greater Trochanteric Bursa: About 4-5 cc of injectate.
Piriformis Muscle: About 5-10 cc.
Hamstring insertions: 2-4 cc injecting into the ischial tuberosity at the level of the insertion of the hamstring insertion. Again, the hamstring insertions are again the semitendinosus, semimembranosus, and biceps femoris.
Posterior injections into the patient's buttocks at the level of the subgluteal crease – when the patient is in prone position.

Sample Dictation/Note:

Sample Dictation for PRP:
The procedure and potential complications were discussed with the patient. After written and verbal consent were obtained, the patient was placed in the seated position. A tourniquet was placed on the right arm and the area was surveyed for large palpable veins. The antecubital area was prepped and draped in the usual sterile fashion using alcohol. Using an 20G needle, approximately [ ] ccs of blood was drawn from the patient and transferred to a specially prepared PRP tube containing anticoagulants. After the needle was removed, and a sterile bandage was placed over the entry site, the tube was vertically rotated back and forth five times.

The tube was placed in a centrifuge with an opposing counter-weight. After five minutes, the tube was removed and inspected. There was a visible gel, a buffy coat, and a golden liquid layer of PRP. The tube was vertically rotated back and forth five times. Afterwards, the PRP and buffy coat were gently extracted and transferred to a 10 cc syringe. The syringe was attached to a 22G 1.5" needle.

[Patient positioning as described above depending on the type of injection and approach]

The _____ was prepped and draped in the usual sterile manner using three coats of betadine. The area of interest was identified using sonography. The area of interest was identified by the following landmarks: _____

With the probe held in place, a ½ a cc of 1% lidocaine was used to create a wheal at the entry site alongside the probe. The needle guidance software package was turned on. After a moment, with the probe held in place, the needle and syringe containing the PRP was advanced through the skin and the deeper tissues towards the target area. Under ultrasound guidance, the PRP was injected. The final image was recorded. The probe was moved, the needle was removed and a sterile gauze was held over the injection site with gentle pressure. A sterile bandage was applied. The patient was repositioned for comfort. The patient tolerated the procedure well with no apparent complications.

CHAPTER 21 - THE HIP

References:

L. Molini et al., Hip Anatomy and US Technique. J Ultrasound. 2011 Jun; 14(2): 99–108.

Tirith Dunn 1, C Ann Heller, Stanley W McCarthy, Cristobal Dos Remedios. Anatomical Study of the "Trochanteric Bursa." Journal of Clinical Anatomy. 2004 May; 16(3): 233-40. DOI: 10.1002/ca. 10084

Jacobsen J. Fundamentals of Musculoskeletal Ultrasound (3rd edition). Page 167. Elsevier, Sep 2017.

Jacobsen J. Fundamentals of Musculoskeletal Ultrasound (3rd edition). Page 168. Elsevier, Sep 2017.

S. Bianchi, S. Martinoli. Hip. S. Bianchi, C. Martinoli (Eds.), Ultrasound of the musculoskeletal system, Springer-Verlag, Berlin (2007), pp. 554-610

Andrea Tufo, OMS IV et al., Psoas Syndrome: A Frequently Missed Diagnosis. The Journal of the American Osteopathic Association, August 2012, Vol. 112, 522-528.

Yeap PM, Robinson P. Ultrasound Diagnostic and Therapeutic Injections of the Hip and Groin. Journal of the Belgian Society of Radiology. 2017;101(S2):6. DOI: http://doi.org/10.5334/jbr-btr.1371

Deshmukh, AJ, Thakur, RR, Goyal, A, Klein, DA, Ranawat, AS and Rodriguez, JA. Accuracy of diagnostic injection in differentiating source of atypical hip pain. Journal of Arthroplasty. 2010; 25: 129–133. DOI: https://doi.org/10.1016/j.arth.2010.04.015

V. Pelsser, E. Cardinal, R. Hobden, et al., Extraarticular snapping hip: sonographic findings. AJR, 176 (2001), pp. 67-73

B.E. Hashimoto, T.M. Green, L. Wiitala. Ultrasonographic diagnosis of hip snapping related to iliopsoas tendon. J Ultrasound Med, 16 (1997), pp. 433

Hopayian K, Song F, Riera R, Sambandan S. The clinical features of the piriformis syndrome: a systematic review. European Spine Journal. 2010 Dec 1;19(12):2095-109.

Wenhua Zhang, MD etc. Ultrasound appears to be a reliable technique for the diagnosis of piriformis syndrome. Muscle Nerve. 2019 Apr; 59(4): 411–416.

Jankovic D, Peng P, van Zundert A. Brief review: piriformis syndrome: etiology, diagnosis, and management. Can J Anaesth 2013;60:1003–1012. [PubMed] [Google Scholar]

Santamato A, Micello MF, Valeno G, Beatrice R, Cinone N, Baricich A, et al Ultrasound guided injection of botulinum toxin type A for piriformis muscle syndrome: a case report and review of the literature. Toxins (Basel) 2015;7:3045–3056.

Fishman LM, Schaefer MP. The piriformis syndrome is underdiagnosed. Muscle Nerve 2003;28:646–649.

Becciolini, Marco MD et al., Ultrasound Features of the Hamstring Muscle-Tendon-Bone Unit. Journal Of Ultrasound Medicine 2019; 38:1367–1382.

Nazarian LN. The top 10 reasons musculoskeletal sonography is an important complementary or alternative technique to MRI. AJR Am J Roentgenol 2008; 190:1621–1626.
Hung CY, Hsiao MY, Özçakar L, et al., Sonographic tracking of the lower limb peripheral nerves: a pictorial essay and video demonstration. Am J Phys Med Rehabil 2016; 95:698–708.

Koski J. Ultrasound-guided injections in rheumatology. J Rheumatol 2000;27:2131-8.

Gray, H. Gray's Anatomy 15th edition by Gray, Henry (1995) (213-216).

Calvillo O., Skaribas I., Turnispeed J., Anatomy and pathophysiology of the SIJ, current science, 2000 (LOE 2A)

Simopoulos T. Manchikanti L. Singh V. Gupta S. Hameed H. Diwan S. Cohen P. A Systematic valuation of Prevalence and Diagnostic Accuracy of Sacroiliac Joint Interventions. Pain Physician 2012; 15:E305-E344 (http://www.painphysicianjournal.com/2012/may/2012;15;E305-E344.pdf)

Patricia Zheng MD, Byron J. Schneider MD, Aaron Yang MD, Zachary L. McCormick MD. Image-Guided Sacroiliac Joint Injections: an Evidence-based Review of Best Practices and Clinical Outcomes. 22 May 2019 https://doi.org/10.1002/pmrj.12191

CHAPTER 22: The Knee

Colin Rigney, Pradeep Albert & Brendan Tarzia

> **CHAPTER PREVIEW**
>
> In this chapter we will cover sonoanatomy of common knee structures as well as patient and probe positions for proper evaluation. Additionally, the chapter will include common pictorial examples and explanations of pathology found with ultrasound as well as basic ultrasound-guided injection techniques.

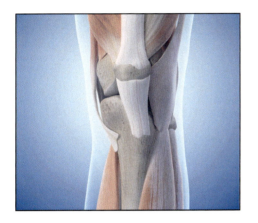

The osseous anatomy of the knee is fairly simple. The knee joint is primarily a hinge joint composed of the femur, tibia, fibula and the patella which is the largest sesamoid bone in the body. We will also be detailing the soft tissue and extra-articular anatomy that can be reliably visualized with musculoskeletal ultrasound.

Quadriceps tendon

The quadriceps muscle group lies anteriorly and comprises four different muscles. The most superficial muscle of the quadriceps is the rectus femoris and the deepest muscle is the vastus intermedius. The vastus lateralis lies laterally and the vastus medialis medially. These four muscles converge into the quadriceps tendon and attach to the superior pole of the patella.

The quadriceps tendon is a common site to examine tendinopathy using musculoskeletal ultrasound to diagnose the tissue with a high degree of sensitivity and specificity (Bianchi et al., 1994). Quadriceps tendinopathy is a clinical diagnosis characterized by significant tenderness at the superior pole of the patella. In many published reports, the name "patellar tendinopathy" is used to describe tendinopathy of the quadriceps tendon; more recently, an association of anterior knee pain and patellar tendinosis in community-based non-athletic patients, who have an increased body mass index (BMI) was found (King et al., 2019). These findings also highlight the importance of surveillance of this entity as a cause of anterior knee pain in the non-athlete or recreational athlete population (King et al., 2019) where overload injuries are the most common mode of pathogenesis in cases of quadriceps tendinopathy. Injury mechanism to the quadriceps tendon usually occurs during activities associated with repetitive loading, stress, and knee extension which is historically labeled as "jumper's knee" (King et al., 2019). Other diagnoses of consideration that often run in tandem, needing to be run for a differential diagnosis with quadriceps tendinosis include chondromalacia patella and patellar tendinopathy; ultrasound is an excellent tool to separate.

Normal sono-anatomy of the quadriceps tendon is characterized by a hyperechoic, linear pattern of echoes attaching to the superior pole of the patella (Figure 5.1 and 5.2). Pathologic departures from normal sono-anatomy include hypoechoic clefting in regions where the tendon should be hyperechoic as well as cortical irregularities at the tendon-bone interface at the superior pole. Historically, the management of quadriceps and patellar tendinopathy typically consists of non-surgical means such as rest and physical therapy. Be mindful when using ultrasound to examine quadriceps tendinopathy on the uninvolved extremity as it is common to find asymptomatic pathology. Regarding the knee extensor mechanism as a whole, there is emerging evidence that the use of orthobiologics can be an excellent treatment option in cases where the quadriceps and patellar tendon does not respond to physical therapy, avoidance therapy or activity modification (Toppi et al., 2014; Filardo et al., 2010).

Suggested injection approach to the quadriceps tendon insertion is to visualize the tendon in short axis, moving the needle from lateral to medial, in-plane with the probe (Figure 5.3 and 5.4).

CHAPTER 22 - THE KNEE

Figure 5.1: Suprapatellar Bursa/Quadriceps Tendon: Transverse/SAX

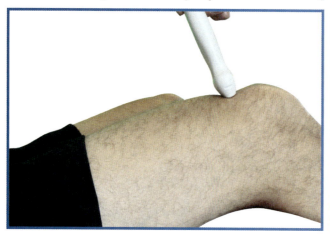 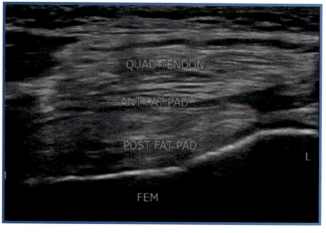

The patient is positioned supine with knee flexed 30-45 degrees. The probe is placed in the short axis to the distal femur and quadriceps tendon where the cross section of the quadriceps tendon can be fully appreciated. The suprapatellar recess is the dark space located in between the anterior and posterior fat pad.

Figure 5.2: Suprapatellar Bursa/Quadriceps Tendon: Longitudinal/LAX

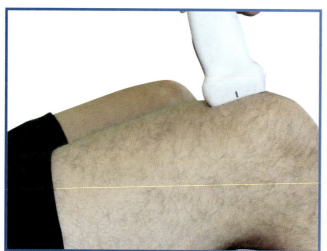 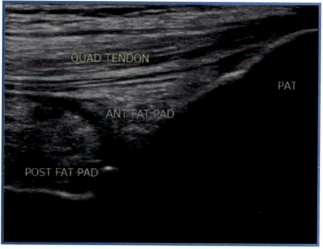

With the patient lying supine, slightly flex the knee 20-30 degrees by placing a small pillow underneath the knee. The probe is placed in the long axis to the distal femur and quadriceps tendon. The superficial, middle and deep layers of the tendon can be appreciated as they attach to the superior pole of the patella. This healthy representation of the suprapatellar recess is visualized as the thin hypoechoic line between the anterior and posterior fat pad.

CHAPTER 22 - THE KNEE

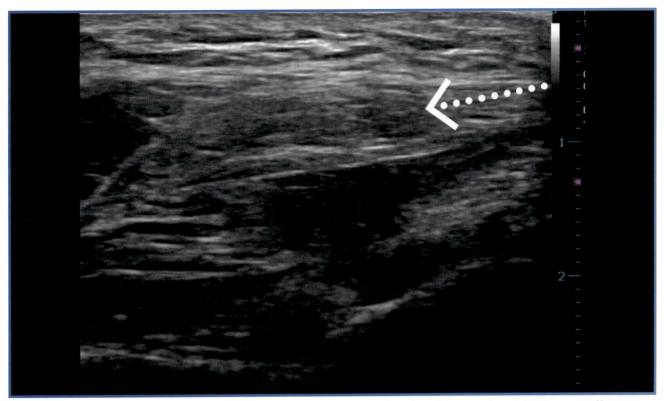

Figure 5.3: Ultrasound image of the quadriceps tendon in short axis with the needle moving lateral to medial in-plane with the probe toward the insertion

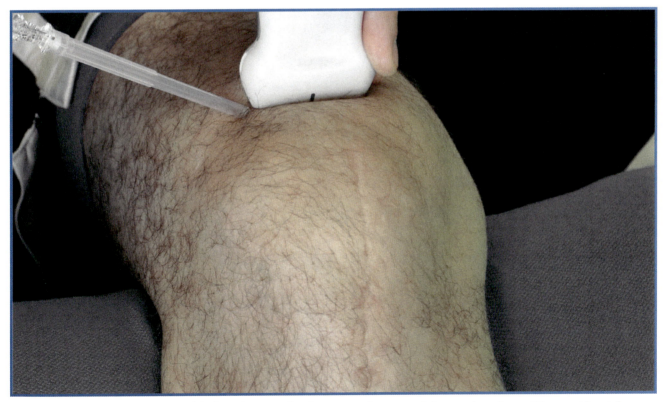

Figure 5.4: Ultrasound injection technique to the quadriceps tendon. The patient is positioned supine with the knee placed over a bolster 25-30 degrees. The tendon is visualized in the short axis and the needle is moved lateral to medial, in-plane with the probe.

Patellar tendon

A common issue treated around the knee in the athletic and recreationally-inclined patient is patellar tendinopathy, commonly known as jumper's knee. Most patellar tendinopathies occur at the tendon-bone interface of the inferior pole of the patella and can be assessed objectively and reliably by using musculoskeletal ultrasound. The patellar tendon is a major force transducer and vitally crucial in the function of the knee extensor mechanism complex. The patellar tendon attaches the patella to the tibial tubercle at the anterior aspect of the knee.

Normal/healthy sonographic characteristics of the patellar tendon are similar to the quadriceps tendon with the main difference being the diameter of the tendon itself (Figure 5.5-5.7). The patellar tendon is smaller in diameter. Similar to the quadriceps tendon at the superior pole patella, most pathologic conditions involving the patellar tendon are located at the tendon-bone interface with the inferior pole of the patella (Figure 5.8). Also similar to the quadriceps tendon, the pathogenesis of patellar tendinopathy is multifactorial and is most likely the result of prolonged repetitive mechanical stresses that involve repeated movements in compromised and uncompromised loading patterns usually without adequate rest between bouts (Walter et al., 1985; Renstrom et al., 1985; Feretti et al., 1983). Obtaining an objective diagnosis is fairly straightforward. Clinically, most patients have significant point tenderness along the tendon as well as history of the pain location being anterior in nature. Sonography is very sensitive in documenting the pathoanatomic features of patellar tendinopathy. Ultrasound characteristics of diseased patellar tendon are very similar to other tendons found in the body and typically consists of tendon thickening, hypoechoic clefting with or without cortical irregularity at the tendon-bone interface at the inferior pole attachment.

Figure 5.5: Patellar Tendon: Longitudinal/long axis

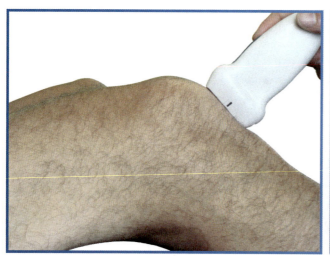
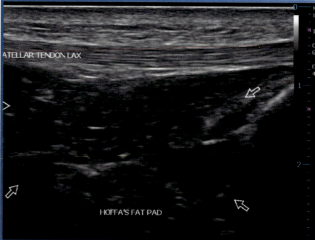
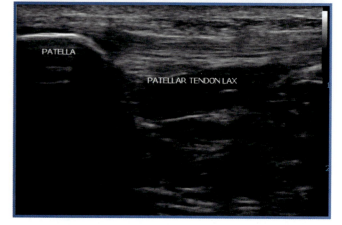

Add a slight bend of the knee and place the probe on the anteromedial aspect of the infrapatellar region, this can be done by resting the extremity over a bolster. The fibrillar patellar tendon can be appreciated running superior to the patellar and inserting distally on to the tibia. The top right image shows arrows pointing to Hoffa fat pad deep to the patellar tendon between the patella and tibia.

Figure 5.6: Patellar Tendon: Transverse/short axis

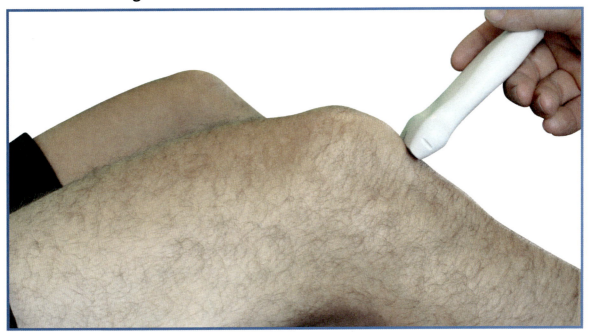

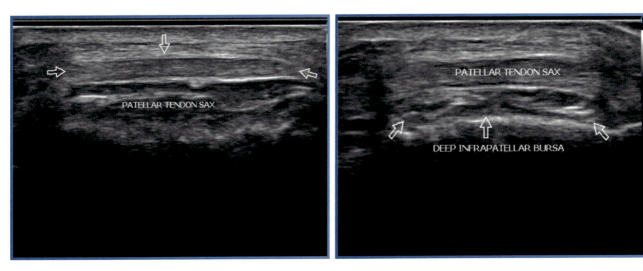

With the same positioning as the long axis view, rotate the probe 90 degrees to appreciate the width and true thickness of the patellar tendon. This view of the top image allows screening for tendinopathy that might not have been in view longitudinally. The bottom image shows arrows pointing to the deep infrapatellar bursa deep to the patellar tendon at the tibial attachment.

CHAPTER 22 - THE KNEE

Figure 5.7: Distal Patellar tendon Infrapatellar Bursae: Longitudinal/LAX

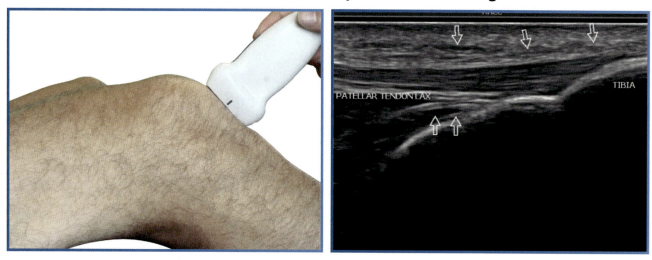

Patient is positioned supine with the knee in 30-45 degrees flexion. Place the probe distal to the patella on the anterior aspect of the knee joint. The ultrasound image details the patellar tendon in the long axis at its tendon-bone junction with the tibia. Top arrows: represent the superficial infrapatellar bursa. Bottom arrows: represent the deep infrapatellar bursa.

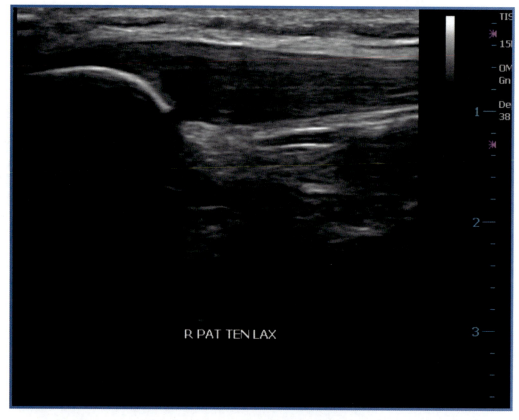

Figure 5.8: Long axis image of patellar tendinopathy at the tendon-bone interface with the inferior patellar pole as evidenced by the increased tendon thickening and hypoechoic clefting

EXOSOMES, PRP, AND STEM CELLS IN MUSCULOSKELETAL MEDICINE ©

CHAPTER 22 - THE KNEE

Historically and prior to innovation in the use of orthobiologics, management of patellar tendinopathy is controversial in the literature. (Charousset et al., 2014; Dragoo et al 2014; Liddle et al., 2014). Similar to tendinopathies in other body regions, conservative management has historically consisted of physical therapy, activity modification, or use of NSAIDS. The administration of orthobiologics has a place in the conservative treatment algorithm for patellar tendinopathy with many studies documenting its efficacy (Charousset et al., 2014; Dragoo et al 2014; Liddle et al., 2014). Provided there is no high grade or full thickness tear of the patellar tendon, PRP and stem cell treatments are an excellent option for patients in cases of refractory patellar tendinopathy.

Injection approach to the patellar tendon is suggested to visualize the tendon in the long axis with the needle moving from distal to proximal, in-plane with the probe (Figure 5.9 and 5.10).

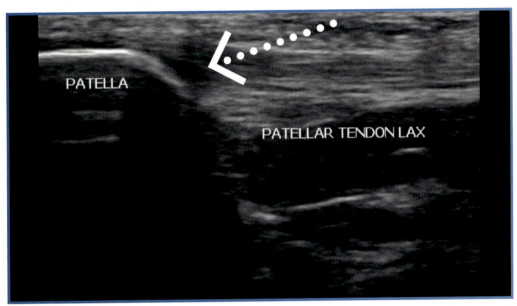

Figure 5.9: Long axis image of the patellar tendon inferior pole attachment with the needle moving distal to proximal in-plane with the probe

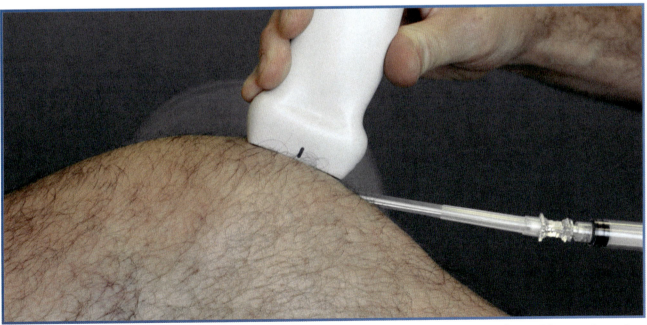

Figure 5.10: Ultrasound-guided injection technique to the patellar tendon. The patient is positioned supine with the knee flexed to 25-30 degrees. The structure is visualized in the long axis with the needle moving distal to proximal, in-plane with the probe.

Medial Knee Structures

The primary medial knee structures we will cover are the medial collateral ligament, medial meniscus, and the pes anserine tendon/bursa.

The medial collateral ligamentous (MCL) complex is the primary stabilizer of the knee against valgus stressors and is commonly injured in sporting events, motor vehicle accidents, or a fall from heights (Indelicato PA. 1995). Be mindful when diagnosing MCL injuries without evaluating additional structures such as the medial meniscus and anterior cruciate ligament (Indelicato et al., 1995) as these structures are often concurrently involved. Medial collateral ligament injuries that involve structural damage to the medial meniscus and anterior collateral ligament is known as the O'Donoghue unhappy triad (Makhamalbaf and Shahpari. 2018) and often require additional imaging (usually MRI) and surgery. Ultrasound can have a high sensitivity and specificity in detecting tears of the anterior cruciate ligament using indirect measures such as measuring abnormal tibial translation and comparing to the opposite side (Jianhong et al., 2018; Chylarecki et al., 1995); however, these studies are highly dependent on the user's expertise with ultrasound detection of tears. Because ultrasound cannot truly visualize the full extent of an anterior cruciate ligament injury and is not the preferred method for pre-operative diagnosis, we will not address the structure of its pathoanatomic features as to do so would fall outside the scope of this book.

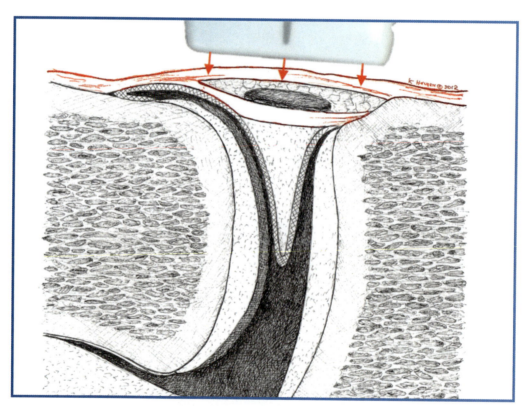

Figure 5.11: Pen and ink long axis image of the medial collateral ligament. Note the deep portion MCL relationship with the medial meniscus forming a capsule

MCL has a most identifiable structure and is usually considered as the most important unit in the treatment process in cases where it is involved (Indelicato, 1995). The MCL is like the sale of a boat, it becomes wider and thinner as it descends towards it's tibial attachment and we can assume that if the mast is not vertical, the sale is not in full mast and not working properly (Indelicato, 1995). The MCL has three layers associated with it that are all identifiable with ultrasound: the superficial, middle and deep (Figure 5.11). The deep layer has a direct attachment to the medial joint line and outer edge of the medial meniscus forming a capsule (Figure 5.12). This capsule is often disrupted in cases of acute injury and degenerative osteoarthritic changes; however, in the case of degenerative osteoarthritis the middle and superficial fibers of the ligament remain intact whereas acute injuries can often involve all three.

Figure 5.11: Medial Collateral Ligament & Medial meniscus: Longitudinal/Long axis

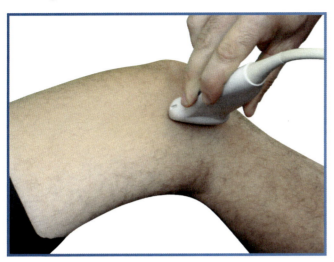
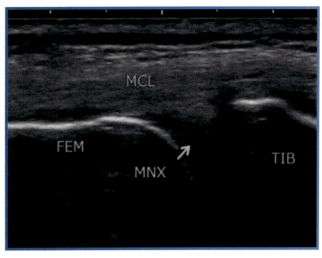

Place the probe on the medial aspect of the knee between the joint space. Appreciate the homogenous medial meniscus between the femur and tibia. The fibrinous medial collateral ligament lies anterior to the medial meniscus. (MCL=Medial Collateral Ligament, FEM=Femur, TIB=Tibia, MNX=Meniscus)

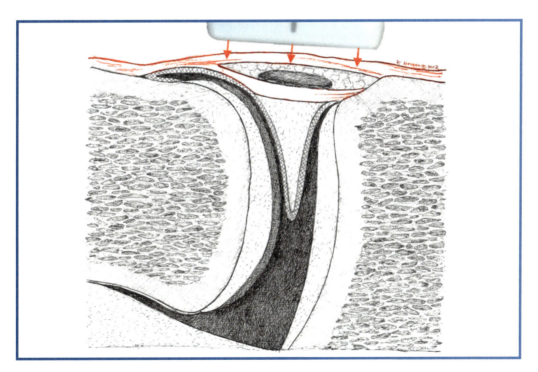

Figure 5.12: Pen and ink Long axis image of the medial collateral ligament. Note the deep portion MCL relationship with the medial meniscus forming a capsule

To inject the medial collateral ligament, the patient is positioned side lying on the affected extremity with the medial aspect of the knee exposed. The medial knee joint is visualized in the long axis with the medial collateral ligament fully visualized at the femoral and/or tibial attachment in the long axis. The injection approach here is a distal to proximal trajectory in-plane with the probe (Figure 5.13 and 5.14). Corticosteroids carry an increased risk for tendon and ligament rupture. Therefore we discourage injecting cortisone into the quadriceps tendon, patellar tendon or medial collateral ligament.

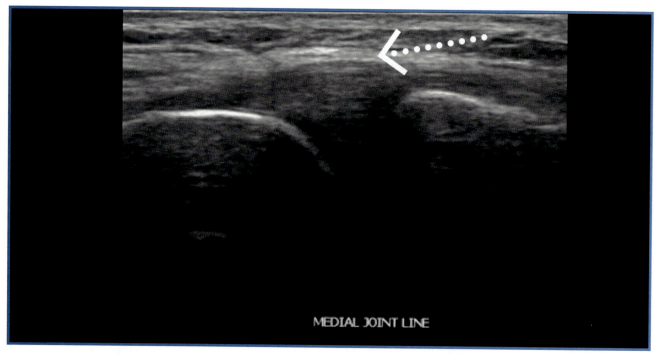

Figure 5.13: Ultrasound image of the medial joint line and medial collateral ligament in long axis. The needle is being moved distal to proximal in-plane with the probe

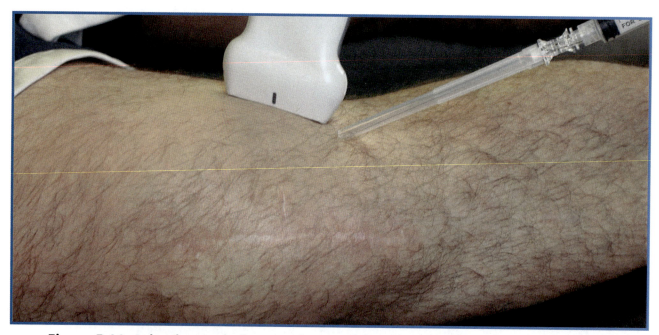

Figure 5.14: Injection technique to the medial collateral ligament. The patient is positioned on the affected side with the medial joint line facing upward. The structure is visualized in long axis and the needle is moved distal to proximal, in-plane with the probe

The outer edge of the meniscal bodies are visible to ultrasound but are not as efficient as MRI in detection of degeneration or tears (Figure 5.15). For tears, the sensitivity and specificity of ultrasound were 90.9% and 63.6% and for MR, 93.3% and 100% respectively (Unlu et al., 2014). With these statistics in mind, we can use ultrasound as a cheap first-line imaging tool to assess whether or not additional soft tissue imaging modalities such as MRI can be utilized in a particular case. The use of ultrasound as a tool to guide needle intervention to the medial knee (and knee structures in general) is extremely valid and efficacious.

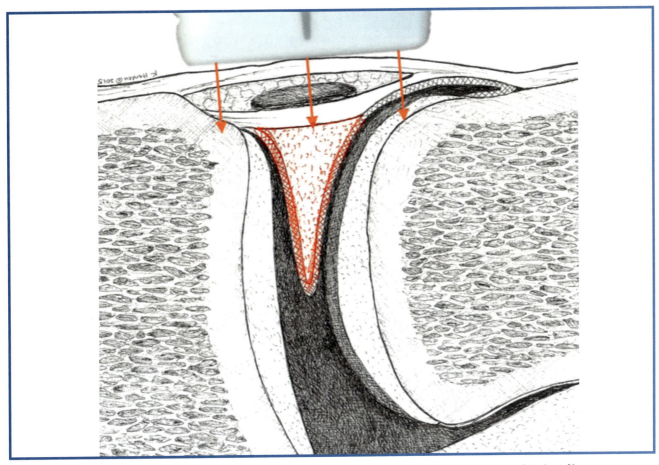

Figure 5.15: Pen and ink illustration of the medial meniscus and joint line

Normal sonographic characteristics of the medial meniscus are consistent with a triangular, homogeneously echogenic "wedge" shaped body with no internal heterogeneous echo changes or differences (78). It should look like a hyperechoic triangle folded in between the joint space. The cortical surfaces of the joint interface of the tibia and femur should be smooth and hyperechoic with adequate spacing to visualize the triangular fold of the meniscus within. The triangular-shaped meniscus should be relatively "flush" with the joint interface and not be extruded beyond it (Figure 5.16). Atypical presentations of the medial meniscus are "bulging" or "ice cream" cone sign protruding beyond the joint interface as well as loss of normal hyperechoic echotexture (Figure 5.17). As opposed to hyaline cartilage, which is full of water, fibrocartilage is not, and thus, appears more hyperechoic on ultrasound. Significant departure from normal echotexture can be consistent with meniscal degeneration and usually runs in tandem with cortical irregularities at the tibial-femoral joint interface and protrusion beyond the normal threshold. Meniscus protrusion beyond the normal threshold is usually coupled with capsule disruption and loss of integrity of the deep layers of MCL.

Figure 5.16: Medial Collateral Ligament & Medial meniscus: Longitudinal/Long axis

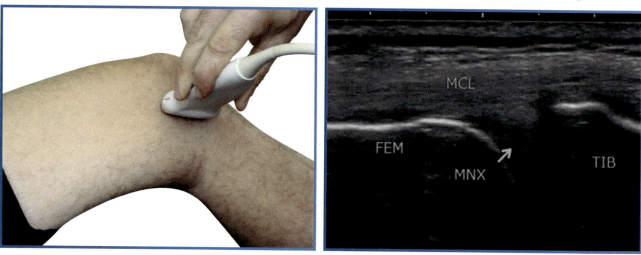

Place the probe on the medial aspect of the knee between the joint space. Appreciate the homogenous medial meniscus between the femur and tibia. The fibrinous medial collateral ligament lies anterior to the medial meniscus. (MCL=Medial Collateral Ligament, FEM=Femur, TIB=Tibia, MNX=Meniscus)

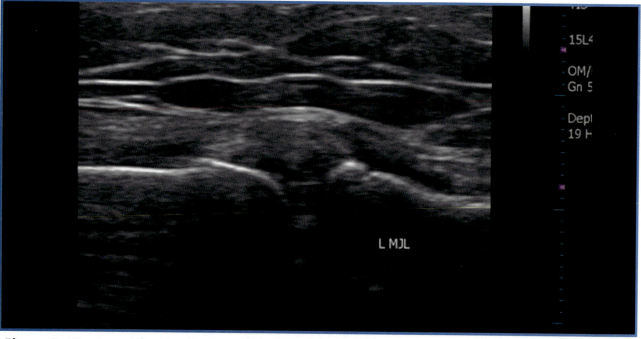

Figure 5.17: Example of a degenerative meniscal extrusion secondary to arthritic changes to the medial knee joint. This is evidenced by the "Ice Cream Cone Sign" as well as space narrowing and bony outgrowth at the femoral and tibial joint interface

If the patient presents with a degenerative meniscal tear; not fragments or bucket-handle tears, correlation with MRI is very important here. As previously mentioned, ultrasound imaging does not detail the entire course of the meniscus. If the pathology is peripheral, it can be visualized sonographically. If the meniscus lesion is located posterior or more internal, ultrasound has a very low sensitivity in reliably detecting. An MRI of the knee will also show areas of cartilage loss to further reconnaissance of what needs to be treated.

When considering injections to this region, the diagnosis needs to be in line with the intervention. PRP and stem cells typically do not help the healing process in cases where there is an unstable meniscus. Having multiple imaging studies or access to in-office arthroscopy can be very important in the diagnostic process in determining if the type of meniscal tear is unstable in nature and what treatment or intervention should be performed.

When a clinician performs a blind injection using a lateral tibial-femoral approach with the patient's knees flexed over the side of the table, the needle is injecting infrapatellar, directed medially, and most likely going to be in the joint space. This approach is not the trajectory of choice when using ultrasound to objectively confirm the needle tip because of limitations of depth and poor visibility of it moving into the intra-articular space.

When using ultrasound guidance to inject the knee joint, the most reliable way to confirm the needle is in the joint space is the direct approach into the suprapatellar recess (Figure 5.18-5.20). The quadriceps and suprapatellar recess are visualized with ultrasound in the short axis and the needle is moved from lateral to medial in-plane with the probe. In the case of osteoarthritis, meniscus tear, and miscellaneous intra-articular derangements, the PRP should address the area of pathology with this approach.

When treating osteoarthritis, meniscal pathology, ACL injury, or a PCL injury with PRP, the main goal is to get the injective into the joint. There are complex fluoroscopy-guided techniques to specifically target the anterior cruciate ligament but due to the advanced training and supervision required to become competent in such techniques, we will not be addressing that in this text.

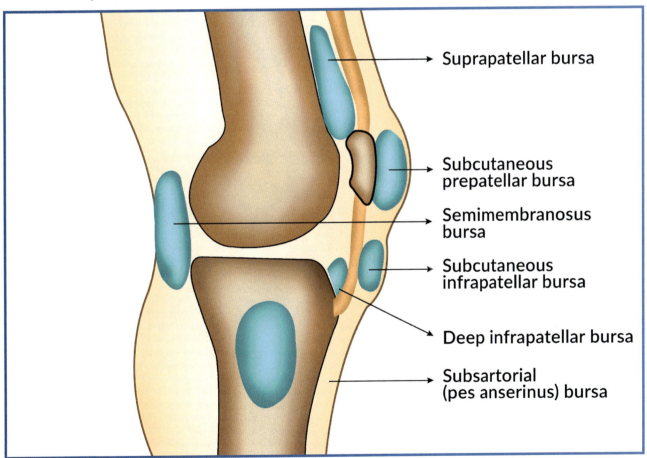

Figure 5.18: Artist rendering of the bursae in the knee. Pay specific attention to the location of the suprapatellar recess as this is the region targeted for intra-articular injection using ultrasound guidance to the majority of internal knee structures.

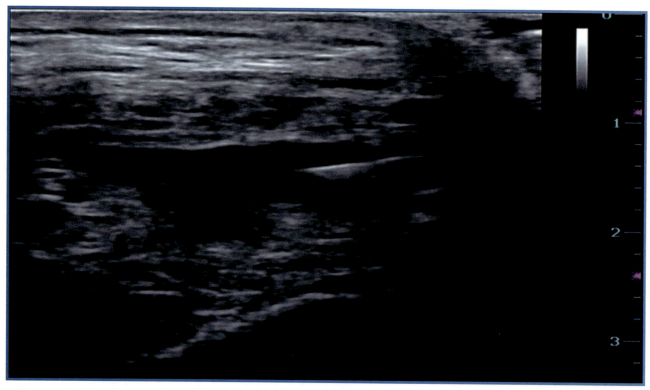

Figure 5.19: Short axis of the quadriceps tendon and suprapatellar recess. The needle is moving lateral to medial (right to left in the image) in-plane with the probe.

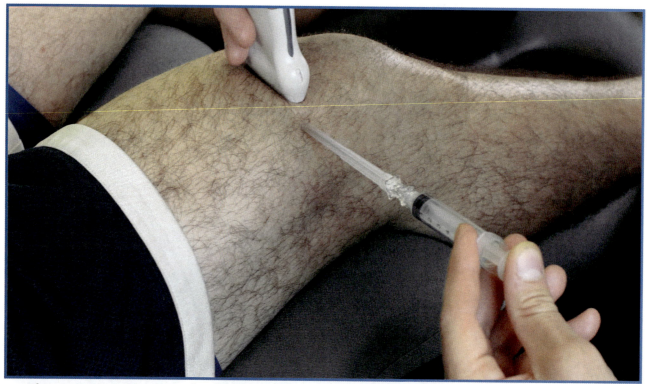

Figure 5.20: Ultrasound guided injection technique via the suprapatellar recess. The patient is positioned supine with the knee flexed 25-30 degrees. The quadriceps tendon and suprapatellar recess are visualized in the short axis and the needle is moved lateral to medial, in-plane with the probe

CHAPTER 22 - THE KNEE

The pes anserine group consists of the tendinous insertions of the sartorius, gracilis, and semitendinosus muscles attaching to the medial side of tibia to generate a shape reminiscent of a "goose's foot", which is the literal meaning of its name (Je-Hun Lee et al., 2014). This structure is clinically important in the reconstructive surgery involving tendons or in the steroid injection for anserine bursitis (Je-Hun Lee et al., 2014). The pes anserine tendon insertion can often mimic medial joint line pain such as meniscus pathology and osteoarthritis so it should be considered in the differential diagnosis due to its location. Pes anserine tendinopathy and/or bursitis occurs frequently in endurance athletes such as long distance biking or running as well as patients who are post-Total Knee Arthroplasty. Its pathogenesis typically is secondary to overuse, such as cases where a bike fitting is poor or suboptimal running mechanics exist, the pes anserine group functions as a medial knee stabilizer and knee flexor. Patients with pes anserine syndrome often complain of medial knee pain during movements of knee flexion-extension. Pain typically is not active at rest or limited to solely weight bearing positions and most often can be replicated by identifying what activities prompt the painful symptoms. This can all be identified with a thorough intake and physical exam. In most cases of pes anserine disorder, the cause is mostly due to chronic insertional tendinopathy rather than bursitis (Rowicki et al., 2014).

The normal sonographic characteristics of the pes anserine tendon insertion is that of a wafer-like, hyperechoic band of tissue inserting longitudinally onto the anterior-medial surface of the tibia (Figure 5.21). Visual confirmation of the tendon and bursa can also be accompanied by identifying anastomoses of the genicular arteries in the area by using Doppler. The pes anserine bursa is poorly visualized in the healthy patient and very rarely is present in the non-symptomatic population. The bursa lies between the bony surface of the tibia and the tendon insertion, it becomes inflamed and distended with chronic friction between the dysfunctional tendon-bone interaction.

Conservative treatment of pes anserine tendinopathy and/or bursitis is historically very successful where typical treatment options typically consist of avoidance therapy, physical therapy, NSAIDS, and cortisone. Recent evidence has shown that orthobiologics can be a superior option than NSAIDS or cortisone without the potentially deleterious side effects (Rowicki et al., 2014).

To inject the pes anserine tendon and bursa, we advocate to visualize the structures in the long axis with the needle moving from distal to proximal, in-plane with the probe (Figure 5.22 and 5.23).

Figure 5.21: Pes Anserinus Bursa: Longitudinal/long axis

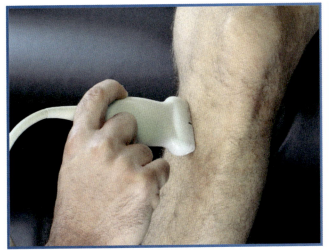
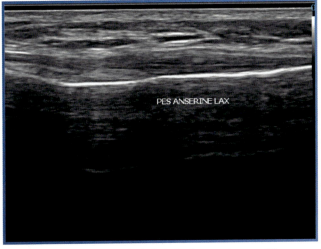

Position the probe on the medial aspect of the knee along the proximal tibia slightly inferior to the positioning of MCL. The sartorius, gracilis and semitendinosus join to form pes anserinus which is appreciated inserting onto the tibia. The pes anserinus bursa will be visualized as a hypoechoic structure deep to the tendons.

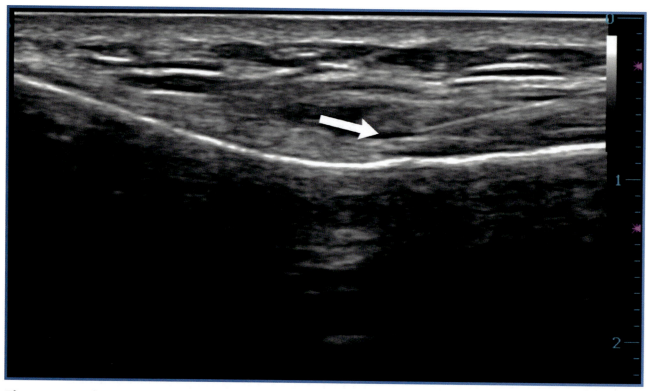

Figure 5.22: long axis image of the pes anserine visualized with the needle moving distal to proximal in plane with the probe

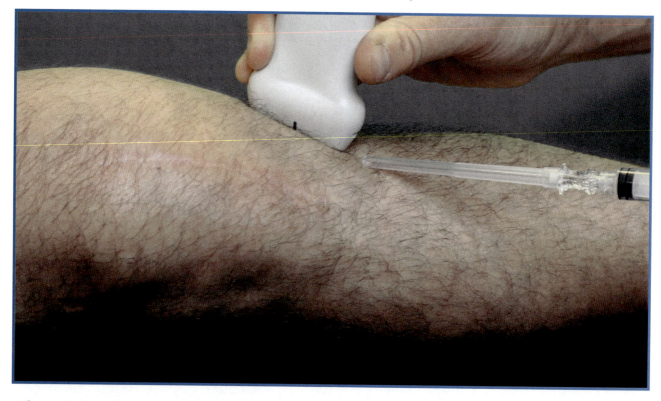

Figure 5.23: Ultrasound guided injection technique to the pes anserine bursa and tendon group. The patient is positioned on the affected extremity with the medial joint line facing upward. The needle is moved distal to proximal, in-plane with the probe.

Lateral Knee Structures

The most common lateral knee structures involved in musculoskeletal conditions are typically the lateral meniscus at the lateral joint line, the iliotibial band, biceps femoris and the lateral collateral ligament.

The iliotibial band is an aponeurosis that originates partially off of the ilium as well as tensor fascia latae and gluteus maximus fascia roughly at the level of the greater trochanter and inserts to Gerdy's tubercle on the proximal lateral aspect of the tibia. Distal Iliotibial band friction syndrome is a common symptom in endurance athletes such as bikers and runners. The two most common locations of iliotibial band friction syndrome typically occur at the lateral femoral condyle and Gerdy's tubercle. Similar to the pes anserine tendon group, patients who are post-TKA also can also be prone to impingement of the iliotibial band at the level of the lateral femoral condyle. Patients with iliotibial band friction syndrome often complain of a palpable "snapping" over the lateral knee, most commonly the lateral femoral condyle that can often be replicated with a thorough physical examination and patient intake. The snapping iliotibial band phenomenon over the lateral femoral condyle can also be evaluated with musculoskeletal ultrasound.

Healthy sonographic characteristics of the iliotibial band are that of a relatively thin, dense, homogeneous hyperechoic band of tissue that moves down the lateral aspect of the thigh and knee that is superficial to all other structures, making it easy to identify (Figure 5.24). Pathologic appearance of the iliotibial band is similar to that of tendinopathic descriptions elsewhere in this text; the fascia becomes thickened and hypoechoic with occasional cortical irregularities visualized at the femoral condyle and Gerdy's tubercle (Federico-Arend et al., 2014). Anatomically speaking, the iliotibial tract is a distinctive anatomical structure but rather a region of the fascia latae connected with the rough line of the femur by the intermuscular septum, which prevents its anteroposterior motion (Fairclough et al., 2007). Given this information, we can now say the pathogenesis of iliotibial syndrome is compressive and not frictional generated as what has been previously accepted. The typical clinical signs in the region of the lateral femoral condyle which become particularly acute at 30° flexion and exacerbated during the physical examination at local knee motion palpation (Fairclough et al., 2006; Fairclough et al., 2007). Given the superficial location of the structure, this can easily be evaluated with musculoskeletal ultrasound.

Injection to the iliotibial band should be performed with the iliotibial band in the long axis with the needle moving distal to proximal in-plane with the probe (Figure 5.25 and 5.26).

Figure 5.24: Iliotibial Band/ ITB: Longitudinal/LAX

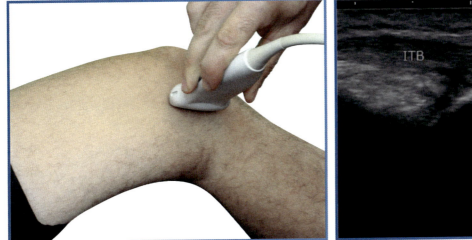

Slightly flex the patient's knee and place the probe superior to the orientation for the lateral meniscus. The iliotibial band can be appreciated running anterior to the lateral femoral condyle. Move the probe slightly inferior to follow the iliotibial band run over the tibia to insert on Gerdi's tubercle.

CHAPTER 22 - THE KNEE

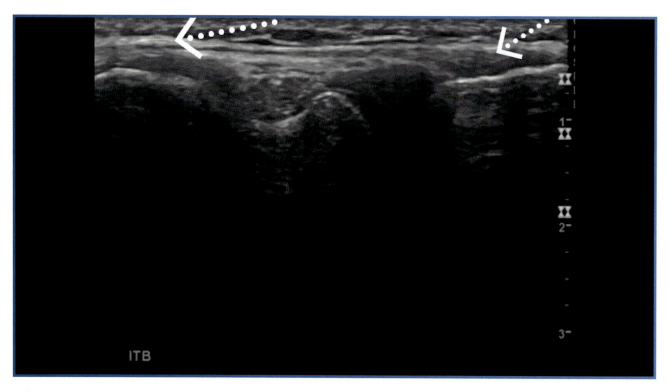

Figure 5.25: Ultrasound image of the lateral joint line with emphasis on the iliotibial band in the long axis. The needle is moved distal to proximal, in-plane with the probe.

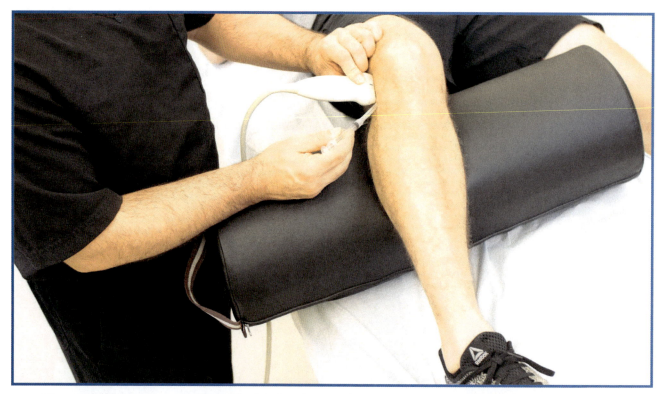

Figure 5.26: Ultrasound guided injection technique to the iliotibial band at Gerdy's Tubercle insertion. The patient is positioned comfortably supine with the affected leg resting over a bolster. The structure is visualized in the long axis while the needle is moved distal to proximal, in-plane with the probe.

Examining the lateral meniscus with ultrasound is very similar to the medial meniscus with a few exceptions. The distal femur at the level of the joint line is hallmarked with the popliteal fossa/recess, making it different in appearance (Figure 5.27). The lateral meniscus compartment biomechanically allows more mobility when compared to the medial meniscus, providing its own set of pathomechanic circumstances for evaluation. In contrast to the medial meniscus, due to the unlocking action of the popliteus as well as the attachments of the ligaments of Humphry and Wrisberg as well as the popliteus muscle, it is thus relatively immune from injury during rotational movements (Last et al., 1950). Injuries to the lateral meniscus often run concurrently with ACL injuries and/or posterior-lateral corner injuries involving the arcuate ligament and the popliteal-fibular ligament.

The normal sonographic appearance of the lateral meniscus is similar to the medial meniscus. It appears as a relatively hyperechoic triangular in-folding that consists of fibrocartilage and the outer layers can be visualized with ultrasound (Figure 5.27). Healthy sonographic characteristics of the lateral joint line are hyperechoic cortical surfaces of the joint interface tibia and femur. The meniscus should be relatively flush with the joint interface as a spacer between the two bones. Atypical findings of the lateral meniscus are protrusions from the joint interface, loss of hyperechoic echotexture as well as dynamic geyser sign when varus pressure is applied. The lateral collateral ligament (LCL) does not form a capsule with the lateral meniscus as the MCL does with the medial meniscus.

Figure 5.27: Lateral Meniscus: Longitudinal long axis

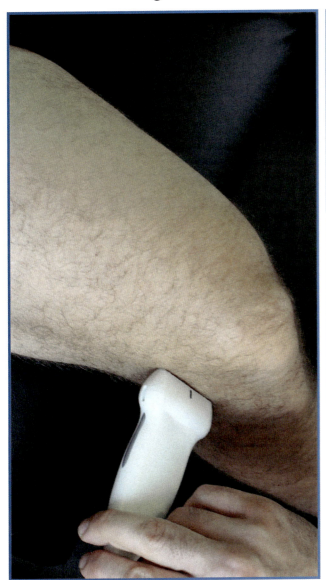
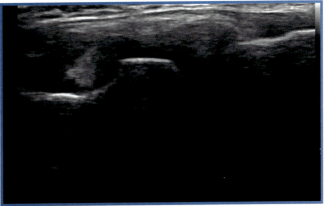
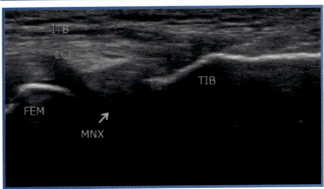

Left: Patient is positioned in supine with the knee flexed 30-45 degrees. The probe is placed across the joint line slightly anterior in the frontal plane. Top Right: The lateral meniscus is the homogenous wedged shaped structure that is seen between the femur and tibia. The popliteal fossa is visualized just proximal (to the left) of the joint line. Bottom Right: The lateral collateral ligament is appreciated lying just superficial to the lateral meniscus with the ITB just above it.

CHAPTER 22 - THE KNEE

As described earlier; when delivering orthobiologics to intra-articular knee structures using ultrasound guidance, including the lateral meniscus, the most efficient non-surgical method to deliver orthobiologics is via the suprapatellar recess. The quadriceps tendon/suprapatellar recess is visualized in the short axis and the needle is moved lateral to medial in-plane with the probe (Figure 5.28 and 5.29).

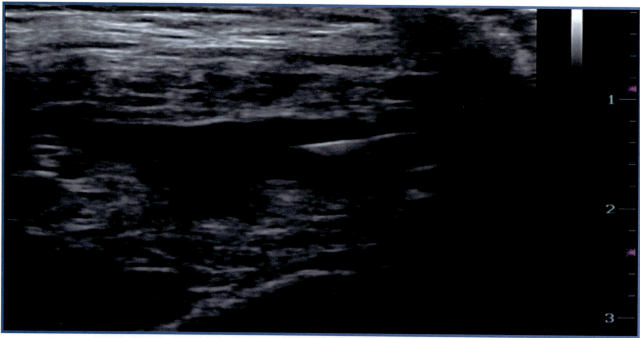

Figure 5.28: Short axis image of the quadriceps tendon and suprapatellar recess. The needle is visualized moving lateral to medial in-plane (right to left within the anechoic recess space) with the probe

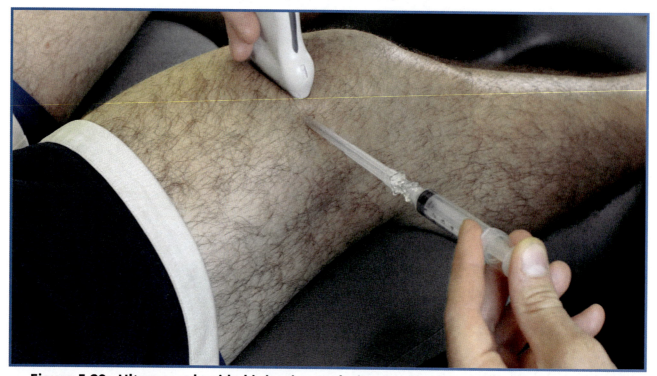

Figure 5.29: Ultrasound guided injection technique to the intra-articular knee via the suprapatellar recess. The patient is positioned supine with the knee flexed 25-30 degrees, the quadriceps tendon and suprapatellar recess are visualized in short axis. The needle is moved lateral to medial, in-plane with the probe.

The distal biceps femoris insertion to the fibula can be a common region of tendinopathy. Like other tendons in the body, the biceps femoris should appear hyperechoic, organized and fibrillar in nature (Figure 5.30). The cortical surface of the tendon-bone attachment site with the biceps femoris should be smooth and homogeneous.

Clinical signs and symptoms associated with distal biceps femoris tendinopathy are palpable pain at the fibular attachment as well as localized pain with tasks or repetitive movements that require knee flexion and activation of the hamstring muscle groups.

Sonographic characteristics of insertional biceps femoris tendinopathy is typically accompanied by increased tendon thickening, hypoechoic clefting as well as loss of homogeneous cortical surface at the tendon-bone interface (cortical irregularity).

Injection techniques to the biceps femoris insertion should be performed with the patient positioned in a side lying position to the unaffected side or in prone. The tendon should be visualized in the long axis with the needle moved from either proximal to distal or distal to proximal in-plane with the probe (Figure 5.31 and 5.32).

Figure 5.30: Biceps Femoris Tendon: longitudinal/long axis

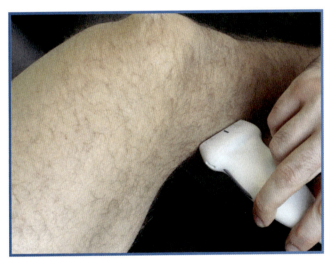
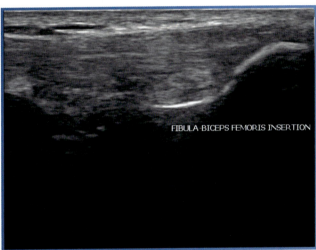

Patient is positioned in supine with the knee flexed between 30-45 degrees. The distal end of the probe is fixed on the fibula and the proximal aspect of the probe is directed more posteriorly toward the hamstrings. The thicker, fibrillar biceps femoris tendon can be differentiated from the lateral collateral ligament with this probe alignment.

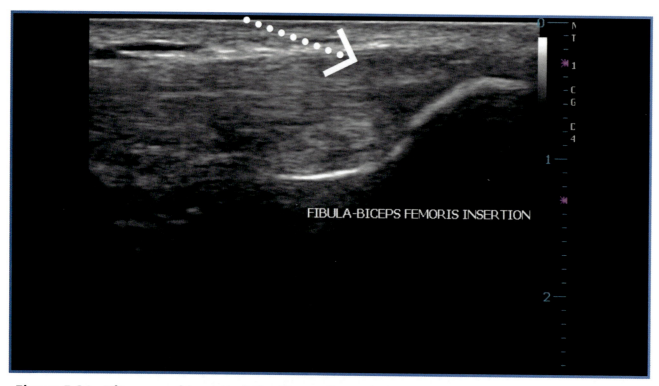

Figure 5.31: Ultrasound image of the biceps femoris in the long axis. The needle is moved from proximal to distal in-plane with the probe.

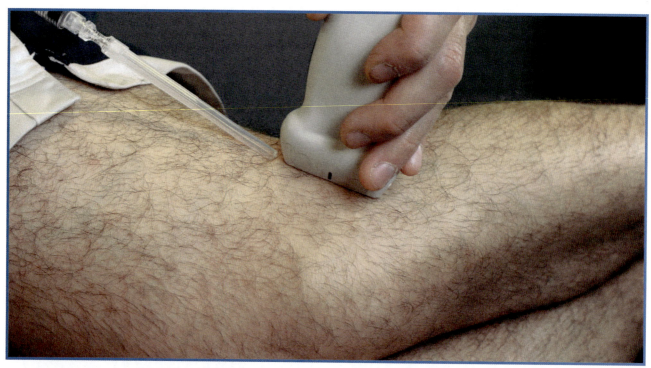

Figure 5.32: Ultrasound guided injection technique to the distal biceps femoris. The patient is positioned in side lying with the knees flexed 20-30 degrees with the affected extremity facing upward. The biceps femoris is visualized in the long axis and the needle is moved proximal to distal, in-plane with the probe.

The lateral collateral ligament (LCL) is a structure that can become damaged with knee injuries. Although not as commonly involved in comparison to the ACL, MCL or meniscus, it can be a region of interest. Most LCL injuries occur in cases of trauma such as collisions on the football field or in motor vehicle accidents. The LCL attaches the femur to the fibula with healthy sonographic characteristics being most consistent with that of a tendon, meaning it appears linear and fibrillar (Figure 5.33). The best patient position to diagnostically capture the image is in supine with the knees flexed 25-30 degrees over a pillow or bolster. The clinician should have a good idea of whether or not the LCL is involved prior to the ultrasound based off of the patient history, mechanism and location of injury. As said earlier, most LCL injuries involve some sort of trauma compromising the varus stress positioning it is intended to protect; and second to the PCL, is the least involved ligament injury in the knee (Majewskia et al., 2006).

Injections to the LCL should be performed with the patient side lying on the unaffected side with the structure visualized in the long axis. The needle should be moved distal to proximal in-plane with the probe.

Figure 5.33: Lateral Collateral Ligament: Longitudinal/long axis

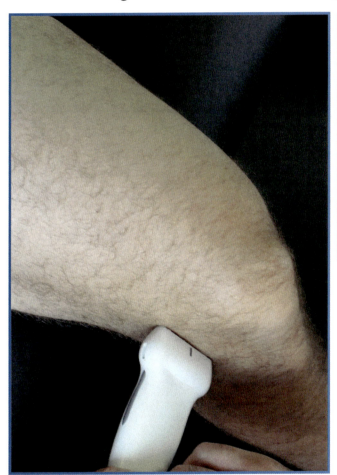
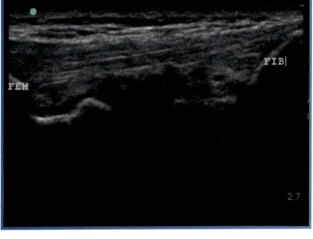

Patient is positioned supine with the knee in 25-30 degrees flexion. The distal aspect of the probe is fixed on the fibula and the proximal end of the probe is directed anteriorly toward the femur. The lateral collateral ligament is a dense, linear/hyperechoic tissue attaching the femur to the fibula

CHAPTER 22 - THE KNEE

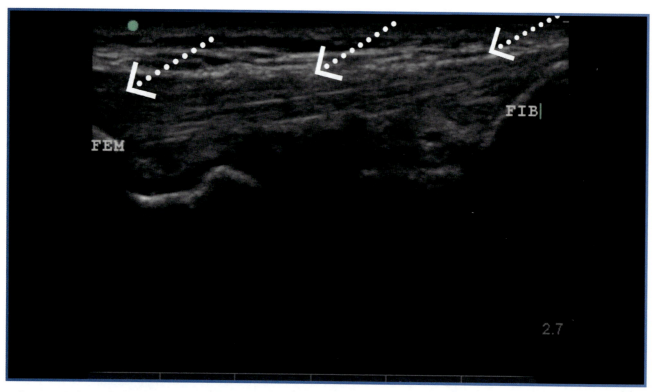

Figure 5.34: Ultrasound image of the lateral collateral ligament (LCL) in the long axis with the needle moved distal to proximal, in-plane with the probe.

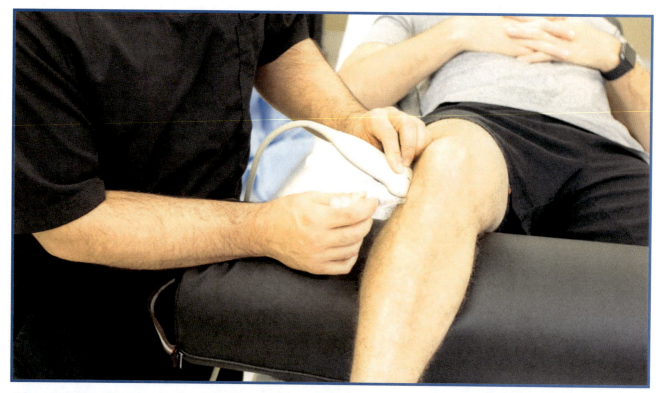

Figure 5.35: Ultrasound guided injection technique to the lateral collateral ligament (LCL). The patient is positioned comfortably in supine with the knees resting over a bolster. The LCL is visualized in the long axis and the needle is moved proximal to distal, in-plane with the probe.

CHAPTER 22 - THE KNEE

Posterior Knee Structures

Baker's cysts are primarily located in the posterior-medial aspect of the knee between the medial head of the gastrocnemius muscle and the semimembranosus tendon (Figure 5.36). Why does this happen? Typically, Baker's cysts most commonly occur when there is intra-articular pathology within the knee and there is a ball-valve phenomenon. The fluid comes in and is going back into the pseudospace or Baker's cyst and stays there; in sense, becomes a one-way ball-valve phenomenon that just keeps filling up with fluid and it does not go back (Figure 5.37). In order to treat, the provider can aspirate Baker's cyst which is fine, but due to the fact it is a full-contained space and any pathology or any effusions that are going to be happening within the knee are going to be coming out there as well. So in this scenario, be aware that injectate placed into the knee joint may end up coming out of the one-way ball-valve phenomena into the Baker's cyst depending on the pressure within the joint.

Popliteal Fossa: Transverse/short axis (Bakers cyst)

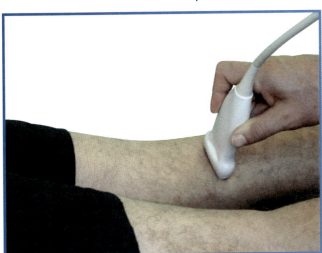
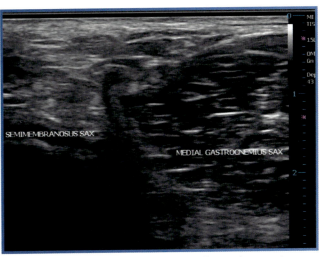

The patient is positioned prone with the knee in full extension. The probe is positioned axially or short axis to the medial gastrocnemius muscle at the proximal third of the calf. Slowly translate the probe proximally until the medial gastrocnemius begins to become smaller; the cross section or short axis view of the semimembranosus tendon will come into view at the level of the posterior joint line. The space between the medial gastrocnemius and semimembranosus tendon is the potential space where Baker's cyst will formulate.

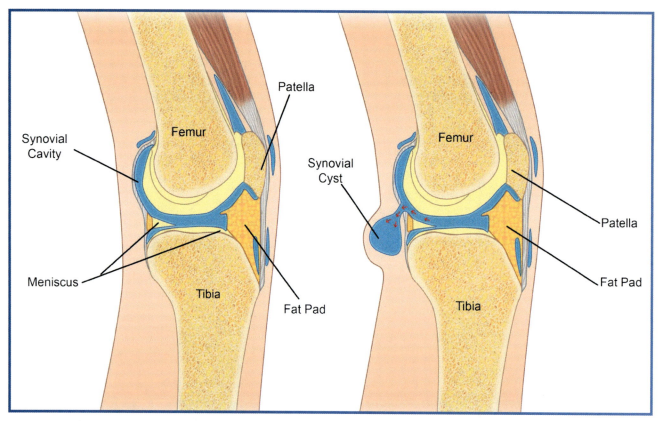

Figure 5.36: Artist depiction of the anatomical formation of a Baker's cyst

Treating the Baker's cyst can be a very complex procedure secondary to intra-articular pathology such as chronic/degenerative meniscus tears and/or osteoarthritic breakdown of the articulating structures that often runs in tandem with it. Practitioners can attempt to burst the Baker's cyst, penetrating the pseudo-epithelial lining around the Baker's cyst. In order to do this, the provider must make multiple fenestrations through the lining and then inject a significant amount of fluid into the potential space in an attempt to get the lining/cyst to scar down so the cyst does not reform. However; after performing this, be aware again that intra-articular knee injections are still prone to leaking out of the ball-valve posteriorly.

Musculoskeletal ultrasound is a valuable tool to diagnostically evaluate the Bakers cyst as well as use for needle guidance. To perform intervention to this region, the anatomic structures medial gastrocnemius and semimembranosus are visualized in short axis while the needle is moved medial to lateral, in-plane with the probe (Figure 5.38 and 5.39). When performing intervention to a Baker's cyst, the provider needs to be aware of the neurovascular structures that typically lie just lateral to its normal location (Figure 5.40) and occasionally, a Baker's cyst can impinge these structures.

CHAPTER 22 - THE KNEE

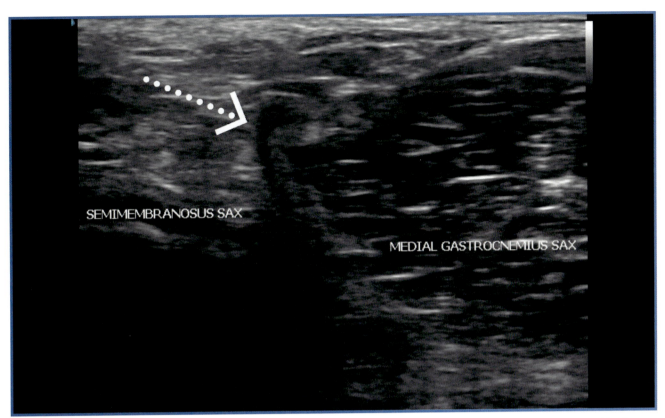

Figure 5.38: Ultrasound image of the bakers cyst location in short axis. The needle is moved from medial to lateral, in-plane with the probe

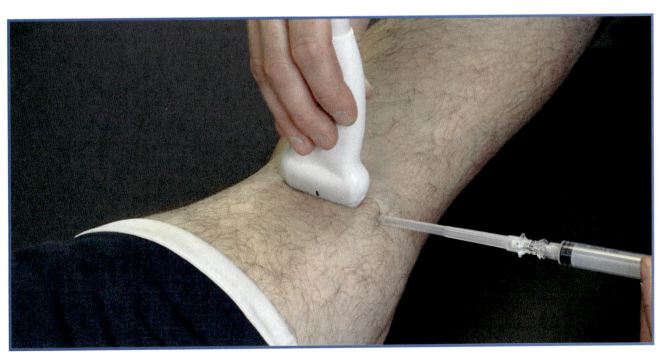

Figure 5.39: Ultrasound guided injection technique to the popliteal recess for Baker's cyst. The patient is positioned prone with the semimembranosus/medial gastrocnemius and the space between visualized in the short axis. The needle is moved medial to lateral, in-plane with the probe.

Figure 5.40: Popliteal Fossa: Transverse/short axis

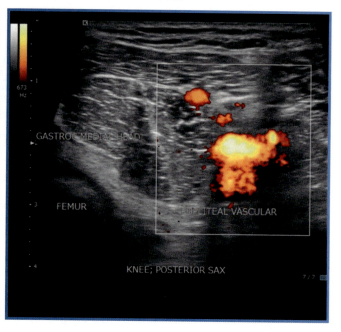

The patient is positioned prone with the knee in full extension. The probe is placed in the short axis to the proximal calf and gastrocnemius musculature. Use power Doppler to assess the venous structures. Add pressure to the probe to check for compressibility of the vein. The inability to compress the vein increases suspicion for a DVT.

CHAPTER 22 - THE KNEE

References:

S Bianchi, A Zwass, I F Abdelwahab and A Banderali. Diagnosis of Tears in the Quadriceps Tendon of the Knee: The Value of Sonography. American Journal of Roentgenology. 1994;162: 1137-1140. 10.2214/ajr.162.5.8165998. Read More: https://www.ajronline.org/doi/abs/10.2214/ajr.162.5.8165998

Dominic King et al., Quadriceps tendinopathy: a review—part 1: epidemiology and diagnosis. Ann Transl Med. 2019 Feb; 7(4): 71.

Toppi J et al., Platelet-rich plasma as a treatment for patellar tendinopathy: a double-blind, randomized controlled trial. Am J Sports Med. 2014 Mar; 42(3):610-8.

Filardo G et al., Use of platelet-rich plasma for the treatment of the refractory jumper's knee. Int Orthop. 2010 Aug; 34(6):909-15.

Walter, S. D., J. R. Sutton, and J. M. McIntosh. The aetiology of sports injuries: a review of methodologies. Sports Med. 2:47–56, 1985.

Renstrom, P. and R. J. Johnson. Overuse injuries in sport: a review. Sports Med. 2:316–322, 1985.
Ferretti, A., E. Ippolito, P. Mariani, and G. Puddu. Jumper's knee. Am. J. Sports Med. 11:58–62, 1983.

Blazina, M. E., R. K. Kerlan, F. W. Jobe, and V. S. Carter. Jumper's knee. Orthop. Clin. North Am. 4:665–672, 1973.

Nichols, C. E. Patellar tendon injuries. Clin. Sports Med. 11:807–813, 1992.

Christophe Charousset, MD et al., Are Multiple Platelet-Rich Plasma Injections Useful for Treatment of Chronic Patellar Tendinopathy in Athletes?: A Prospective Study. American Journal of Sports Medicine. Volume: 42 issue: 4, page(s): 906-911. 2014.
Ferretti A, Ippolito E, Mariani P, Puddu G. Jumper's Knee. The American Journal of Sports Medicine. 1983;11(2):58-62. doi:10.1177/036354658301100202

Jason L. Dragoo, MD et al., Platelet-Rich Plasma as a Treatment for Patellar Tendinopathy: A Double-Blind, Randomized Controlled Trial. American Journal of Sports Medicine. Volume: 42 issue: 3, page(s): 610-618. 2014

Alexander D. Liddle, BSc, MRCS et al., Platelet-Rich Plasma in the Treatment of Patellar Tendinopathy: A Systematic Review. American Journal of Sports Medicine. Volume: 43 issue: 10, page(s): 2583-2590. 2014

Indelicato PA. Isolated Medial Collateral Ligament Injuries in the Knee. J Am Acad Orthop Surg. 1995 Jan; 3(1):9-14.

Hadi Makhmalbaf, MD and Omid Shahpari, MD. Medial Collateral Ligament Injury; A New Classification Based on MRI and Clinical Findings. A Guide for Patient Selection and Early Surgical Intervention. Arch Bone Jt Surg. 2018 Jan; 6(1): 3–7.

Wang Jianhong et al., The role of ultrasonography in the diagnosis of anterior cruciate ligament injury: A systematic review and meta-analysis. Sports and Exercise Medicine and Health. Pages 579-586 | Published online: 21 Feb 2018.

Chylarecki C, Hierholzer G, Klose R. Ultrasound diagnosis of acute rupture of the anterior cruciate ligament. An experimental and clinical study. Der Unfallchirurg, 31 Dec 1995, 99(1):24-30

Indelicato PA. Isolated Medial Collateral Ligament Injuries in the Knee. J Am Acad Orthop Surg. 1995 Jan; 3(1):9-14.
Elif Nisa Unlu et al., The role of ultrasound in the diagnosis of meniscal tears and degeneration compared to MRI and arthroscopy. Acta Med Anatol 2014;2(3):80-87

Je-Hun Lee et al., Pes anserinus and anserine bursa: anatomical study. Anatomy Cell Biology. 2014 Jun; 47(2): 127–131.

Krzysztof Rowicki 1, Janusz Płomiński, Artur Bachta. Evaluation of the effectiveness of platelet rich plasma in treatment of chronic pes anserinus pain syndrome. Traumatology Rehabilitation. May-Jun 2014;16(3):307-18.

Carlos Frederico Arend. Sonography of the Iliotbial Band: A Spectrum of Findings. Radiologia Brasileira. vol.47 no.1 São Paulo Jan./Feb. 2014

Fairclough J, Hayashi K, Toumi H, et al., Is iliotibial band syndrome really a friction syndrome? J Sci Med Sport. 2007;10:74-8.

Fairclough J, Hayashi K, Toumi H, et al., The functional anatomy of the iliotibial band during flexion and extension of the knee: implications for understanding iliotibial band syndrome. J Anat. 2006;208:309-16.

Fairclough J, Hayashi K, Toumi H, et al., Is iliotibial band syndrome really a friction syndrome? J Sci Med Sport. 2007;10:74-8. R. J. Last. The Popliteus Muscle and the Lateral Meniscus. The Journal of Bone and Joint Surgery. British Vol. 32-B No. 1. 93-99

M.Majewskia, Habelt Susanneb, Steinbrück Klausc. Epidemiology of athletic knee injuries: A 10-year study. The Knee. Volume 13, Issue 3, June 2006, Pages 184-188

CHAPTER 23: The Foot and Ankle

Colin Rigney, Pradeep Albert, Rock Positano & Rock Positano Jr.

> **CHAPTER PREVIEW**
>
> This chapter will cover sonoanatomy of the foot and ankle complex as well as patient and probe positions for proper evaluation. The chapter will also include common pictorial examples and explanations of sono-pathology found as well as basic ultrasound-guided injection techniques.

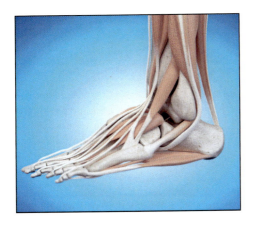

Osseous anatomy of the ankle includes the tibia, the fibula, talus and the calcaneus. From superior-medial to inferior-lateral, the mid-foot osseous anatomy consists of the navicular which abuts the medial cuneiform inferiorly which interfaces with the first metatarsal, lateral and adjacent to the medial cuneiform is the middle cuneiform which is adjacent to the second metatarsal, and the lateral cuneiform adjacent to it interfaces with the third metatarsal. The cuboid is lateral-adjacent to the lateral cuneiform and interfaces with the fourth and fifth metatarsal. This section will break down ultrasound anatomy and intervention in four compartments of the ankle/foot complex: posterior, lateral, medial, and anterior.

Posterior Compartment

Two very common soft tissue disorders in the posterior ankle occur in the Achilles and the plantar fascia. Imaging the Achilles tendon and its insertion at the calcaneus is one of the easier anatomical regions to learn how to scan with musculoskeletal ultrasound because it is very superficial and accessible. The most common soft tissue disorders in the Achilles region are retrocalcaneal bursitis, retro-Achilles bursitis, insertional and midsubstance tendinopathy or edema/calcification along the course of the Achilles.

The Achilles tendon, although very strong, is one of the most frequently injured tendons in the body (Maffulli et al., 1999; Maffulli et al., 1999). It is a common tendon shared between the gastrocnemius and soleus muscles of the lower-posterior leg. The Achilles tendon is a connection of muscle groups that are collectively known as the triceps surae (consisting of the medial and lateral gastrocnemius and soleus), attaching to the posterior aspect of the calcaneus. Generally the tendon winds 90 degrees perpendicular to the supporting surface on its path towards the heel, such that the gastrocnemius attaches laterally and the soleus attaches medially. The Achilles tendon provides an attachment site for the gastrocnemius muscles as well as the soleus and inserts onto the posterior surface of the calcaneus. The primary function of the Achilles is to provide force in plantar flexion and also provide both elasticity and shock absorbance for eccentric control in the sagittal plane (89). The Achilles tendon is the largest and strongest tendon in the body and is capable of supporting tensional forces produced by movement of the lower limb (Del Buono et al., 2013). The retro-Achilles bursa is a superficial subcutaneous calcaneal bursa that permits movement of the skin over the flexed tendon as well as providing a lubricant during dorsiflexion-plantar flexion (Figure 6.1). The retrocalcaneal bursa is located deep to the Achilles tendon at the proximal aspect of the calcaneus and reduces friction to allow free movement of the tendon over the bone. Normal sonographic appearance of the Achilles tendon at the calcaneus is similar to other tendons in the body, it should appear hyperechoic, linear, homogeneous in shape and the cortical surface of the calcaneus should be smooth and uninterrupted (Figure 6.2-6.4).

CHAPTER 23 - THE FOOT AND ANKLE

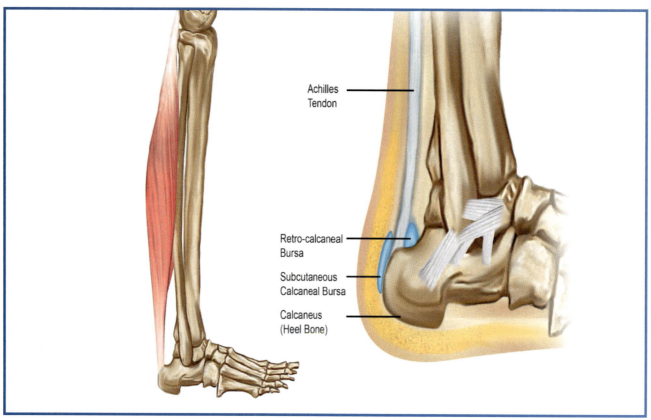

Figure 6.1: Artist depiction of distal Achilles anatomy with retrocalcaneal and retro Achilles bursa locations

Figure 6.2: Posterior Ankle: Distal Achilles Tendon Attachment

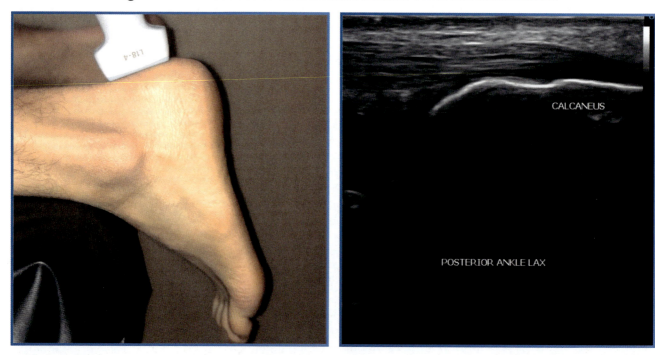

With the patient prone, place the foot comfortably hanging off the examination table. With the patient prone, place the foot comfortably hanging off the examination table. The normal appearance of the Achilles tendon insertion is linear, fibrillar, homogeneous in shape and hyperechoic. The tendon-bone interface with the calcaneus should be smooth and uninterrupted.

Figure 6.3: Posterior Ankle: Achilles Tendon Mid-Portion

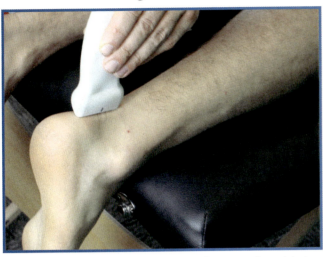 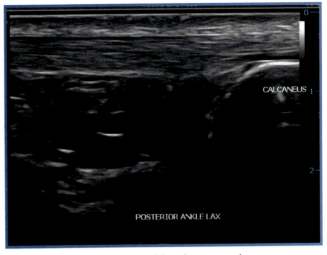

With the patient prone, place the foot comfortably hanging off the examination table. The normal appearance of the Achilles tendon is linear, fibrillar, homogeneous in shape and hyperechoic. The tendon-bone interface at the calcaneus should be smooth and uninterrupted. The most common location of Achilles tendon ruptures is this region encompassing 2-3cm proximal to the insertion point.

Figure 6.4: Posterior Ankle Achilles Tendon (short axis)

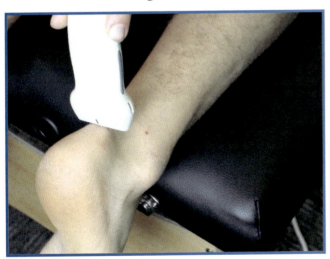 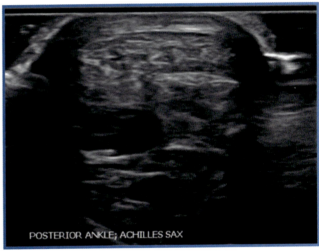

With the patient prone, place the foot comfortably hanging off the examination table. Palpate the distal part of the Achilles tendon. Place probe transverse plane in the short axis overwhere the tendon inserts at the posterior portion of the calcaneus. Visualize the more superficial Achilles tendon insert onto the calcaneus. This view allows for a more accurate measurement of the thickness of the Achilles tendon.

The plantar fascia originates from the plantar surface of the calcaneus as a strong layer of dense fibrous tissue (Figure 6.5). It is made of up three "cords" originating from the medial plantar calcaneal surface and extends distally as medial, central and lateral cords that envelopes the flexor digitorum brevis muscle (Jacobsen et al., 2017). Just proximal to the level of the metatarsal-phalangeal junction, the aponeurotic band of the plantar fascia further divides into five sections, each of which extends into a toe and straddles the flexor tendons where the superficial layer of each section attaches to deep skin fold between toes and the sole (Gray et al., 1995) while the deep layer blends with the fibrous flexor tendon sheaths on each proximal phalanx and sends septa to the deep transverse metatarsal ligament of the sole forming a series of arches through which tendons of the short and long flexors pass through (Gray et al., 1995). The main function of the plantar fascia is to stabilize the arch of the foot and provide significant stability to the first metatarsal phalangeal joint and arch through what is known as the Windlass Mechanism. This mechanism can be disrupted and when it does, plantar flexion does not occur efficiently enough during normal walking to transfer load and therefore weight is then transferred to the metatarsals 2 through 5 which can result in pain and dysfunction. Normal sonographic appearance of the plantar fascia is linear, hyperechoic and have a smooth bony interface with the calcaneus attachment (Figure 6.6). It is fairly easy to objectively measure plantar fasciosis using musculoskeletal ultrasound. With the patient either prone or supine on the table, the foot lying over and ankle roughly 90 degrees, the operator should take a diameter measurement using a long axis image of the plantar fascia. The normal diameter is between 3-4mm and anything greater than 4-5mm with a mean measurement of 5.7mm +/- 0.3 in symptomatic patients usually falls in line with the diagnosis of plantar fasciosis (Figure 6.7) (Kornfeld R. 2010).

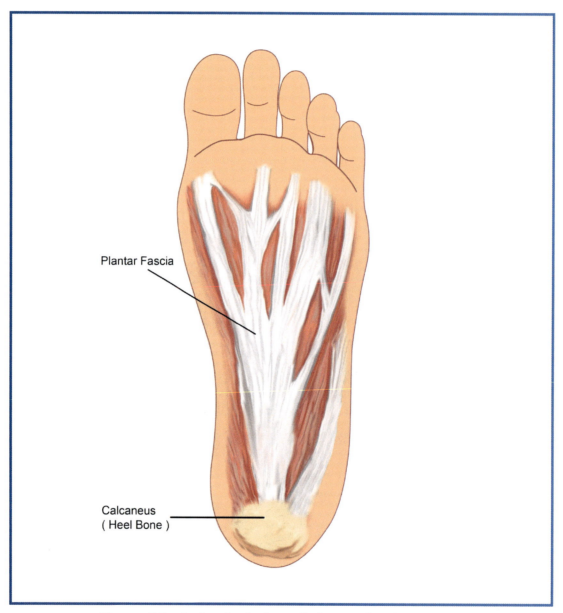

Figure 6.5: Artist depiction of plantar fascia anatomy

CHAPTER 23 - THE FOOT AND ANKLE

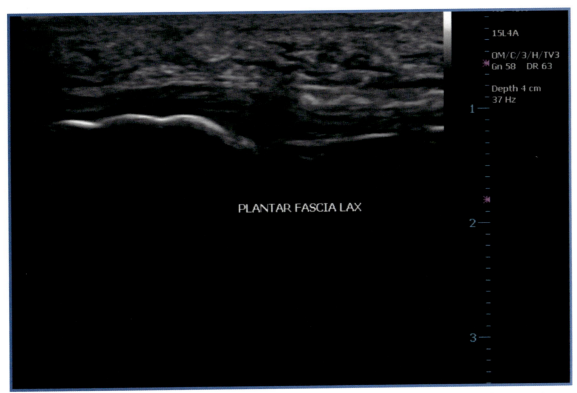

Figure 6.6: Normal ultrasound image of the plantar fascia in the long axis

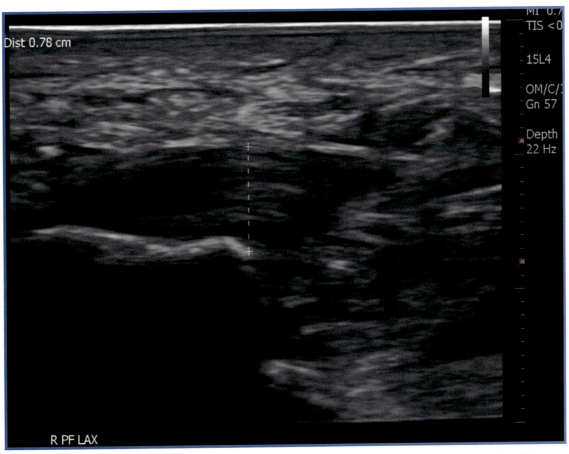

Figure 6.7: Long axis image of plantar fasciosis (PF=Plantar Fascia). Note the diameter of 7.8mm

When considering intervention in the Achilles tendon region, it is important to locate the specific area of pathology utilizing musculoskeletal ultrasound. It is also incumbent on the provider to critically evaluate the surrounding structures to grade the severity of pathology in cases where non-surgical intervention may not be enough. There are two classifications of Achilles tendon pathology: insertional or midsubstance (watershed zone) and each has its own set of challenges when considering treatment. Insertional tendinopathy often includes what is commonly known as "bone spurs" or enthesophytes where the attachment of the tendon attachment "tugs" on the bony interface causing cortical abnormalities to form (Figure 6.8). MIdsubstance Achilles tendinopathy of the Achilles is marked by hypoechoic clefting and thickening of the tendon, giving it a fusiform appearance (Figure 6.9). Small enthesophytes or bone spurs can be treated percutaneously with a large bore needle and the tendon adjacent to it by fenestrating and/or aspirating the diseased portion of the tendon-bone interface in an attempt to break up the tissue. Injecting the orthobiologic of choice after percutaneous tenotomy is the preferred method in this intervention. The US-guided needle approach for this technique is best visualized with the Achilles insertion in the short axis with the needle guided from medial to lateral or lateral to medial, both in-plane with the probe.

Treating midsubstance Achilles tendinopathy is slightly less complex than insertional tendinopathy because the bony interface isn't involved. The typical appearance of Achilles tendinopathy in the mid-portion/watershed zone appears hypoechoic, thickened and has a general fusiform heterogeneous appearance. Needle guided intervention to this region of the Achilles can be taken in multiple angles and is largely dependent on the comfort and skill set of the provider. The needle approach when targeting the Achilles tendon and can be visualized in the short axis and the needle is moved from lateral to medial or medial to lateral depending on the provider's comfort level and expertise (Figure 6.10 and 6.11).

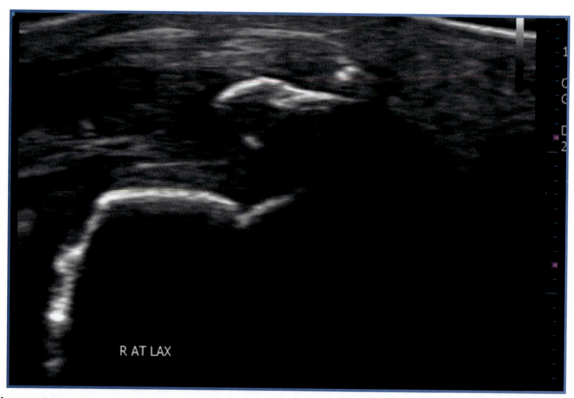

Figure 6.8: Long axis ultrasound image of severe insertional Achilles tendinosis as evidenced with a large, linear spur with significant fiber discordance at the tendon-bone interface.

CHAPTER 23 - THE FOOT AND ANKLE

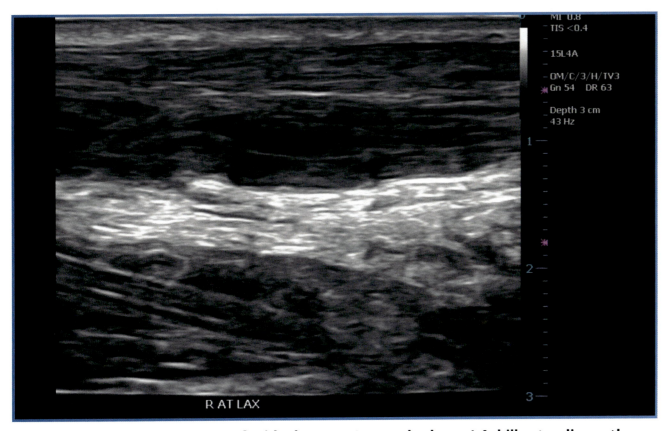

Figure 6.9: Long axis image of midsubstance (watershed zone) Achilles tendinopathy. Note the diffuse hypoechoic clefting, tendon thickening and sound artifact deep to the tendon with what is known as "Increased through transmission" where the soundwaves are penetrating the diseased Achilles with ease and thus highlighting the deeper structure of Kager's fat pad more prominently than normal.

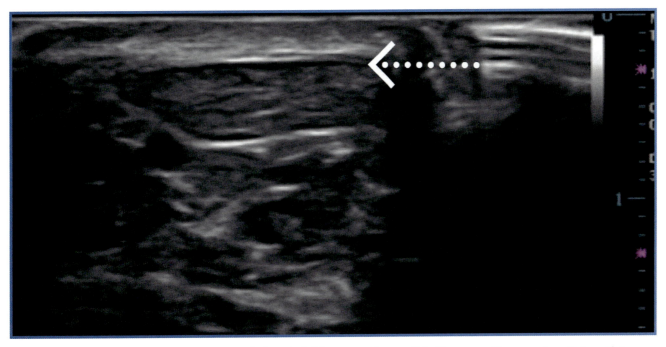

Figure 6.10: Short axis image of the Achilles tendon with the needle moving lateral to medial, in-plane with the probe

A COMPLETE GUIDE TO REGENERATIVE MEDICINE ©

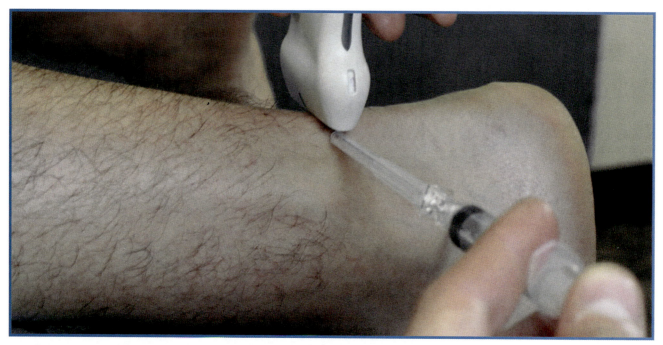

Figure 6.11: Ultrasound guided injection technique to the Achilles tendon. The patient is positioned prone with the affected foot hanging off of the table. The Achilles tendon is visualized in the short axis with the needle moving lateral to medial, in-plane with the probe

Treating plantar fasciitis can be fairly difficult to do percutaneously because it is a sensitive region with dense sensory nerve endings. Because of this, we recommend a short axis view of the plantar fascia with the needle moving medial to lateral, in-plane with the probe so we avoid the plantar surface as the point of entry.

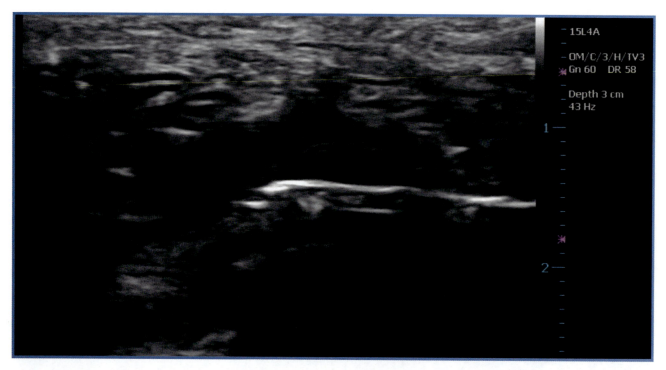

Figure 6.12: Ultrasound-guided Image of the percutaneous procedure to the plantar fascia in the short axis. The needle is visualized moving medial to lateral (right to left) in-plane with the probe

CHAPTER 23 - THE FOOT AND ANKLE

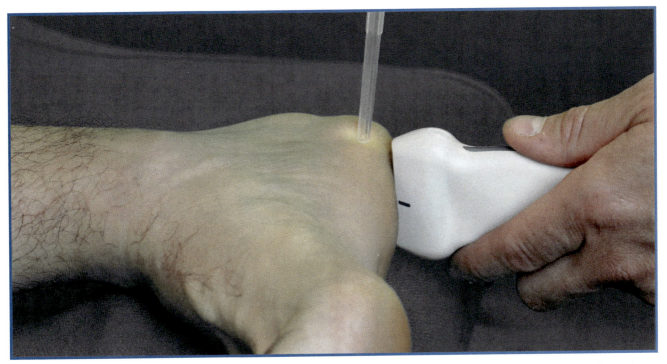

Figure 6.13: Ultrasound guided injection technique to the plantar fascia. The patient is positioned in sidelying on the affected extremity with the medial ankle facing upward. The plantar fascia is visualized in the short axis and the needle is moved medial to lateral, in-plane with the probe.

Medial Compartment:

The medial compartment houses the posterior tibialis, flexor digitorum longus tendon, flexor hallucis and the posterior tibial nerve, artery and vein (Figure 6.14 and 6.15). Evaluation of the tarsal tunnel is important when evaluating the medial ankle, most specifically the posterior tibialis tendon. The posterior tibialis tendon is the primary dynamic stabilizer of the foot arch; and in conjunction with the plantar fascia, provides the "truss" of which the arch is supported and is the most common tendon pathology in the medial compartment of the ankle. It is most common to find zones of inflammation and tendon pathology in the posterior tibial tendon starting at the medial malleolar zone extending distally to the tendon-bone insertion at the interface with the navicular and medial cuneiform (Figure 6.16). The primary function of the posterior tibialis tendon is to invert the foot and ankle as well as to provide dynamic stability to the arch of the foot. Gray's anatomy describes the muscle originating from lateral part of the posterior surface of the tibia, medial of the fibula as well as the interosseous membrane and major tendon inserts to the navicular and also has slips attach to the sustentaculum tali of calcaneus as well as plantar surface of the three cuneiforms.

CHAPTER 23 - THE FOOT AND ANKLE

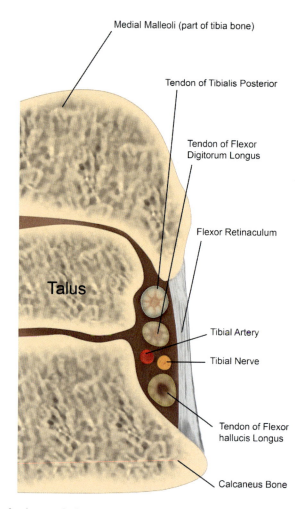

Figure 6.14: Artist depiction of the cross sectional anatomy of the tarsal tunnel

Figure 6.15: Medial Ankle: Tarsal Tunnel SAX

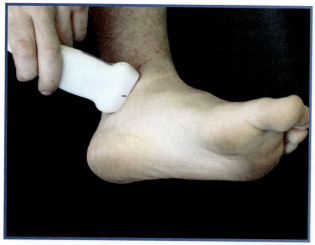 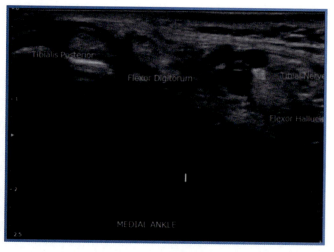

Place the probe at the distal portion of the medial ankle with the inferior edge pointing toward the heal. The medial malleolus is the bony landmark. From right to left starting at the medial malleolus: tibialis posterior tendon, flexor digitorum tendon, artery, vein, nerve and flexor hallucis longus to the bottom left of the ultrasound image.

306 EXOSOMES, PRP, AND STEM CELLS IN MUSCULOSKELETAL MEDICINE ©

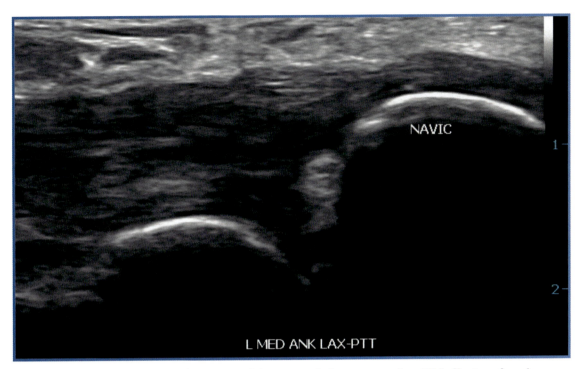

Figure 6.16: Long axis ultrasound image of the posterior tibialis tendon insertional tendinopathy at the navicular insertion as evidenced with intratendinous and insertional hypoechoic clefting and disorganization

Posterior tibialis tendon failure typically occurs in three stages and can be graded with a high degree of reliability with musculoskeletal ultrasound. Stage I is where acute or subacute tendinitis is present but the tendon remains its normal shape, length and diameter. If this occurs in a young patient the provider should consider the possibility of an accessory navicular. Treatment of Stage I posterior tibialis tendon failure can vary across individuals and practitioners but can be treated fairly reliably with a combination of orthobiologics, footwear modification, rehabilitation and in some cases, immobilization. In the case of acute or subacute tendinitis also be careful to evaluate the peritenon sheath for thickening or effusion. Stage II posterior tibialis tendinopathy occurs where the inflammation is becoming chronic in nature. Ultrasound characteristics of tendon failure at this stage are visible tenosynovitis, thickening with loss of intratendinous fibrillar pattern and elongation of the tendon. Treatments and management of Stage I can vary across individuals. Stage II is often accompanied by flattening of the foot arch in a loaded position and with the removal of weight, the foot resumes its normal arch and therefore the hallmark differentiating factor between Stage II failure vs Stage III tendon failure. This stage can be treated conservatively and reliably with a combination of orthobiologics, rehabilitation, footwear modification and immobilization. Stage III posterior tibialis tendon failure is typically precipitated by chronic tendinopathy and strain to failure of the tendon itself. Following lengthening or even rupture of the posterior tibialis tendon, the patient usually develops what is known as a fixed hindfoot deformity with hindfoot valgus and forefoot abduction. Conservative treatment of Stage III posterior tibialis tendon failure is typically associated with poor conservative outcomes so it becomes incumbent to evaluate and grade the level of pathology accurately and reliably using musculoskeletal ultrasound (Tome et al., 2006; Johnson et al., 1989).

Treating the posterior tibialis tendon with orthobiologics should be combined with footwear modifications and rehabilitation as it is important to restore the mechanics of the foot in order for the orthobiologics to do their job in remodeling the diseased tissue. When injecting this area, the tendon is best visualized in the long axis with the needle moving in plane with the probe from either distal to proximal or proximal to distal. If the main pathology is located at the navicular insertion or to a tendon-bone interface, moving the needle from proximal to distal in the long axis with the probe would be the best approach. Below is an example of needle guidance to address mild-moderate Stage II posterior tibialis tendinopathy at the navicular insertion (Figure 6.17 and 6.18).

CHAPTER 23 - THE FOOT AND ANKLE

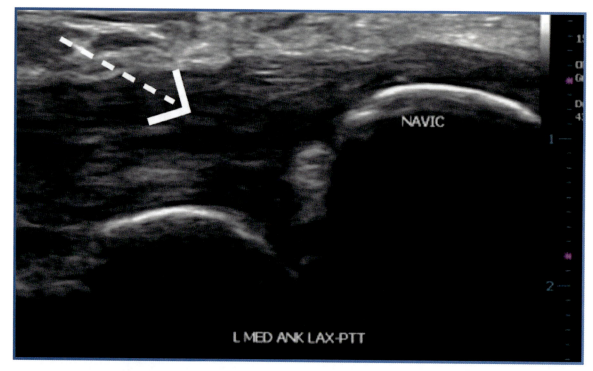

Figure 6.17: Ultrasound image of the posterior tibialis tendon at the navicular attachment. This image displays signs of tendinopathy at the bony interface as evidenced by loss of fibrillar pattern, hypoechoic clefts and atypical thickening of the tendon. The needle is moving proximal to distal, in-plane with the probe.

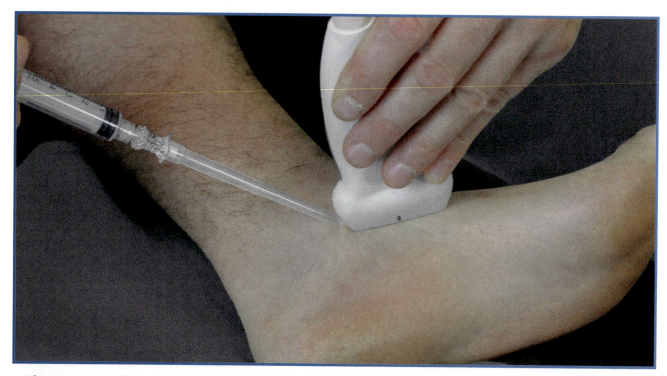

Figure 6.18: Ultrasound guided injection technique to the posterior tibialis tendon. The patient is positioned side lying with the affected extremity with the medial aspect of the ankle facing upward. The needle is moved proximal to distal, in-plane with the probe

CHAPTER 23 - THE FOOT AND ANKLE

Another common pathology found in the medial ankle compartment is tarsal tunnel syndrome. Tarsal tunnel syndrome typically consists of posterior tibial nerve inflammation secondary to compression of some sort; this can also be accompanied by vascular compression as well. This can occur from tenosynovitis of the flexor digitorum or more often the flexor hallucis longus because of where they sit on either side of the neurovascular structures within the tunnel. A combination of tenosynovitis and/or tendinopathy with tendon thickening of the flexor digitorum or the flexor hallucis longus significantly reduces the neurovascular structures ability to move freely within the confined space thus impingement occurs (Figure 6.19). The use of orthobiologics, with or without hydrodissection technique of the posterior tibial nerve using needle guided placement into this region is paramount. The structures in the tarsal tunnel are best visualized in short axis while the needle is moved posterior to anterior, in-plane with the probe (Figure 6.21 and 6.22).

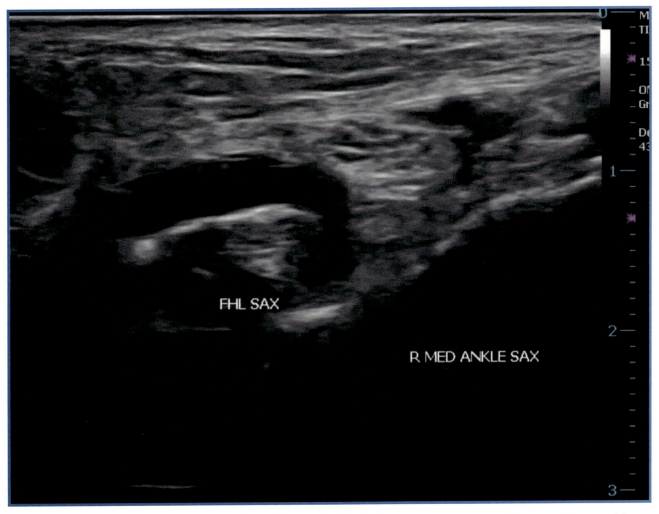

Figure 6.19: Short axis image of the flexor hallucis longus tenosynovitis as evidenced by the hypoechoic "halo" surrounding the tendon and compressing the posterior tibial nerve in tarsal tunnel syndrome

A COMPLETE GUIDE TO REGENERATIVE MEDICINE ©

CHAPTER 23 - THE FOOT AND ANKLE

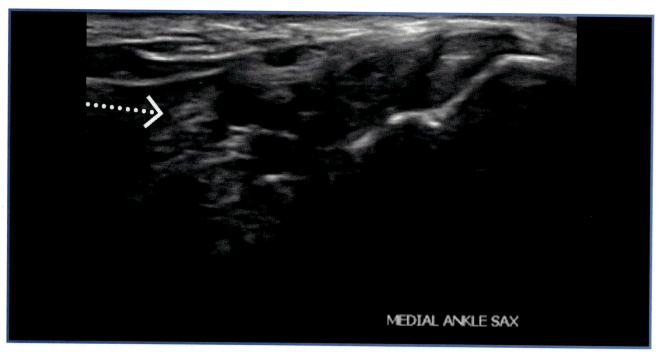

Figure 6.20: Short axis image of the tarsal tunnel. The needle is moving medial to lateral, in-plane with the probe. The arrow tip demonstrating the needle track is pointing to the tibial nerve.

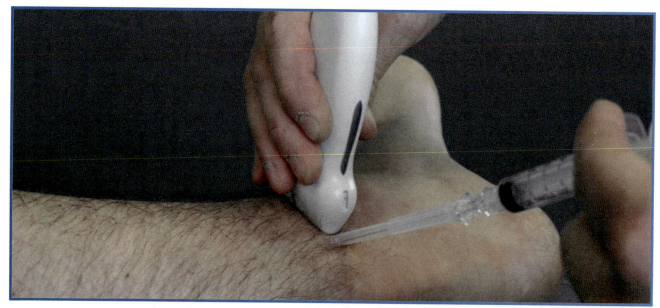

Figure 6.21: Ultrasound guided injection technique to the tarsal tunnel for tibial nerve block or hydrodissection. The patient is positioned in sidelying on the affected extremity with the medial ankle facing upward. The structures are visualized in the short axis and the needle is moved posterior to anterior, in-plane with the probe

The flexor hallucis longus and flexor digitorum both cross underneath the plantar surface of the foot and form what is known as the Knot Of Henry (Figure 6.22). Tendinitis or tenosynovitis in this region can mimic plantar fasciitis so it is important to rule this out as a differential diagnosis. Tenosynovitis at the Knot of Henry will not elicit pain at the calcaneal tubercle like plantar fasciitis does; however, it can mimic mid-band plantar fasciitis. This is where the use of musculoskeletal ultrasound is a great tool where the provider can perform the contralateral exam in cases to confirm the suspicion.

CHAPTER 23 - THE FOOT AND ANKLE

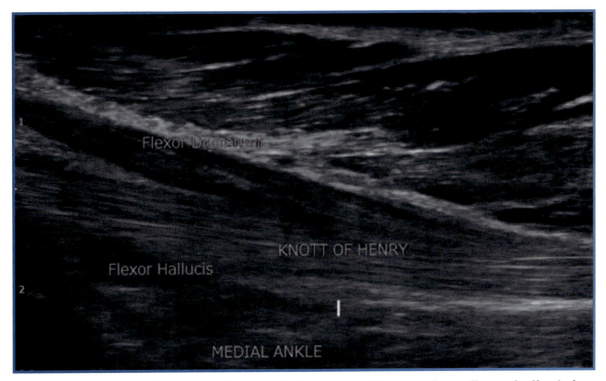

Figure 6.22: Long axis ultrasound image of the Knot of Henry where flexor hallucis longus and flexor digitorum cross over each other at the medial plantar surface of the foot

Anterior Compartment:

The anterior compartment consists of the anterior tibialis tendon, extensor hallucis longus tendon, extensor digitorum longus tendon and dorsalis pedis artery (Figure 6.23-6.25). The anterior compartment is primarily the dorsiflexion compartment of the ankle. A complete ankle exam of the anterior compartment will always evaluate all 3 tendons as well as the cortical surfaces of the talocrural joint, the intertarsal joints and the tarsal-metatarsal joints.

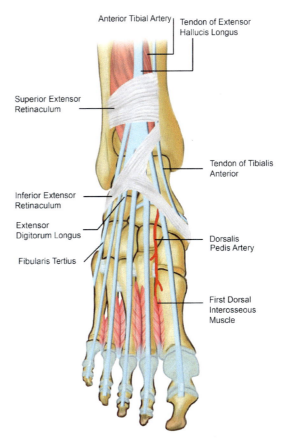

Figure 6.23: Artist depiction of dorsal foot-ankle soft tissue anatomy

A COMPLETE GUIDE TO REGENERATIVE MEDICINE ©

CHAPTER 23 - THE FOOT AND ANKLE

Figure 6.24: Anterior Ankle: Transverse/SAX

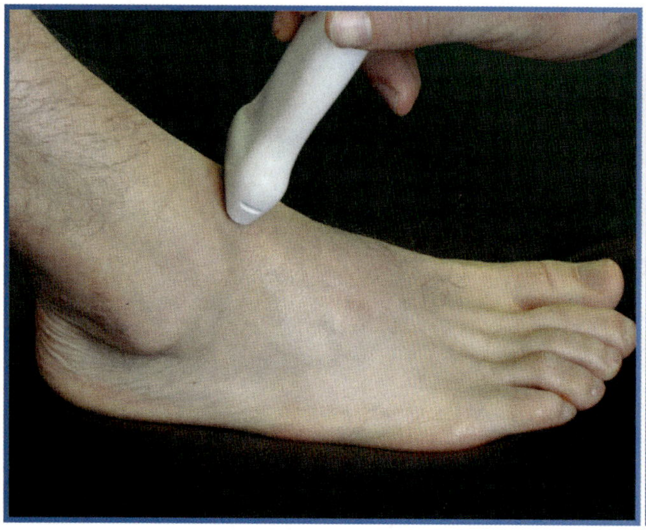

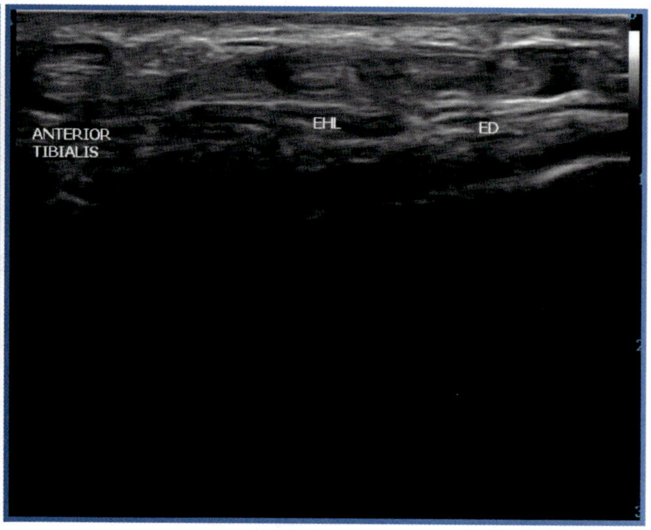

The patient is placed supine and the probe is placed over the anterior aspect of the ankle. This may also be performed with the patient's knee bent and foot lying flat. The extensor digitorum longus can be seen most lateral, and moving medial is the extensor hallucis longus followed by the tibialis anterior tendon. Medially and posterior to the tendons is the tibialis anterior artery and the anterior tibial vein lateral to the artery.

Figure 6.25: Anterior Ankle/Tibialis Anterior: Longitudinal/long axis

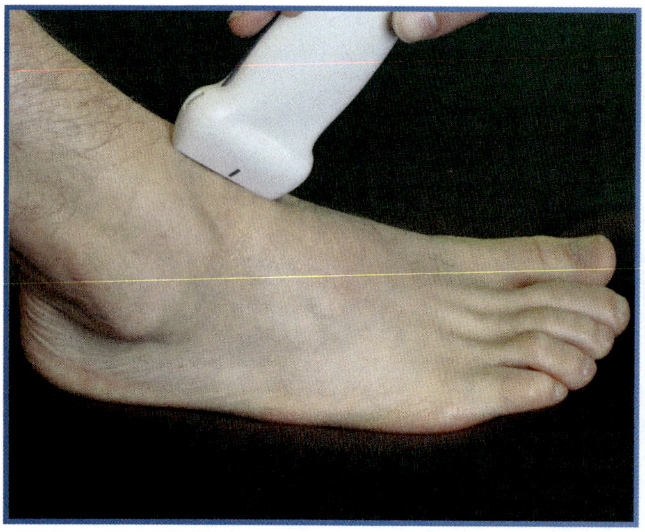

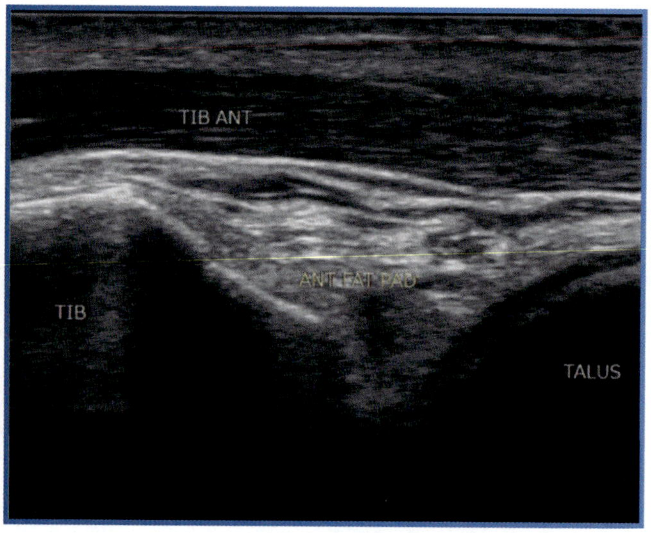

The patient is placed supine and the probe is placed longitudinally over the anterior aspect of the ankle. This may also be performed with the patient's knee bent and foot lying flat in slight plantar flexion. (TIB=Tibia, ANT FAT PAD=Anterior Fat Pad, TIB ANT=Tibialis Anterior)

CHAPTER 23 - THE FOOT AND ANKLE

Chronic tendinopathies in the anterior ankle compartment aren't as common as the other ankle compartments and the use of orthobiologics in the anterior ankle/foot complex typically involve the talocrural joint or the smaller midfoot joints as described in the osseous anatomy in the first section of the foot/ankle. A common joint injection is the large talocrural joint where cases of osteoarthritis and small chondral defects are two of the most common pathologies in this region. A reliable approach to take after the clinician has chosen to perform intervention here is an in-plane injection while the joint itself is visualized in the long axis where the needle is moved obliquely, medial to lateral underneath the tendon compartments and into the joint space (Figure 6.26 and 6.27).

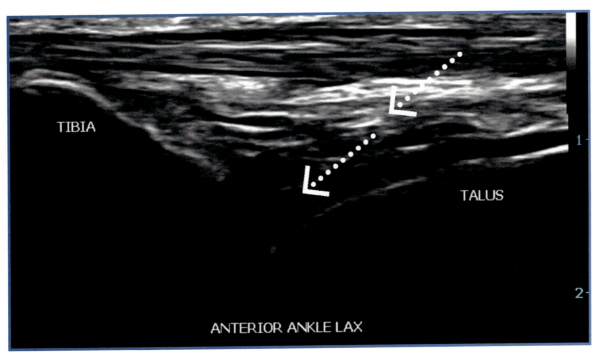

Image: 6.26 Long axis image of the tibial-talar joint. The needle is moved oblique-lateral to medial in-plane with the probe.

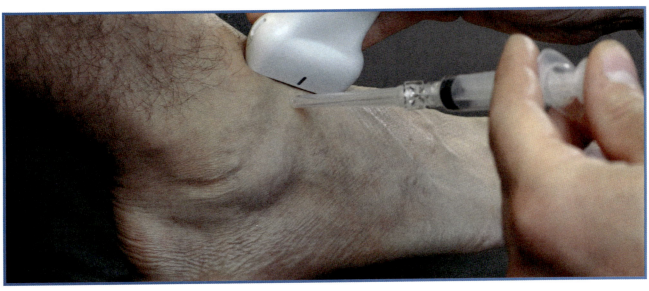

Figure 6.27: Ultrasound guided injection technique to the talocrural joint. The patient is positioned supine with the foot in slight plantar flexion. The joint and tibialis anterior are visualized in the long axis and the needle is moved oblique distal to proximal in plane with the probe.

Lateral Compartment

The lateral compartment structures we will cover involve the peroneus longus, peroneus brevis tendons and the anterior talofibular ligament. The peroneal tendons provide secondary stability in dynamic positions as well as functioning as the primary evertors of the foot. Henry Gray describes the peroneal tendons originating from the lateral condyle of the tibia, head and proximal 2/3 of the lateral surface of the fibula, intermuscular septa and adjacent deep fascia. The peroneus longus inserts to the base of the first metatarsal and medial cuneiform while the peroneus brevis inserts to the base of the fifth metatarsal (Gray et al., 1995).

Normal sonographic appearance of the peroneal longus and brevis tendons on ultrasound are similar to anywhere else in the body; they should appear hyperechoic, fibrillar and homogeneous in shape (Figure 6.28-6.30).

Figure 6.28: Lateral ankle: peroneal tendons short axis

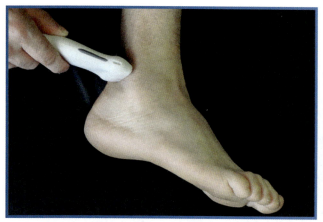
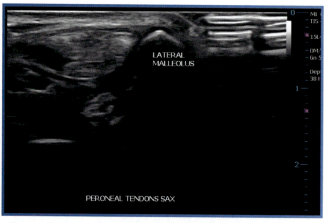

With the patient prone and the foot off the table place the probe posterior to the lateral malleolus in the transverse plane. With the lateral malleolus visualized in the short axis, slide the probe slightly posterior and the peroneus brevis and longus will come into view. The brevis is visualized deep and closer to the malleolus and the peroneus is superficial and further away from the malleolus.

Figure 6.29: Lateral ankle: peroneal tendons long axis

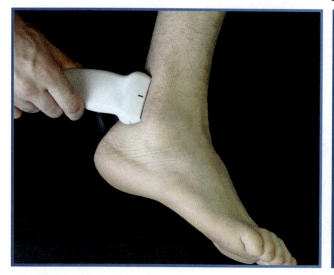
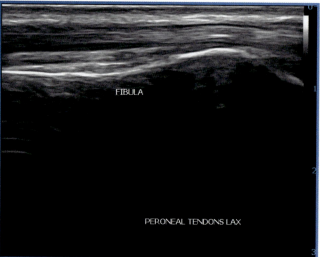

With the patient prone and the foot off the table place the probe posterior to the lateral malleolus. The long axis shows the fibrinous peroneus longus superior to the peroneus brevis tendon, both of which lay superior to the lateral malleolus.

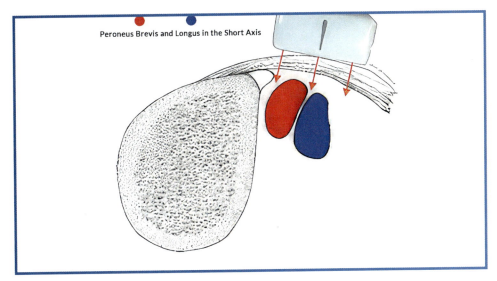

Figure 6.30: Pen and Ink illustration of peroneus brevis and longus in the short axis

Pathologies of the peroneus brevis are more common than peroneus longus and can occur anywhere within the lateral malleolar zone to the level of peroneal tubercle of the calcaneus where the longus and brevis split and travel to their respective insertions. Another common region to evaluate peroneus brevis pathology is its insertion to the base of the 5th metatarsal. Peroneal brevis tendinopathy within the malleolar zone is fairly common because it lies close to the bone and is more exposed to the lateral malleolus and its bony prominence (Figure 6.31). This is pronounced during movements such as inversion-eversion motions in athletic positions and in cases of chronic ankle instability where the peroneus brevis is prone to fraying and tendinopathy along this bony prominence. Peroneal longus tendinopathy typically occurs at the level of the peroneal tubercle and at the level of the cuboid. In young patients presenting with peroneal longus tendinitis, be careful to evaluate for accessory os peroneum as this predisposes the anatomy for problems.

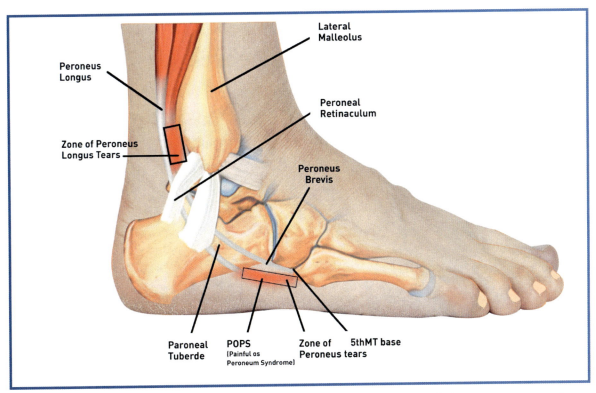

Figure 6.31: Artist depiction of the lateral ankle structures and the common regions of peroneal brevis and longus pathologies

There are different injection approaches for peroneal brevis tendinopathy with small tears in the malleolar zone. We advocate to visualize the peroneal tendons in short axis here and move the needle from lateral to medial in-plane with the probe to the area of concern (Figure 6.32 and 6.33) It is very important when performing and incorporating interventions with orthobiologics into your practice to have an idea of which patients will respond well. This is where the use of ultrasound not only as a tool to guide the needle comes in but knowing how to use the tool as a diagnostic measurement. Being able to critically evaluate the tissues you are considering to treat is equally as important as delivering the orthobiologic. Conservative outcomes for management of peroneus brevis tendinopathy goes down significantly if the patient has chronic subluxation or dislocation of the tendons around the lateral malleolus so be careful to do a thorough static and dynamic assessment utilizing ultrasound. With the peroneal tendons visualized in the short axis, ask the patient to actively or the provider passively move the ankle in-out of eversion to elicit tendon subluxation or dislocation.

Be careful when considering percutaneous needle tenotomy to the peroneal tendons as well as tendons that lie within the medial and anterior compartment. These tendons don't have the bulk, diameter or footprint attachment strength of tendons elsewhere in the body such as the patellar tendon, common extensor, quadriceps tendon, rotator cuff or the Achilles tendon. We do not advise percutaneous tenotomies in the ankle compartments unless the rendering provider is aware of the risks. For instance, a high risk scenario is when a provider is using an assistive percutaneous tenotomy machine. A low risk clinical scenario is to fenestrate an ankle tendon such as the peroneus brevis or longus when the provider incidentally or intentionally makes passes through the peroneal tendon to deliver the orthobiologic with or without a dry needle 18g or 22g. This is because fenestrating a needle through a chronically inflamed tendon can have positive benefits as it can generate healthy inflammation and a subsequent healing cascade similar to PRP. Percutaneous tenotomy has been described to be very effective for many regions in the body such as the common extensor tendon, plantar fascia, Achilles tendon, patellar tendon as well as successful case reports on this being performed in the peroneus brevis but there is no consensus in the literature on the number of passes for each case, so erring on the side of caution here is prudent (Sussman et al., 2019).

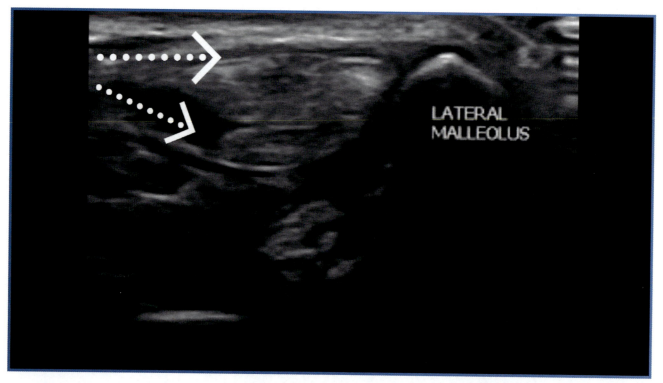

Figure 6.32: Short axis view of the peroneus brevis, peroneus longus and the lateral malleolus. The needle is moving lateral to medial, in-plane with the probe. The bottom arrow is directed toward the peroneus brevis and the superficial arrow is pointing toward the peroneus longus

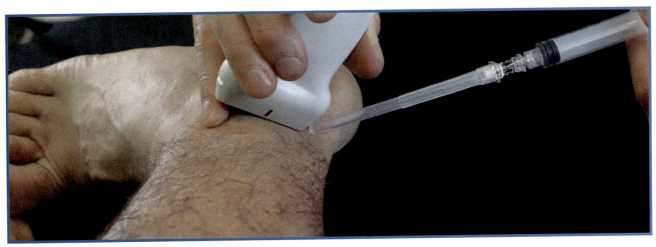

Figure 6.33: Ultrasound guided injection technique to the peroneal tendons in the malleolar zone. The patient is positioned supine with the lateral aspect of the affected extremity facing upward. The peroneal tendons are visualized in short axis and the needle is visualized moving posterior to anterior, in-plane with the probe

Anterior talofibular ligament (ATFL) injury is the most frequent cause of acute ankle pain and in cases of chronic ankle pain, often finds its cause in its laxity (Golano et al., 2010). Understanding the anatomy of the ligament structure is important for correct diagnosis and treatment. The ATFL is a dense band of fibrous tissue that connects on the anterior-medial talus to the anterior margin of the lateral malleolus of the distal fibula. Normal sonographic appearance of the ATFL is a hyperechoic band of tissue connecting the talus and fibula that appears homogeneous (Figure 6.34). The cortical surfaces of the attachment points along the talus and fibula should also be smooth and uninterrupted.

The most frequent mechanism of injury to the ATFL is an inversion sprain. In addition to competitive and recreational athletics, Inversion sprains can occur in most activities of daily living which include stepping off a curb wrong, slipping in the house or walking the dog. Injuries to the ATFL have multiple classification systems, we will use the American Medical Association's system (AMA) which is graded by clinical presentation systems of patients who experience anterior talofibular ankle sprains (Balduini et al., 1987; Easley and Wiesel. 2010):

Grade I
- ligament stretch

Grade II
- partial tear
- partial loss of movement
- mild to moderate joint instability

Grade III
- complete tear
- inability to bear weight
- significant joint instability

The ultrasound characteristics of a grade I sprain to the ATFL typically do not reveal much evidence beyond what is normally found with the exception of fluid or effusion collection if the sprain is acute. Sonographic evidence of grade II ATFL tears typically are accompanied by visible disruptions in ligamentous fibers while leaving some fibers still intact. Dynamic evidence of grade II tears often include atypical joint gapping, leaving some fibers intact. Sonographic characteristics of grade III ATFL tears are typically accompanied with full thickness disruption of fibers, atypical dynamic joint gapping with inversion stress and cortical irregularities at the lateral malleolar attachment site (Figure 6.35).

CHAPTER 23 - THE FOOT AND ANKLE

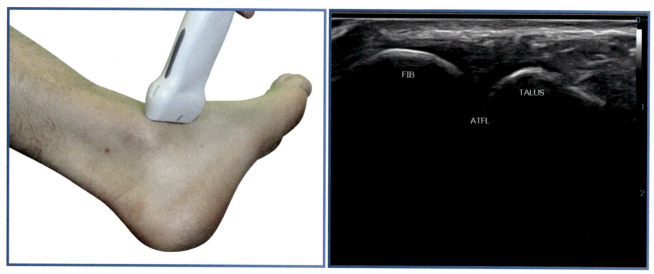

Figure 6.34: Lateral Ankle/ATFL: Longitudinal/LAX

Have the patient lay supine with the foot slightly inverted. Place the probe slightly anterior to the lateral malleolus. The anterior talofibular ligament should be seen as a fibrous, linear structure connecting the talus to the fibula

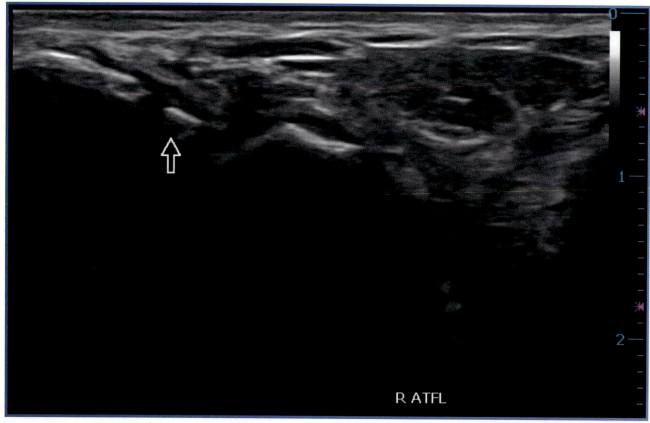

Figure 6.35: Long axis ultrasound image of a grade III anterior talofibular ligament tear as evidenced by the hypoechoic space in the middle of the joint and the arrow pointing to an avulsion of the distal fibula

Performing intervention to the anterior talofibular ligament with orthobiologics can be done in a number of ways. With the patient positioned sidelying on the unaffected extremity, we advocate for an out-of-plane approach with the ligament visualized in the long axis (Figure 6.36 and 6.37).

EXOSOMES, PRP, AND STEM CELLS IN MUSCULOSKELETAL MEDICINE ©

CHAPTER 23 - THE FOOT AND ANKLE

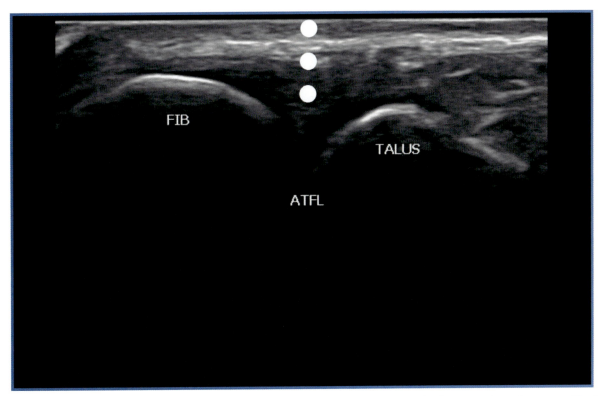

6.36: Ultrasound image of the anterior talofibular ligament in long axis. The needle is moved out of plane along the ligamentous track connecting the talus and the fibula

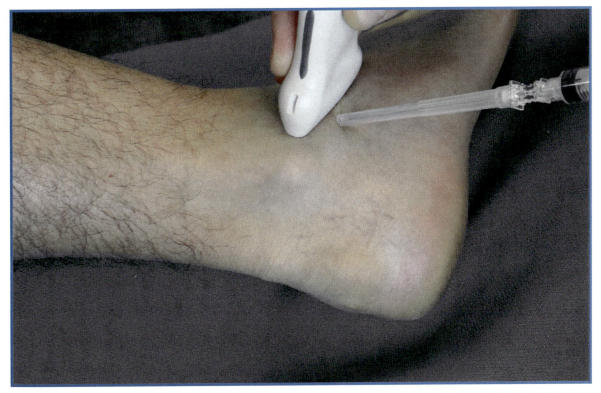

Figure 6.37: Ultrasound guided injection technique to the anterior talofibular ligament (ATFL). The patient is positioned in sidelying with the affected extremity facing upward. The ATFL is visualized in long axis and the needle is moved lateral to medial, out of plane with the probe.

Plantar Plate

The plantar plate is a fibrocartilaginous support system located on the volar surface of the metatarsal phalangeal joints and interphalangeal joints to help support the weight of the body (Figure 6.38). The plantar plate is a broad ribbon-like disc, firm but flexible, with a form ranging from rectangular to trapezoidal (Deland et al., 1995; Gregg et al., 2007). Its plantar surface is smooth, and grooved at its outer borders to provide a gliding plane for the flexor tendons. Its vessels appear to enter peripherally, mainly plantarly, and are part of the loose connective tissue septae (endotenon) that surround the collagen fascicles (Gregg et al., 2007).

Its primary function is to bear load and passively restrict dorsiflexion in weight bearing positions. The most common plantar plate injuries occur at the second metatarsal phalangeal joint. Most of the plantar plate fibers are oriented longitudinally, in the same direction as the plantar fascia, and the plate can thus sustain substantial tensile loads in this direction. The lone anatomical exception in the foot digits is the MTP joint of the first toe; it differs from those of the other toes in that other muscles act on the joint due to the two sesamoid bones and flexor hallucis longus that act as weight distributor and load bearers. Injuries to the plantar plate typically don't occur in acute fashion and are most common in active individuals who partake in recreational or competitive running and endurance sport where the injury typically occurs from repetitive and chronic use.

Normal sonographic appearance of the plantar plate should be relatively hyperechoic, linear fibers attaching the metatarsal head to the proximal phalanx (Figure 6.39). Dynamic stress testing of the plantar plate can be performed by placing the affected digit into dorsiflexion-plantarflexion motion; this is a fast method of determining the integrity of the structure.

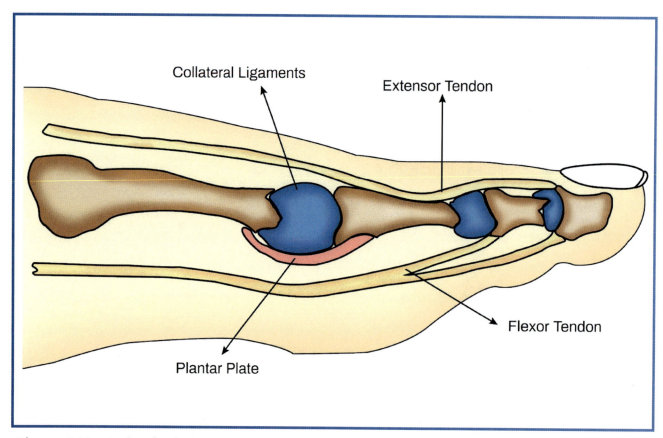

Figure 6.38: Artist depiction of metatarsal-phalangeal anatomy of digits two through five. Note the plantar plate and its location

Figure 6.39: Plantar Foot: Plantar Plate

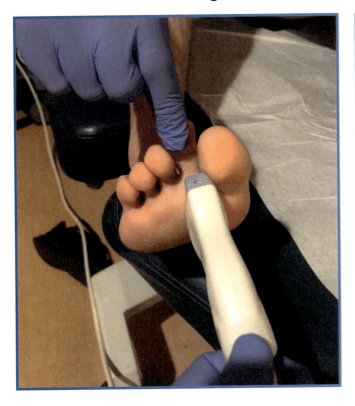

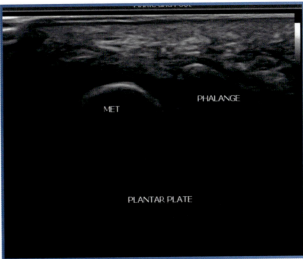

The probe should be placed at the plantar surface of the foot with the toes extended to view the where the flexor hallucis longus inserts at the base of the distal phalanx of the hallux. The plantar plate is the supportive, ligamentous structure between the metatarsal and phalange where the most often affected is the second digit.

Treating plantar plate injuries with orthobiologics using ultrasound guidance can be a difficult task. This is a delicate area with a lot of nerve endings. For proper visualization of anatomy and needle placement, we advise the patient to be placed in supine with the affected digit (most often the 2nd) in slight dorsiflexion. The plantar plate and metatarsal phalangeal joint are visualized in the long axis with the needle moving from distal to proximal, in-plane with the probe (Figure 6.40 and 6.41).

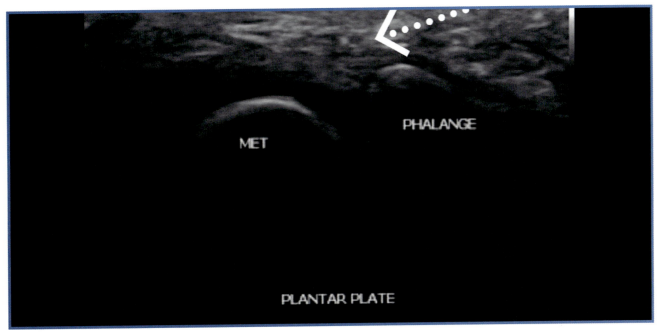

Figure 6.40: Long axis image of the plantar plate at the second metatarsal phalangeal joint. The needle is moving from distal to proximal, in-plane with the probe.

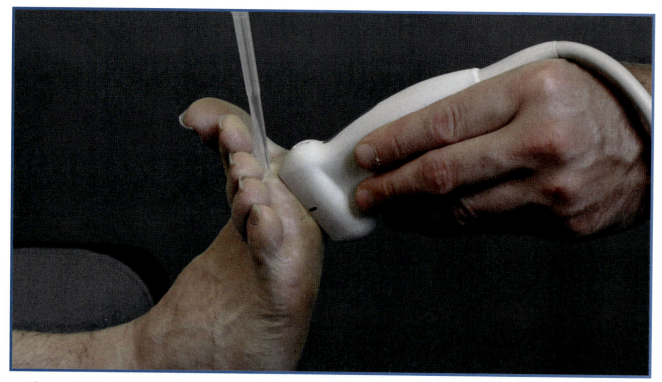

Figure 6.41: Ultrasound guided injection technique to the plantar plate. The patient is positioned supine. The plantar plate is visualized in the long axis with the needle moving distal to proximal, in-plane with the probe.

Morton's Neuroma

The term "Morton's Neuroma" has some controversy in the literature (Nikolaos et al., 2019). Morton himself described in 1876 a painful syndrome of the fourth metatarsophalangeal joint, rather than a nerve problem (Morton 1876), whereas others before him had described a 'painful clinical syndrome of the forefoot' (Dicaprio et al., 2017). Thus, the widely used terminology of 'Morton's neuroma' may represent an oversimplification of a clinical condition that may be misleading for doctors and patients. It is important that clinicians who deal with this condition realize the issue is not a benign tumour of the nerve (as the terminology would imply), but rather neurogenic pain syndrome in the forefoot that is associated with the interdigital nerve (most commonly the one between the third and fourth metatarsal heads), and to educate their patients accordingly (Figure 6.42) (DiCaprio et al., 2017). The etiology of Morton's neuroma is also somewhat controversial. There are functional and biomechanical sources to be mindful of when treating the condition in conjunction with needle-guided intervention. The most common working theory as to the biomechanical pathogenesis of Morton's neuroma development is that it is associated with abnormal pressure distribution in the forefoot secondary to deformity and/or tight calf development (Nikolaos et al., 2019)

Normal sonographic appearance of digital nerves within the web spaces should be benign and poorly visible because of its small diameter. Atypical appearance of an inflamed interdigital nerve in the web space, most commonly between the third and fourth digit, is abnormally large in circumference and can be replicated dynamically with ultrasound using the Mulder squeeze test where the operator should feel a click with the corresponding image replicating the special test maneuver on the screen. When treating the Morton neuroma percutaneously, we advise an out of plane approach using a step down technique from dorsal to volar. The probe is placed on the volar surface of the interweb space, care should be taken to not translate the needle to the volar portion of the skin surface with this technique (Figure 6.44 and 6.45).

CHAPTER 23 - THE FOOT AND ANKLE

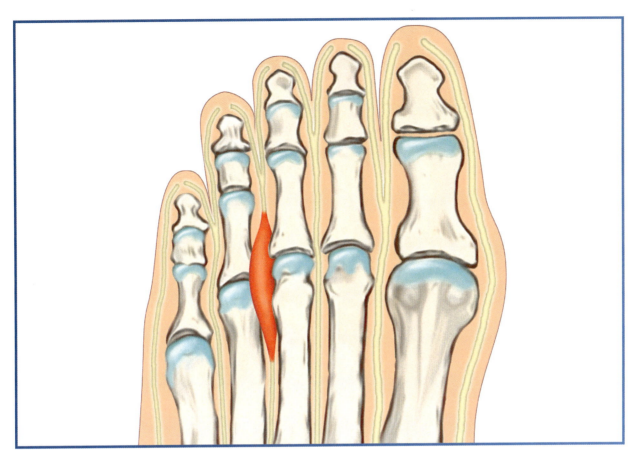

Figure 6.42: Artist depiction of Morton's neuroma location

Figure 6.43: Morton's Neuroma short axis

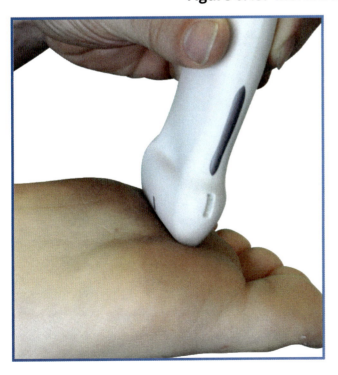

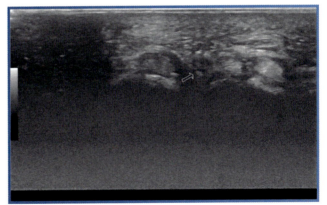

The patient is positioned in either prone or supine with the affected foot hanging off of the table. Place the probe in the short axis to the metatarsal heads and specifically between the third and fourth web space. The arrow is pointing to an enlarged digital nerve consistent with Morton's Neuroma finding.

CHAPTER 23 - THE FOOT AND ANKLE

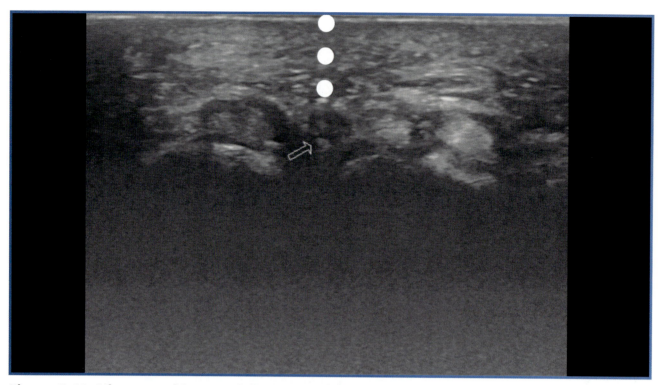

Figure 6.44: Ultrasound image of the interweb space in short axis. The arrow is pointing to a Morton's neuroma in short axis, the needle is moved from dorsal to plantar, out of plane with the probe.

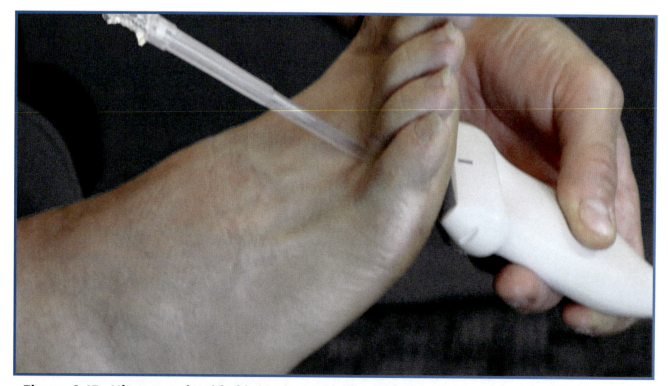

Figure 6.45: Ultrasound guided injection technique for Morton's neuroma. The interweb space and Morton neuroma is visualized in short axis and the needle is moved dorsal to plantar, out of plane with the probe.

References:

Maffulli N. Rupture of the Achilles tendon. J Bone Joint Surg Am. 1999;81: 1019–1036.

Maffulli N, Waterston SW, Squair J, Reaper J, Douglas AS. Changing incidence of Achilles tendon rupture in Scotland: a 15-year study. Clin J Sport Med. 1999;9: 157–160

Angelo Del Buono, Otto Chan, and Nicola Maffulli. Achilles tendon: functional anatomy and novel emerging models of imaging classification. Int Orthop. 2013 Apr; 37(4): 715–721.

Jacobsen J. Fundamentals of Musculoskeletal Ultrasound (3rd edition). Page 263. Elsevier, Sep 2017.

Gray, Henry. Gray's Anatomy (15th edition). Page 418-419. Barnes and Noble. 1995

Robert Kornfeld, DPM. Diagnostic Ultrasound: Can It Have An Impact For Plantar Fasciitis? Podiatry Today. Volume 23 - Issue 11 - Pages 30-34. November 2010.

Tome J, Nawoczenski DA, Flemister A, Houck J. Comparison of Foot Kinematics Between Subjects With Posterior Tibialis Tendon Dysfunction and Healthy Controls, Journal of Orthopaedic Sports Physical Therapy 36(12):986. 2006

Johnson KA, Strom DE. Tibialis posterior tendon dysfunction. Clin Orthop Rel Res 1989;239:196-206. 1989

Gray, Henry. Gray's Anatomy (15th edition). Page 416-417. Barnes and Noble. 1995

Walter I Sussman, Kurt Hofmann. Treatment of Insertional Peroneus Brevis Tendinopathy by Ultrasound-Guided Percutaneous Ultrasonic Needle Tenotomy: A Case Report. Ankle Surgery. 2019 Nov; 58 (6): 1285-1287.

Pau Golanó, et al., Anatomy of the ankle ligaments: a pictorial essay. Knee Surg Sports Traumatol Arthrosc. 2010 May; 18(5): 557–569.

Balduini FC, Vegso JJ, Torg JS, Torg E. Management and rehabilitation of ligamentous injuries to the ankle. Sports medicine (Auckland, N.Z.). 4 (5): 364-80. 1987. Pubmed.

Mark E. Easley, Sam W. Wiesel. Operative Techniques in Foot and Ankle Surgery. 2010. ISBN: 9781608319046

Deland JT, Lee KT, Sobel M, DiCarlo EF Anatomy of the plantar plate and its attachments in the lesser metatarsal phalangeal joint. Foot Ankle Int. 1995 Aug; 16(8):480-6.

Gregg J, Marks P, Silberstein M, Schneider T, Kerr J. Histologic anatomy of the lesser metatarsophalangeal joint plantar plate. Surg Radiol Anat. 2007;29(2):141–7

Deland JT, Lee KT, Sobel M, DiCarlo EF Anatomy of the plantar plate and its attachments in the lesser metatarsal phalangeal joint. Foot Ankle Int. 1995 Aug; 16(8):480-6.

Johnston RB, 3rd, Smith J, Daniels T. The plantar plate of the lesser toes: An anatomical study in human cadavers. Foot Ankle Int. 1994;15(5):276–282
Gregg J, Marks P, Silberstein M, Schneider T, Kerr J. Histologic anatomy of the lesser metatarsophalangeal joint plantar plate. Surg Radiol Anat. 2007;29(2):141–7

Nikolaos Gougoulias,1 Vasileios Lampridis,1 and Anthony Sakellariou. Morton's interdigital neuroma: instructional review. EFORT Open Rev. 2019 Jan; 4(1): 14–24.

Morton TG. A peculiar and painful affection of the fourth metatarso-phalangeal articulation. Am J Med Sci 1876;71:37–45

Di Caprio F, Meringolo R, Eddine MS, Ponziani L. Morton's interdigital neuroma of the foot: a literature review. Foot Ankle Surg 2017;24:92–98.

Nikolaos Gougoulias,1 Vasileios Lampridis,1 and Anthony Sakellariou. Morton's interdigital neuroma: instructional review. EFORT Open Rev. 2019 Jan; 4(1): 14–24.

ADDENDIX
Kinesiologic Planes of Motion
Pradeep Albert

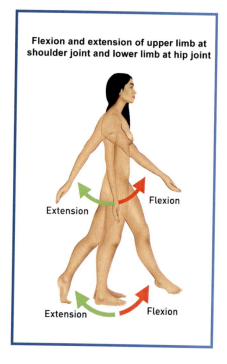

Flexion and extension of upper limb at shoulder joint and lower limb at hip joint

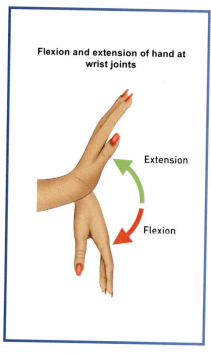

Flexion and extension of hand at wrist joints

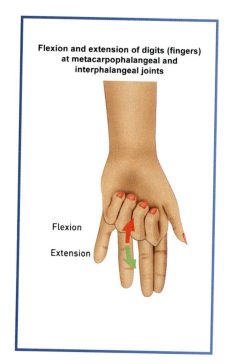

Flexion and extension of digits (fingers) at metacarpophalangeal and interphalangeal joints

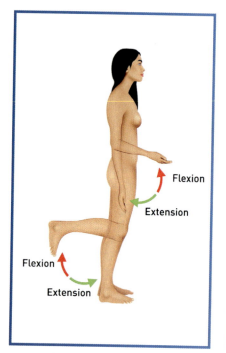

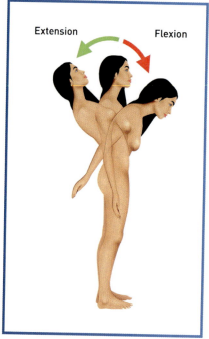

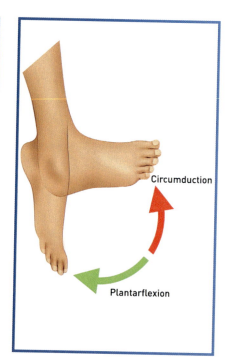

CHAPTER 24 - THE HAND AND WRIST

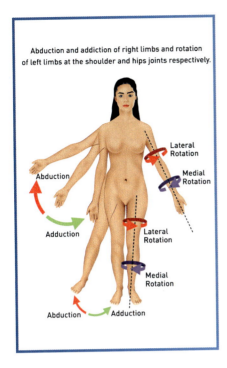

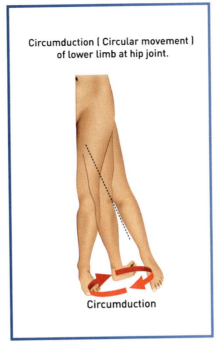

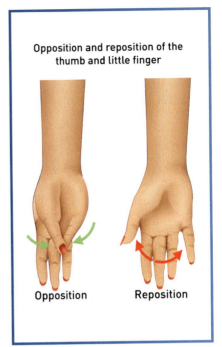

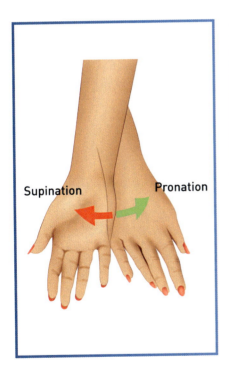

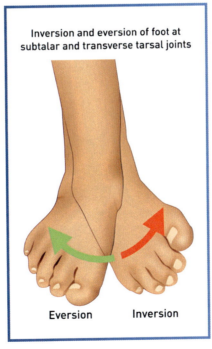

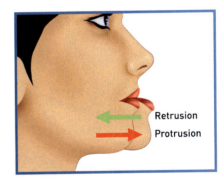

A COMPLETE GUIDE TO REGENERATIVE MEDICINE ©

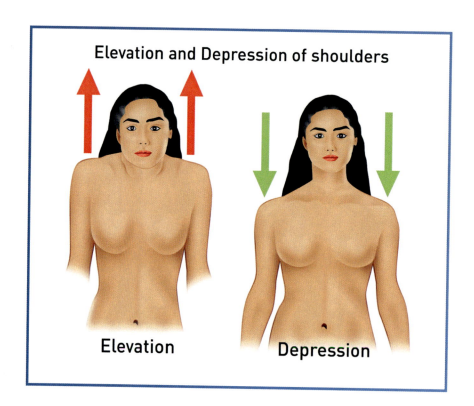